Methods in Molecular Biology

Series Editor
John M. Walker
School of Life and Medical Sciences
University of Hertfordshire
Hatfield, Hertfordshire, AL10 9AB, UK

For further volumes:
http://www.springer.com/series/7651

Urothelial Carcinoma

Methods and Protocols

Edited by

Wolfgang A. Schulz, Michèle J. Hoffmann and Günter Niegisch

Department of Urology, Heinrich Heine University, Düsseldorf, Germany

Humana Press

Editors
Wolfgang A. Schulz
Department of Urology
Heinrich Heine University
Düsseldorf, Germany

Michèle J. Hoffmann
Department of Urology
Heinrich Heine University
Düsseldorf, Germany

Günter Niegisch
Department of Urology
Heinrich Heine University
Düsseldorf, Germany

ISSN 1064-3745 ISSN 1940-6029 (electronic)
Methods in Molecular Biology
ISBN 978-1-4939-7233-3 ISBN 978-1-4939-7234-0 (eBook)
DOI 10.1007/978-1-4939-7234-0

Library of Congress Control Number: 2017948666

Printed on acid-free paper

This Humana Press imprint is published by Springer Nature
The registered company is Springer Science+Business Media LLC
The registered company address is: 233 Spring Street, New York, NY 10013, U.S.A.

Preface

Urothelial carcinoma is the major histological subtype of bladder cancer in most regions of the world, except where endemic schistosomiasis causes another subtype, squamous cell carcinoma. Outside the field of urology, the incidence and impact of urothelial carcinoma are often underestimated, but in fact, it is the fourth most common cancer in males in many countries, albeit with a lower incidence in women. One reason for this underestimate may be that a large fraction of urothelial carcinomas are papillary tumors with a low tendency toward progression to invasive and metastatic cancers. However, while rarely life-endangering, these tumors require surgery, may progress to higher stages, and, not least, have a nasty tendency to recur, thus necessitating long-term monitoring and treatment. Moreover, the 20–30% of urothelial carcinomas, which are invasive at first presentation or have progressed from papillary tumors, are as dangerous as any carcinoma in other tissues. Despite radical surgery and multimodal cytotoxic chemotherapy, only about half of the patients survive for more than 5 years. Worse, no major improvements have been achieved in the therapy of invasive urothelial carcinoma over the last two decades and in particular, none of the novel molecularly targeted drugs has yielded significant benefit in this cancer type and, accordingly, none has entered routine clinical practice.

Obviously, a better understanding of the biology of urothelial carcinoma is a fundamental prerequisite to develop more appropriate approaches for therapy. Another evident key issue for this heterogeneous disease is the development of biomarkers, especially for monitoring following initial therapy and for prognostication of its progression risk. For urothelial carcinoma, analysis of urine offers a unique access. A third important issue is prevention, which could be improved by further insights into the mechanisms of carcinogenesis. Prevention may be neglected in cancer research in general, but this would be particularly ironic in the case of urothelial carcinoma, where specific chemical carcinogens have been known to be involved for many years.

It has been felt by many that, like progress in its treatment, research on urothelial carcinoma was proceeding at a much too slow pace. Fortunately, now, it has reached a turning point. To some extent, this development owes to the outpour of data from large-scale high-throughput investigations, as in other tumor types. Nevertheless, large amounts of data obtained by generic approaches provide only the basis for investigations. In order to translate insights into pathomechanisms and application in diagnostics and therapy, further dedicated and specific analyses tailored to the particular disease are crucial. As documented by this volume, these are forthcoming in urothelial carcinoma. Based on these considerations, in addition to standard techniques for the characterization of urothelial carcinoma, methods to investigate mechanisms of carcinogenesis constitute one focus of this volume. Another main focus is on cellular and animal models for urothelial carcinoma and related diseases. The fourth major section comprises molecular analyses from body fluids, but especially from urine. New approaches to therapy constitute the final section.

We hope that the concepts and techniques described in this volume will contribute to the current upturn in research on urothelial carcinoma and to the application of its results in clinical practice. Moreover, we are confident that many techniques described here in the context of urothelial carcinoma may be valuable also for colleagues whose research aims at better understanding, prevention, diagnostics, and treatment of other cancers.

Düsseldorf, Germany

Wolfgang A. Schulz
Michèle J. Hoffmann
Günter Niegisch

Contents

Part III Cellular and Animal Models

Part IV Biomarkers

Part V Therapy Development

Contributors

MUSTAFA ALAMYAR • *Department of Pathology, Erasmus MC, Rotterdam, The Netherlands*

REGINA ARANTES-RODRIGUES • *Department of Veterinary Sciences, University of Trás-os-Montes and Alto Douro (UTAD), Vila Real, Portugal; Center for the Research and Technology of Agro-Environmental and Biological Sciences (CITAB), Vila Real, Portugal*

ANGELA BENTIVEGNA • *School of Medicine and Surgery, University of Milano-Bicocca, Monza (MB), Italy*

CARINA BERNARDO • *Experimental Pathology and Therapeutics Group—Research Center, Portuguese Oncology Institute—Porto (IPO-Porto), Porto, Portugal; Institute for Biomedicine (IBiMED), University of Aveiro, Porto, Portugal*

AHMAD BESARATINIA • *Department of Preventive Medicine, USC Keck School of Medicine, University of Southern California, Los Angeles, CA, USA*

SAMIR BIDNUR • *Department of Urologic Sciences, University of British Columbia, Vancouver, BC, Canada*

PETER C. BLACK • *Department of Urologic Sciences, University of British Columbia, Vancouver, BC, Canada*

MEINOLF BLASZKEWICZ • *Leibniz Research Centre for Working Environment and Human Factors at TU Dortmund (IfADo), Dortmund, Germany*

VLADIMIR BOBEK • *Department of Laboratory Genetics, University Hospital Kralovske Vinohrady, Prague, Czech Republic*

CHANCHAI BOONLA • *Department of Biochemistry, Faculty of Medicine, Chulalongkorn University, Bangkok, Thailand*

DONATELLA CONCONI • *School of Medicine and Surgery, University of Milano-Bicocca, Monza (MB), Italy*

RUI M. GIL DA COSTA • *Department of Veterinary Sciences, University of Trás-os-Montes and Alto Douro (UTAD), Vila Real, Portugal; Center for the Research and Technology of Agro-Environmental and Biological Sciences (CITAB), Vila Real, Portugal*

LEANDRO S. D'ABRONZO • *VA Northern California Health Care System, University of California at Davis, Sacramento, CA, USA; Department of Urology, University of California at Davis, Sacramento, CA, USA*

DIMO DIETRICH • *Institute of Pathology, University Hospital of Bonn, Bonn, Germany; Department of Otolaryngology, Head and Neck Surgery, University Hospital Bonn, Bonn, Germany*

HIROKO ENDO • *Department of Biochemistry, Osaka International Cancer Institute, Osaka, Japan*

KATI ERDMANN • *Department of Urology, Technische Universität Dresden, Dresden, Germany*

SUSANNE FUESSEL • *Department of Urology, Technische Universität Dresden, Dresden, Germany*

HIDEKI FURUYA • *Clinical and Translational Research Program, University of Hawaii Cancer Center, Honolulu, HI, USA*

NADINE T. GAISA • *Institute of Pathology, RWTH Aachen University, Aachen, Germany*

PARAMITA M. GHOSH • *VA Northern California Health Care System, University of California at Davis, Sacramento, CA, USA; Department of Urology, University of California at Davis, Sacramento, CA, USA; Department of Biochemistry and Molecular*

Medicine, University of California at Davis, Sacramento, CA, USA; Department of Urology, University of California Davis School of Medicine, Sacramento, CA, USA

WOLFGANG GOERING • *Department of Urology, Medical Faculty, Heinrich Heine University Düsseldorf, Düsseldorf, Germany; Institute of Pathology, Medical Faculty, Heinrich Heine University Düsseldorf, Düsseldorf, Germany*

KLAUS GOLKA • *Leibniz Research Centre for Working Environment and Human Factors at TU Dortmund (IfADo), Dortmund, Germany*

AKIHIRO GORIKI • *The Vancouver Prostate Centre, University of British Columbia, Vancouver, BC, Canada*

JIRI HATINA • *Faculty of Medicine in Pilsen, Institute of Biology, Charles University in Prague, Plzen, Czech Republic*

DIETER HÄUSSINGER • *Clinic for Gastroenterology, Hepatology, and Infectiology, Medical Faculty, Heinrich Heine University Düsseldorf, Düsseldorf, Germany*

RAKESH HEER • *Solid Tumour Target Discovery Laboratory, Newcastle Cancer Centre, Northern Institute for Cancer Research, Medical School, Newcastle University, Newcastle Upon Tyne, UK*

ANASTASIA HEPBURN • *Solid Tumour Target Discovery Laboratory, Newcastle Cancer Centre, Northern Institute for Cancer Research, Medical School, Newcastle University, Newcastle Upon Tyne, UK*

MICHÈLE J. HOFFMANN • *Department of Urology, Medical Faculty, Heinrich Heine University Düsseldorf, Düsseldorf, Germany*

MICHAEL H. HSIEH • *Children's National Medical Center, Washington, DC, USA; Biomedical Research Institute, Rockville, MD, USA*

MASAHIRO INOUE • *Department of Biochemistry, Osaka International Cancer Institute, Osaka, Japan; Department of Clinical and Experimental Pathophysiology, Osaka University Graduate School of Pharmaceutical Sciences, Osaka, Japan*

WOLFGANG JÄGER • *Department of Urology and Paediatric Urology, Johannes Gutenberg-Universität Mainz, Mainz, Germany*

ANANDA AYYAPPAN JAGUVA VASUDEVAN • *Clinic for Gastroenterology, Hepatology, and Infectiology, Medical Faculty, Heinrich Heine University Düsseldorf, Düsseldorf, Germany; Department of Urology, Medical Faculty, Heinrich Heine University Düsseldorf, Düsseldorf, Germany*

TAKASHI KOBAYASHI • *Department of Urology, Kyoto University Graduate School of Medicine, Kyoto, Japan*

KATARINA KOLOSTOVA • *Department of Laboratory Genetics, University Hospital Kralovske Vinohrady, Prague, Czech Republic*

MICHAELA KRIPNEROVA • *Faculty of Medicine in Pilsen, Institute of Biology, Charles University in Prague, Plzen, Czech Republic*

ERIC A. KURZROCK • *Department of Urology, University of California, Davis School of Medicine, Sacramento, CA, USA; Stem Cell Program, Institute for Regenerative Cures, University of California, Davis Medical Center, Sacramento, CA, USA*

ANDREA LOHSE-FISCHER • *Department of Urology, Technische Universität Dresden, Dresden, Germany*

EVARISTUS C. MBANEFO • *Children's National Medical Center, Washington, DC, USA; Biomedical Research Institute, Rockville, MD, USA*

MARGARITA MELNIKOVA • *Institute of Cell Biology (Cancer Research), University of Duisburg-Essen Medical School, Essen, Germany*

LOURDES MENGUAL • *Laboratory and Department of Urology, Centre de Recerca Biomèdica CELLEX, Hospital Clínic, Universitat de Barcelona, IDIBAPS, Barcelona, España*
GEORG MICHAEL • *Steinen, Germany*
IGOR MOSKALEV • *The Vancouver Prostate Centre, University of British Columbia, Vancouver, BC, Canada*
CARSTEN MÜNK • *Clinic for Gastroenterology, Hepatology, and Infectiology, Medical Faculty, Heinrich Heine University Düsseldorf, Düsseldorf, Germany*
ROMAN NAWROTH • *Department of Urology, Klinikum rechts der Isar, Technische Universität München, Munich, Germany*
GÜNTER NIEGISCH • *Department of Urology, Medical Faculty, Heinrich Heine University Düsseldorf, Düsseldorf, Germany*
PÉTER NYIRÁDY • *Department of Urology, Semmelweis University, Budapest, Hungary*
OSAMU OGAWA • *Department of Urology, Kyoto University Graduate School of Medicine, Kyoto, Japan*
HIROAKI OKUYAMA • *Department of Biochemistry, Osaka International Cancer Institute, Osaka, Japan*
MIREIA OLIVAN • *Group of Biomedical Research in Urology, Vall d'Hebron Research Institute (VHIR), Universitat Autònoma de Barcelona (UAB), Barcelona, Spain*
PAULA A. OLIVEIRA • *Department of Veterinary Sciences, University of Trás-os-Montes and Alto Douro (UTAD), Vila Real, Portugal; Center for the Research and Technology of Agro-Environmental and Biological Sciences (CITAB), Vila Real, Portugal*
STEPHANIE L. OSBORN • *Department of Urology, University of California, Davis School of Medicine, Sacramento, CA, USA; Stem Cell Program, Institute for Regenerative Cures, University of California, Davis Medical Center, Sacramento, CA, USA*
CHONG-XIAN PAN • *VA Northern California Health Care System, University of California at Davis, Sacramento, CA, USA; Department of Urology, University of California at Davis, Sacramento, CA, USA; Division of Hematology and Oncology, Department of Internal Medicine, University of California at Davis, Sacramento, CA, USA*
HAMENDRA SINGH PARMAR • *Faculty of Medicine in Pilsen, Institute of Biology, Charles University in Prague, Plzen, Czech Republic*
SUCHITTRA PHOYEN • *Department of Biochemistry, Faculty of Medicine, Chulalongkorn University, Bangkok, Thailand*
MARIA PINKERNEIL • *Department of Urology, Medical Faculty, Heinrich Heine University Düsseldorf, Düsseldorf, Germany*
PETER RAVEN • *The Vancouver Prostate Centre, University of British Columbia, Vancouver, BC, Canada*
MICHAEL ROSE • *Institute of Pathology, RWTH Aachen University, Aachen, Germany*
CHARLES J. ROSSER • *Clinical and Translational Research Program, University of Hawaii Cancer Center, Honolulu, HI, USA*
KARSTEN SALOMO • *Department of Urology, Technische Universität Dresden, Dresden, Germany*
LÚCIO LARA SANTOS • *Experimental Pathology and Therapeutics Group—Research Center, Portuguese Oncology Institute—Porto (IPO-Porto), Porto, Portugal; Department of Surgical Oncology, Portuguese Oncology Institute—Porto (IPO-Porto), Porto, Portugal*
ANUJA SATHE • *Department of Urology, Klinikum rechts der Isar, Technische Universität München, Munich, Germany*
SILVIA SELINSKI • *Leibniz Research Centre for Working Environment and Human Factors at TU Dortmund (IfADo), Dortmund, Germany*

GOTTFRID SJÖDAHL • *Division of Urological Research, Department of Translational Medicine, Lund University, Lund, Sweden*
TIBOR SZARVAS • *Department of Urology, Semmelweis University, Budapest, Hungary*
RICARDA THIER • *Leibniz Research Centre for Working Environment and Human Factors at TU Dortmund (IfADo), Dortmund, Germany; School of Medicine, Griffith University, Southport, Australia*
JÜRGEN THOMALE • *Institute of Cell Biology (Cancer Research), University of Duisburg-Essen Medical School, Essen, Germany*
STELLA TOMMASI • *Department of Preventive Medicine, USC Keck School of Medicine, University of Southern California, Los Angeles, CA, USA*
DANA VU VAN • *Department of Urology, Technische Universität Dresden, Dresden, Germany*
CÁRMEN VASCONCELOS-NÓBREGA • *Centre for the Study of Education, Technologies and Health, Polythecnic Institute of Viseu, Viseu, Portugal*
PATCHARAWALAI WHONGSIRI • *Department of Biochemistry, Faculty of Medicine, Chulalongkorn University, Bangkok, Thailand*
MANFRED P. WIRTH • *Department of Urology, Technische Universität Dresden, Dresden, Germany*
TAKAHIRO YOSHIDA • *Department of Urology, The James Buchanan Brady Urological Institute, The Johns Hopkins University School of Medicine, Baltimore, MD, USA*
ELLEN C. ZWARTHOFF • *Department of Pathology, Erasmus MC, Rotterdam, The Netherlands*

Part I

Molecular Characterization

Chapter 1

Analysis of Chromosomal Alterations in Urothelial Carcinoma

Donatella Conconi and Angela Bentivegna

Abstract

Here, we describe the use of complementary techniques applicable to different types of samples to analyze chromosomal alterations in urothelial carcinoma. By a conventional chromosome analysis on fresh biopsies, it is possible to delineate the status of ploidy and rough chromosomal aberrations. The multi-target fluorescence in situ hybridization (FISH) UroVysion test, for the rapid detection of chromosomal aneusomy of chromosomes 3, 7, and 17 and/or deletion of 9p21 locus, is applicable to urine specimens as well as to formalin-fixed paraffin-embedded (FFPE) specimens and fresh biopsies. Finally, array comparative genomic hybridization (array-CGH) gives the possibility of analyzing the DNA in a single experiment from a biopsy of the tumor but also from FFPE specimens; this technique is able to detect alterations at the genome level not excluding any chromosome.

Key words Urothelial carcinoma, Chromosome aberrations, Fluorescence in situ hybridization (FISH), UroVysion test, Comparative Genomic Hybridization (Array-CGH), DNA copy number variations, Urine specimens, Fresh biopsies, Formalin-fixed paraffin-embedded (FFPE) specimens

1 Introduction

The biological differences among the two different clinical and prognostic subtypes of transitional cell carcinoma (TCC, also urothelial cell carcinoma)—non-muscle-invasive, and muscle-invasive bladder cancers—reflect the underlying genetic heterogeneity that leads to specific pathways of tumor development and progression and they consequently influence the prognosis, the choice of treatment, and the survival rate. Innumerable studies have traced the status of known oncogenes and tumor suppressor genes and have revealed several recurring chromosomal changes associated with the pathologic stage and/or outcome of the tumor [1, 2]. On one hand, based on the well-known genetic alterations of bladder cancer, a multi-target fluorescence in situ hybridization (FISH) assay has been developed for the detection of TCC in urine specimens [3]. The UroVysion FISH test, approved by the U.S.

Wolfgang A. Schulz et al. (eds.), *Urothelial Carcinoma: Methods and Protocols*, Methods in Molecular Biology, vol. 1655, DOI 10.1007/978-1-4939-7234-0_1, © Springer Science+Business Media LLC 2018

Food and Drug Administration, is based on three centromeric probes specific for chromosomes 3, 7, and 17 and a fourth probe to the 9p21 region, for the detection of chromosomal aneusomy and/or deletion of 9p21 locus, which are common genetic alterations in TCCs [4, 5]. On the other hand, the development of array comparative genomic hybridization (array-CGH) led to the possibility of analyzing the whole genome in a single experiment, suggesting its possible application in screening/surveillance programs of cancer patients. With the use of the high-resolution mapping of array-CGH, novel copy number alterations were identified in many small genomic regions that had not been detected in previous studies [6–8].

Here, in order to analyze chromosomal alterations in urothelial carcinoma, we describe the use of complementary techniques applicable to different types of samples: starting from conventional chromosome analysis on TCC biopsies in order to delineate the status of ploidy in bulk tumors and rough chromosomal aberrations, moving to array-CGH and FISH. These are complementary techniques, as array-CGH is able to detect alterations at the genome level not excluding any chromosome across a sample, whereas FISH is able to reveal information for individual cells, but focuses on few genomic regions. Array-CGH provides the possibility of analyzing the DNA from a biopsy of the tumor but also from formalin-fixed paraffin-embedded (FFPE) specimens; in addition to these two resources, the UroVysion FISH test is also applicable to urine specimens.

2 Materials

2.1 Cytogenetic Analysis from Fresh Tumor Biopsies

2.1.1 Solutions

1. Transport solution: 30 ml of HBSS (Hank's Balanced Salt Solution) and 0.2 ml of heparin under sterile conditions. Store at 4 °C.
2. Hank's Balanced Salt Solution.
3. Complete culture medium: RPMI 1640 supplemented with 20% of fetal calf serum and 1% of penicillin/streptomycin. Store at 4 °C, pre-warm before the use.
4. Colcemid solution (10 μg/ml). Store at 4 °C, pre-warm before the use.
5. Sodium citrate tribasic dihydrate 1% solution: dissolve 1 g of sodium citrate tribasic dihydrate in 100 ml of sterile distilled water. Store at 4 °C, pre-warm before the use.
6. Fixative solution for fragments: acid acetic: ethanol absolute 3:1 solution. The fixative solution must be made fresh.

7. Dissociating solution (acid acetic aqueous solution 60%): 3 ml of acid acetic and 2 ml of sterile distilled water. The dissociating solution must be made fresh.
8. Potassium chloride solution: 0.56 g of KCl in 100 ml of sterile distilled water. Store at 4 °C, pre-warm before the use.
9. Fixative solution for cell suspension: methanol: acid acetic 3:1 solution. The fixative solution must be made fresh.
10. Quinacrine mustard solution: dissolve 5 mg in 100 ml of sterile distiller water. Store at 4 °C in the dark. Use at room temperature.
11. McIlvaine's buffer: dissolve 3.8 g of citric acid monohydrate and 29.15 g of disodium phosphate dihydrate in 1 l of sterile distilled water. Store at 4 °C, use at room temperature.

2.1.2 Laboratory Equipment

1. Multipurpose container for tissue culture, with lid, sterile.
2. Sterile nippers.
3. Cell culture dishes (35 mm).
4. Sterile scissors.
5. Microliter pipettors (100–1000 μl) and clean tips.
6. Pasteur glass pipettes.
7. Paper towel.
8. Microscope slides.
9. Spreader.
10. Conical centrifuge tubes (15 ml).
11. Serological pipettes (5 ml).
12. Glass coverslip (22 × 50 mm).
13. Vertical Staining Jar with Cover.

2.1.3 Laboratory Facilities

1. Laminar flow hood.
2. CO_2 incubator.
3. Fume hood.
4. Agglutinoscope or instrument for automated smearing.
5. Bench-top centrifuge.
6. Phase-contrast microscope.
7. Fluorescent microscope equipped with a charge coupled device camera.
8. Software for cytogenetic analyses.

2.2 Fluorescent In Situ Hybridization on Urine Specimens (Urovysion Bladder Cancer kit)

2.2.1 Solutions

1. UroVysion® Bladder Cancer Kit composed of:
   - (a) UroVysion DNA Probe Mixture (*see* datasheet for details). Store at −20 °C.
   - (b) DAPI II Counterstain (*see* datasheet for details). Store at −20 °C.
   - (c) NP-40 (*see* datasheet for details). Store at −20 °C.
   - (d) 20× SSC (*see* datasheet for details). Store at −20 °C.
2. PBS 1×.
3. Fixative solution: methanol: acid acetic 3:1 solution. The fixative solution must be made fresh.
4. Acid acetic aqueous solution: 3 ml of acid acetic and 2 ml of sterile distilled water. The solution must be made fresh.
5. 2× SSC: 100 ml of 20× SSC and 900 ml of distilled H_2O. Store at room temperature.
6. Pepsin solution (Zytovision, ES-00001-4).
7. Ethanol solutions: prepare dilutions of 70% and 85% using 100% ethanol and purified water. Store at room temperature in tightly capped containers when not in use.
8. 0.4× SSC + 0.3% NP-40: 20 ml of 20× SSC, 877 ml of distilled H_2O and 3 ml of NP-40. Adjust pH to 7.5 and adjust volume to 1 l with water. Store at room temperature.
9. 2× SSC + 0.1% NP-40: 100 ml of 20× SSC, 849 ml of distilled H_2O and 1 ml of NP-40. Adjust pH to 7.0 and adjust volume to 1 l with water. Store at room temperature.

2.2.2 Laboratory Equipment

1. Conical centrifuge tubes (15 and 50 ml).
2. Serological pipettes (5 ml).
3. Pasteur glass pipettes.
4. Microscope slides.
5. Diamond Tip Glass Engraving Pen.
6. Vertical Staining Jar with Cover.
7. Microliter pipettors (2–20 μl) and clean tips.
8. Glass coverslip (size depending to the size of selected area).
9. Humidified hybridization chamber.

2.2.3 Laboratory Facilities

1. Bench-top centrifuge.
2. Refrigerator.
3. Phase-contrast microscope.
4. Laboratory water bath (73 °C).
5. HYBrite System (Vysis).
6. Vortex mixer.

7. Microcentrifuge.
8. Laboratory oven (39 °C).
9. Fluorescence microscope equipped with a 100-watt mercury lamp and recommended filters.

2.3 Fluorescent In Situ Hybridization on Tumor-Isolated Cells (Urovysion Bladder Cancer kit)

2.3.1 Solutions

1. UroVysion® Bladder Cancer Kit composed of:
   (a) UroVysion DNA Probe Mixture (*see* datasheet for details). Store at −20 °C.
   (b) DAPI II Counterstain (*see* datasheet for details). Store at −20 °C.
   (c) NP-40 (*see* datasheet for details). Store at −20 °C.
   (d) 20× SSC (*see* datasheet for details). Store at −20 °C.
2. 2× SSC: 100 ml of 20× SSC and 900 ml of distilled H_2O. Store at room temperature.
3. Pepsin solution (Zytovision, ES-00001-4).
4. PBS 1×.
5. Post-fixative solution: 37.1 ml of PBS 1×, 1.9 ml of MgCl2 and 1 ml of formaldehyde solution 37%. Store at 4 °C.
6. Ethanol solutions: prepare dilutions of 70% and 85% using 100% ethanol and purified water. Store at room temperature in tightly capped containers when not in use.
7. 0.4× SSC + 0.3% NP-40: 20 ml of 20× SSC, 877 ml of distilled H_2O and 3 ml of NP-40. Adjust pH to 7.5 and adjust volume to 1 l with water. Store at room temperature.
8. 2× SSC + 0.1% NP-40: 100 ml of 20× SSC, 849 ml of distilled H_2O and 1 ml of NP-40. Adjust pH to 7.0 and adjust volume to 1 l with water. Store at room temperature.

2.3.2 Laboratory Equipment

1. Microscope slides.
2. Diamond Tip Glass Engraving Pen.
3. Vertical Staining Jar with Cover.
4. Glass coverslip (size depending to the size of selected area).
5. Microliter pipettors (2–20 μl) and clean tips.
6. Humidified hybridization chamber.

2.3.3 Laboratory Facilities

1. Phase-contrast microscope.
2. Laboratory water bath (73 °C).
3. HYBrite System (Vysis).
4. Vortex mixer.
5. Microcentrifuge.
6. Laboratory oven (39 °C).

7. Refrigerator.
8. Fluorescence microscope equipped with a 100-watt mercury lamp and recommended filters.

2.4 Fluorescent In Situ Hybridization on Formalin-Fixed, Paraffin-Embedded (FFPE) Tissues (Urovysion Bladder Cancer Kit)

2.4.1 Solutions

1. UroVysion® Bladder Cancer Kit composed by:
   (a) UroVysion DNA Probe Mixture (*see* datasheet for details). Store at −20 °C.
   (b) DAPI II Counterstain (*see* datasheet for details). Store at −20 °C.
   (c) NP-40 (*see* datasheet for details). Store at −20 °C.
   (d) 20× SSC (*see* datasheet for details). Store at −20 °C.
2. Xylene.
3. Ethanol solutions: prepare dilutions of 70% and 85% using 100% ethanol and purified water. Store at room temperature in tightly capped containers when not in use.
4. Distilled H_2O.
5. Heat pre-treatment solution citric (Zytovision, PT-00001-500). Store at 4 °C.
6. Pepsin solution (Zytovision, ES-00001-4). Store at 4 °C.
7. Propidium iodide stain.
8. 0.4× SSC + 0.3% NP-40: 20 ml of 20× SSC, 877 ml of distilled H_2O and 3 ml of NP-40. Adjust pH to 7.5 and adjust volume to 1 l with water. Store at room temperature.
9. 2× SSC + 0.1% NP-40: 100 ml of 20× SSC, 849 ml of distilled H_2O and 1 ml of NP-40. Adjust pH to 7.0 and adjust volume to 1 l with water. Store at room temperature.

2.4.2 Laboratory Equipment

1. Diamond Tip Glass Engraving Pen.
2. Vertical Staining Jar with Cover.
3. Microliter pipettors (2–20 μl) and clean tips.
4. Glass coverslip (size depending to the size of selected area).
5. Humidified hybridization chamber.

2.4.3 Laboratory Facilities

1. Laboratory oven (39–60 °C).
2. Laboratory water bath (95 °C).
3. HYBrite System (Vysis).
4. Vortex mixer.
5. Microcentrifuge.
6. Fluorescence microscope equipped with a 100-watt mercury lamp and recommended filters.

2.5 Array Comparative Genomic Hybridization (Array-CGH)

Solution, laboratory equipment and facilities according to the Agilent Technologies instructions (http://www.agilent.com/cs/library/usermanuals/Public/G4410-90020_CGH_ULS_3.5.pdf).

3 Methods

3.1 Cytogenetic Analysis from Fresh Tumor Biopsies

3.1.1 Biopsy Sample Preparation

1. Prepare transport solution and put in a multipurpose container for tissue culture under sterile conditions.
2. Put the biopsy in the container for tissue culture using sterile nipper.

   Work under a laminar flow hood for **steps 3–6**.
3. Remove the biopsy from container and transfer in a 35 mm cell culture dish with 2 ml of HBSS (Hank's Balanced Salt Solution).
4. Cut the biopsy with sterile scissors into small pieces.
5. Move some pieces with a sterile nipper into a new 35 mm cell culture dish that contains 2.5 ml of complete culture medium. Incubate cells in a 37 °C, 5% CO_2 incubator.
6. After at least 2 h add 100 μl of Colcemid and leave in a CO_2 incubator overnight at 37 °C.

   Work under a laboratory fume hood for points 3.1.2 and 3.1.3. Perform these points at the same time.

3.1.2 Chromosome Preparation from Biopsy Fragments.

1. Transfer the fragments with a Pasteur glass pipette in a dish that contains 2.5 ml of Sodium citrate tribasic dihydrate 1% solution (hypotonic solution), pre-warmed at 37 °C and incubate for 30 min at room temperature.
2. Transfer the fragments with a Pasteur glass pipette in a 35 mm dish that contains 3 ml of fixative solution for 1 min.
3. Transfer the fragments with a Pasteur glass pipette in a 35 mm dish that contains 3 ml of fixative solution for 15 min.
4. Aspirate only fixative solution with a Pasteur glass pipette, remove the excess with a paper towel and add a few drops of dissociating solution on fragments (*see* **Note 1**).
5. Put the slide on agglutinoscope, drop two or three drops of dissociating cells on a slide with a Pasteur glass pipette and smear the drops onto a slide surface with a spreader (make a spreader from disposable Pasteur glass pipette). Alternatively use an instrument for automated smearing.

   Leave the slides to air-dry. Check the slide for the presence and quality of metaphases by a phase-contrast microscope (*see* **Note 2**).
6. Store the remaining pellet in fixative solution at −20 °C. Store slides at room temperature.

3.1.3 Chromosome Preparation from Cell Suspension

1. Transfer the complete culture medium deprived of fragments in a 15 ml conical tube. Centrifuge at 750 × *g* for 10 min.
2. Remove the supernatant and resuspend completely the cell pellet in 5 ml of pre-warmed 37 °C hypotonic solution KCl 0.56%. Incubate for 20 min at room temperature.
3. Add 1 ml of fixative solution for 1 min, shaking the tube. Centrifuge at 750 × *g* for 5 min.
4. Remove the supernatant and resuspend completely the cell pellet in 5 ml of fixative solution. Incubate for 20 min at room temperature. Centrifuge at 750 × *g* for 5 min.
5. Remove the supernatant and add a few drops of fixative solution. Drop (from a height of about 5–10 cm) two or three drops of cells on a slide with a Pasteur glass pipette to obtain a cell smear. Leave the slides to air-dry. Examine the slides for the presence and quality of metaphases under a Phase-contrast microscope (*see* **Note 3**).
6. Store cell pellet in fixative solution at +4 °C for short time or −20 °C for long time. Store slides at room temperature.

3.1.4 Staining of the Slides

Stain the slides by immersion in quinacrine mustard solution for 5 min. Remove the slides from the stain and put in McIlvaine's buffer for few seconds. Mount the slide with a coverslip.

3.1.5 Acquisition of the Images

Photograph the metaphases using a fluorescent microscope equipped with a charge coupled device camera (Fig. 1, *see* **Note 4**) and analyze them by means of a software for cytogenetics.

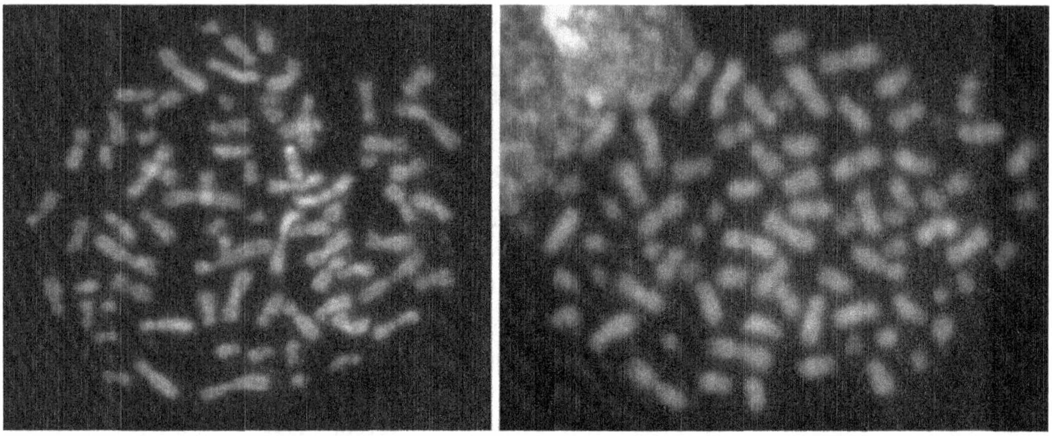

Fig. 1 Examples of QFQ banded metaphases obtained from fresh tumor biopsies. As expected, there are polyploid and rearranged metaphases

3.2 Fluorescent In Situ Hybridization (UroVysion Bladder Cancer Kit)

The UroVysion® Bladder Cancer Kit is FDA approved and designed to detect aneuploidy for chromosomes 3, 7, 17 and loss of the 9p21 locus in urine specimens from persons with hematuria suspected of having bladder cancer or for surveillance of recurrence in patients previously diagnosed with bladder cancer (https://www.abbottmolecular.com/us/products/urovysion.html).

This probe consists of three alpha-satellite repeat sequence probes: CEP 3 SpectrumRed, CEP 7 SpectrumGreen, and CEP 17 SpectrumAqua that hybridize to the centromere regions of chromosomes 3, 7, and 17, respectively and a unique sequence probe, LSI p16 (9p21) SpectrumGold, that hybridizes to the *CDKN2A*/p16 gene.

3.2.1 Fluorescent In Situ Hybridization on Urine Specimens

1. Centrifuge the urine specimens at 750 × *g* for 10 min in a 50 ml tube.
2. Remove the supernatant and resuspend the pellet in 10 ml of PBS 1×. Transfer the contents to a 15 ml conical tube.
3. Centrifuge the urine specimens at 750 × *g* for 10 min.
4. Remove the supernatant leaving about 500 μl of supernatant. Slowly add 5 ml of fixative solution.
5. Let fixed specimens at −20 °C for a minimum of 30 min (maximum 10 days).
6. Centrifuge at 750 × *g* for 5 min. Carefully remove the supernatant and resuspend the pellet in 5 ml of fixative solution.
7. Centrifuge at 750 × *g* for 5 min. Carefully remove the supernatant and resuspend the pellet in few drops of fixative solution. Put one drop of cell suspension on a slide with a Pasteur glass pipette and leave to air-dry. Examine the slide under a phase-contrast microscope for choosing the hybridization area in which at least 100 cells are visible in the field (use a diamond tip glass engraving pen). Avoid overlapping cells.
8. Immerse slide in the acid acetic aqueous solution 60% for 5 min at room temperature. Leave the slides to air-dry.
9. Put slide in the pre-warmed 2× SSC solution for 2 min at 73 °C in a water bath.
10. Leave the slides to air-dry for a few minutes, then place on a HYBrite plate at 37 °C, and put a few drops of pepsin on the target area, for 5 min.
11. Wash the slide in 2× SSC for 1 min at room temperature.
12. Wash the slide in PBS 1× for 5 min at room temperature.
13. Immerse the slide in fixative solution for 5 min at room temperature.
14. Allow the slide to completely dry at room temperature.

15. Remove the UroVysion probe from −20 °C storage and allow warming to room temperature. Vortex and spin briefly.
16. Put 2–10 μl of probe (depending on the size of the selected area) to the slide and place a coverslip over the probe. Apply light pressure to the coverslip to allow the probe to distribute under the coverslip. Avoid air bubbles.
17. Use HYBrite instrument to perform co-denaturation of slide and probe at 73 °C for 2 min.
18. Wait that the temperature decreases to 39 °C, and then place slide in a pre-warmed humidified hybridization chamber. Incubate at 39 °C overnight in the dark.
19. Remove the coverslip and immediately immerse the slide in a pre-warmed 0.4× SSC + 0.3% NP-40 solution at 73 °C for 2 min.
20. Immerse the slide in the pre-warmed 2× SSC + 0.1% NP-40 solution at room temperature for 1 min.
21. Remove the slide from the wash solution and allow it to dry completely.
22. Apply 10–20 μl (depending on the size of the selected area) of DAPI II on the target area and place a coverslip. Avoid air bubbles. Leave the slide in the dark at 4 °C for some minutes before count. Store the slide in the dark at 4 °C for short times, at −20 °C for long periods.
23. Count 100 nuclei signals with a fluorescence microscope equipped with a 100-watt mercury lamp and recommended filters capable of detecting the emission spectrum of the probes used (*see* **Note 5**).

3.2.2 Fluorescent In Situ Hybridization on Tumor-Isolated Cells

1. Follow the protocol for cytogenetic analysis at **steps 3.1.2–3.1.3**. Examine the slide under a Phase-contrast microscope for choosing the hybridization area in which at least 100 cells are visible in the field (use a diamond-tip glass-engraving pen). Avoid overlapping cells.
2. Put the slide in the pre-warmed 2× SSC solution for 2 min at 73 °C in a water bath.
3. Leave the slides to air-dry for a few minutes, and then place on the HYBrite plate at 37 °C and put a few drops of pepsin on the target area, for 20 min.
4. Wash the slide in PBS 1× for 5 min at room temperature.
5. Immerse the slide in the post-fixative solution for 5 min at room temperature.
6. Wash the slide in PBS 1× for 5 min at room temperature.
7. Dehydrate the slide in 70% ethanol solution at room temperature for 1 min. Repeat with 85% ethanol, followed by 100% ethanol.

8. Allow the slide to completely dry at room temperature.
9. Remove the UroVysion probe from −20 °C storage and allow warming to room temperature. Vortex and spin briefly.
10. Put 2–10 μl of probe (depending on the size of the selected area) to the slide and place a coverslip over the probe. Apply light pressure to the coverslip to allow the probe to distribute under the coverslip. Avoid air bubbles.
11. Use HYBrite instrument to perform co-denaturation of slide and probe at 73 °C for 2 min.
12. Wait that the temperature decreases to 39 °C, and then place the slide in a pre-warmed humidified hybridization chamber. Incubate at 39 °C overnight in the dark.
13. Remove the coverslip and immediately immerse the slide in the pre-warmed 0.4× SSC + 0.3% NP-40 solution at 73 °C for 2 min.
14. Immerse the slide in the pre-warmed 2× SSC + 0.1% NP-40 solution at room temperature for 1 min.
15. Remove the slide from the wash solution and allow it to dry completely.
16. Apply 10–20 μl (depending on the size of the selected area) of DAPI II on the target area and place a coverslip. Avoid air bubbles. Leave the slide in the dark at 4 °C for some minutes before count. Store the slide in the dark at 4 °C for short times, at −20 °C for long periods.
17. Count 100 nuclei signals with a fluorescence microscope equipped with a 100-watt mercury lamp and recommended filters capable of detecting the emission spectrum of the probes used (*see* **Note 6** and Fig. 2).

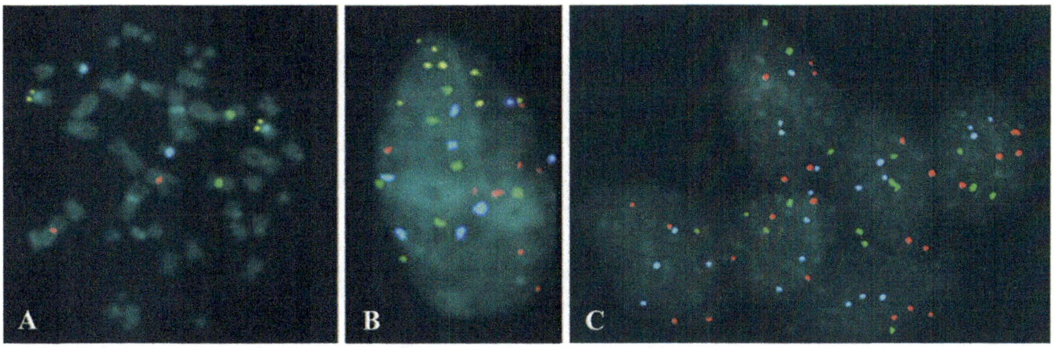

Fig. 2 Examples of UroVysion FISH test on a metaphase (**a**), an isolated cell (**b**), and a cell cluster (**c**). (**a**) Metaphase shows a normal/disomic signals pattern (*2 red, 2 green, 2 aqua, 2 yellow*). (**b**) Isolated cell shows an aberrant signals pattern with multiple copies of each probe. (**c**) Cell cluster shows multiple copies of CEP3, CEP7, and CEP17 signals, but a complete loss of 9p21 locus (*yellow probe*) [9]

3.2.3 Fluorescent In Situ Hybridization on Formalin-Fixed, Paraffin-Embedded (FFPE) Tissues

1. Use 4–5 μm thick section from formalin-fixed, paraffin-embedded tissues. Examine the slides under a phase-contrast microscope for choosing the hybridization area in which at least 100 tumoral cells are visible in the field (use a diamond-tip glass-engraving pen). The slides must be baked overnight vertically in an oven at 60 °C before use.
2. Deparaffinize tissue section in xylene two times for 30 min each.
3. Hydrate the slide in two changes of 100% ethanol at room temperature, 10 and 5 min respectively, two changes of 85% ethanol, and two changes of 70% ethanol, 5 min each.
4. Immerse the slide in distilled H_2O for at least 10 min (better overnight).
5. Incubate the slide in the pre-warmed pretreatment solution for 10 min at 95 °C. After 10 min, leave the slide in the solution for 7 min at room temperature.
6. Rinse the slide in two changes of distilled H_2O, 3 min each.
7. Leave the slide to air-dry, then place on HYBrite plate at 37 °C and put a few drops of pepsin on the target area, for 7–12 min. Time depends on fixation, age of section, and type of tissue (*see* **Note 7**).
8. Rinse the slide in two changes of distilled H_2O, 3 min each.
9. Apply 10–20 μl (depending on the size of tissue section) of propidium iodide on the target area and place a coverslip. Check the tissue digestion (*see* **Note 8**) with a fluorescent microscope, eventually remove the coverslip and repeat **steps 6–8**.
10. Remove the coverslip and rinse the slide in three changes of distilled H_2O, 3 min each.
11. Dehydrate slide in 70% ethanol solution at room temperature for 2 min. Repeat with 85% ethanol, followed by 100% ethanol.
12. Allow slides to completely dry at room temperature.
13. Remove the UroVysion probe from −20 °C storage and allow warming to room temperature. Vortex and spin briefly.
14. Put 2–10 μl of probe (depending on the size of section) to the tissue section and place a coverslip over the probe. Apply light pressure to the coverslip to allow the probe to distribute under the coverslip. Avoid air bubbles.
15. Use HYBrite instrument to perform co-denaturation of slide and probe at 75 °C for 10 min.
16. Wait that the temperature decreases to 39 °C, then place slide in a pre-warmed humidified hybridization chamber. Incubate at 39 °C overnight in the dark.

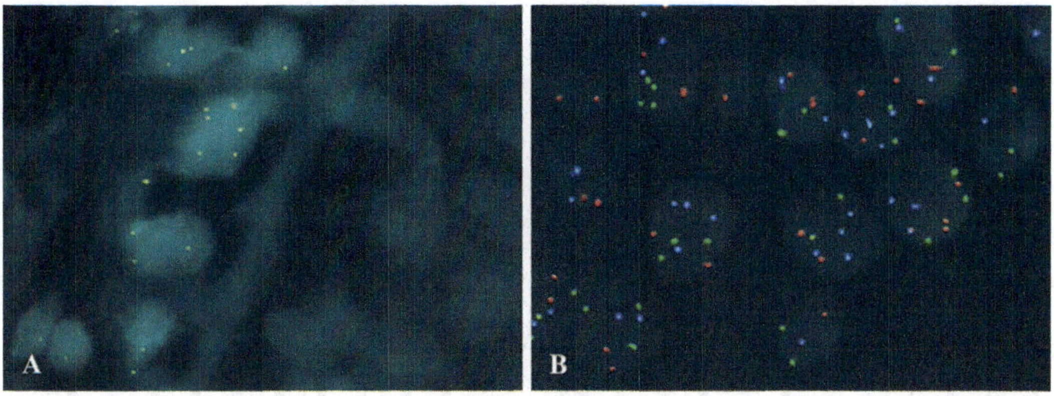

Fig. 3 Examples of UroVysion FISH test on formalin-fixed paraffin-embedded tissues. (**a**) Clear distinction between neoplastic and normal tissue divided by the stromal axis. Neoplastic tissue is recognizable by the complete loss of 9p21 locus (*yellow probe*) present in normal tissue (*left*). (**b**) Cells with an aberrant pattern of signals, characterized by the complete loss of 9p21 signal (*yellow probe*) and the presence of multiple copies of CEP3 (*red*), CEP7 (*green*), and CEP17 (*aqua*)

17. Remove the coverslip and immediately immerse slide in the pre-warmed 0.4× SSC + 0.3% NP-40 solution at 73 °C for 2 min.
18. Immerse the slide in the pre-warmed 2× SSC + 0.1% NP-40 solution at room temperature for 1 min.
19. Remove the slide from the wash solution, briefly dry, and immediately apply 10–20 μl (depending on the size of section) of DAPI II on the tissue section and place a coverslip. Avoid air bubbles. Leave slide in the dark at 4 °C for some minutes before count. Store the slide in the dark at 4 °C for short times, at −20 °C for long periods.
20. Count 100 nuclei signals with a fluorescence microscope equipped with a 100-watt mercury lamp and recommended filters capable of detecting the emission spectrum of the probes used (*see* **Note 6** and Fig. 3).

3.3 Array Comparative Genomic Hybridization (Array-CGH)

Perform array-CGH following the Agilent Technologies instructions faithfully (http://www.agilent.com/cs/library/usermanuals/Public/G4410-90020_CGH_ULS_3.5.pdf).

This technique gives the possibility of analyzing the DNA from blood, cells, and FFPE tissues.

For results interpretation we apply a filtering option of a minimum of 3 aberrant consecutive probes and a minimum absolute average log2 ratio that differs among all samples and depends on DLRS values, so it is related to the quality of experiment.

Somatic mosaicism is a typical condition of cancer, which is a mixture of different subpopulations. For this reason, also mosaic gains and losses must be discovered. In particular, non-mosaic gains

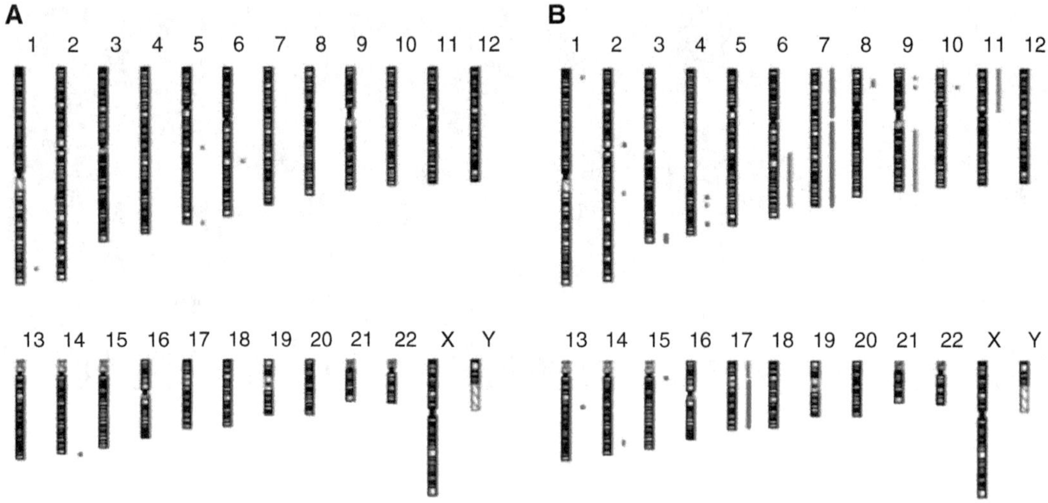

Fig. 4 Examples of array-CGH results analyzed using Agilent Genomic Workbench v5.0 software (*red*: gains, *green*: losses). (**a**) Low-grade non-muscle-invasive transitional cell carcinoma. (**b**) High-grade muscle-invasive transitional cell carcinoma

and losses are identified by standard log2 ratios values for all samples: values over 0.6, which correspond to 3 copies, identify non-mosaic gains; values under −1, which correspond to 1 copy, identify non-mosaic losses. Accordingly, log2 ratios values for mosaic gains range between DLRS value and 0.6 and for mosaic losses between DLRS value and −1 [10] (Fig. 4).

4 Notes

1. Leave the dissociating solution for a few minutes, gently resuspending with a Pasteur glass pipette.
2. If the slide is too full of nuclei and the metaphases are too closed, add more drops of dissociating solution and repeat point 5.
3. If metaphases are too closed, put the slide above a hot vapor for a few seconds (use the laboratory water bath). If metaphases are too open, put the slide under a lamp for a few seconds.
4. Select metaphases with a good banding resolution. Avoid metaphases with overlapping chromosomes.
5. Count only morphologically abnormal cells; do not count morphologically normal, overlapping or damaged cells.
6. Count only morphologically abnormal cells; do not count morphologically normal, overlapping or damaged cells. For FFPE tissue sections, it is also important to avoid cells that are truncated during the sectioning process.

7. 7–12 min are recommended for bladder cancer FFPE; different types of tissues might require various tests to identify the best condition.
8. If the nuclei are visible with distinct cell borders from one another, the digestion of the stroma/matrix can be considered adequate. Holes in the tissue or a pale staining of nuclei indicate an over-digestion. In this case, restart from point 1 with a new slide.

Acknowledgment

The authors want to gratefully acknowledge Professor Leda Dalprà for her help in revising the manuscript. This work was supported by Gianluca Strada Association for research and treatment of urological cancer.

References

1. Fadl-Elmula I (2005) Chromosomal changes in uroepithelial carcinomas. Cell Chromosome 4:1
2. Höglund M, Säll T, Heim S et al (2001) Identification of cytogenetic subgroups and karyotypic pathways in transitional cell carcinoma. Cancer Res 61:8241–8246
3. Sokolova IA, Halling KC, Jenkins RB et al (2000) The development of a multitarget, multicolor fluorescence in situ hybridization assay for the detection of urothelial carcinoma in urine. J Mol Diagn 2:116–123
4. Tsai YC, Nichols PW, Hiti AL et al (1990) Allelic losses of chromosomes 9, 11, and 17 in human bladder cancer. Cancer Res 50:44–47
5. Sandberg AA, Berger CS (1994) Review of chromosome studies in urological tumors. Ii. Cytogenetics and molecular genetics of bladder cancer. J Urol 151:545–560
6. Veltman JA, Fridlyand J, Pejavar S et al (2003) Array-based comparative genomic hybridization for genome-wide screening of DNA copy number in bladder tumors. Cancer Res 63:2872–2880
7. Hurst CD, Fiegler H, Carr P et al (2004) High-resolution analysis of genomic copy number alterations in bladder cancer by microarray-based comparative genomic hybridization. Oncogene 23:2250–2263
8. Blaveri E, Brewer JL, Roydasgupta R et al (2005) Bladder cancer stage and outcome by array-based comparative genomic hybridization. Clin Cancer Res 11:7012–7022
9. Panzeri E, Conconi D, Antolini L et al (2011) Chromosomal aberrations in bladder cancer: fresh versus formalin fixed paraffin embedded tissue and targeted fish versus wide microarray-based CGH analysis. PLoS ONE 6(9):e24237
10. Conconi D, Redaelli S, Bovo G et al (2016) Unexpected frequency of genomic alterations in histologically normal colonic tissue from colon cancer patients. Tumour Biol. doi:10.1007/s13277-016-5181-0

Chapter 2

Analysis of Point Mutations in Clinical Samples of Urothelial Carcinoma

Mustafa Alamyar and Ellen C. Zwarthoff

Abstract

In the last two decades specific point mutations in oncogenes have been identified in urinary bladder cancers. Identification of these mutations in clinical samples (e.g., urine or tumor tissue) can be of use for diagnostic or prognostic purposes. In this chapter we describe how mutations in multiple oncogenes can be identified with a simple assay.

Key words Oncogenic mutations, FGFR3, TERT, PIK3CA, RAS, DNA isolation, Mutation analysis

1 Introduction

1.1 Oncogenic Mutations in Bladder Tumors

In bladder tumors specific point mutations have been found in the *FGFR3, TERT, PIK3CA, HRAS, KRAS,* and *NRAS* oncogenes. Except for *TERT,* the mutations lead to the incorporation of another amino acid in the corresponding protein. This results in a more active protein, and since these proteins are all involved in cell growth and proliferation, the end result is tumor growth. Mutations in the *TERT* gene occur instead in the promoter region and result in more mRNA and more protein and hence active lengthening of telomeres at the end of chromosomes, which is thought to immortalize cells. Table 1 gives an overview of the common mutations in these genes [1–3].

FGFR3 mutations occur in about 60% of bladder tumors, with the highest prevalence in stage Ta (65%,) with 33% in stage T1 (both non-muscle invasive (NMIBC)) and 22% in MIBC. Because of this distribution *FGFR3* together with Ki-67 can be used to predict progression in NMIBC tumors [1]. *TERT* mutations were found in 60–80% of tumors, regardless of stage and grade [1, 2, 4, 5]. Mutations in *PIK3CA* are found in 24% of bladder tumors, with a similarly equal distribution over stage. Finally,

Wolfgang A. Schulz et al. (eds.), *Urothelial Carcinoma: Methods and Protocols*, Methods in Molecular Biology, vol. 1655, DOI 10.1007/978-1-4939-7234-0_2, © Springer Science+Business Media LLC 2018

Table 1
Overview of the relevant genes and their mutation sites

Genes	Mutation sites
HRAS	G12C/S, G12D/V, G13C/R, Q61K, Q61L/R
KRAS	G12C/R/S, G12A/D/V, Q61E
NRAS	Q12R, Q61L/R
PIK3CA	E542K, E545K/Q, E545G, H1047L/R
FGFR3	R248C, S249C, G372C, S373C, Y375C, G382R, A393E, K652E/Q, K652 T/M
TERT[a]	-124 C > T/A; −138 C > T; −146 C > T

[a]Mutations in *TERT* are respective to the ATG start codon

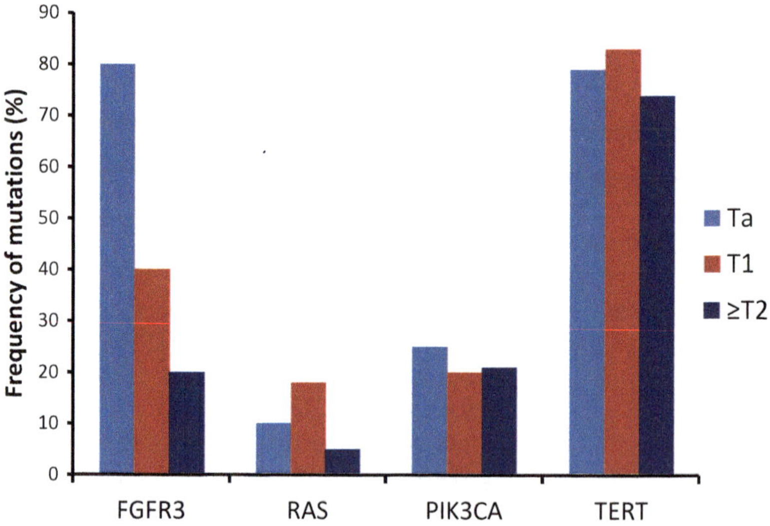

Fig. 1 Frequencies of *FGFR3, RAS, PIK3CA* and *TERT* mutations according to stage

mutations in the three *RAS* genes are relatively uncommon (6–10%) [1]. Figure 1 gives an overview of frequencies according to stage [1–3].

1.2 The Use of Oncogenic Mutations in Clinical Practice

Analyses of the mutations in DNA isolated from tumor tissue is important for predicting possible progression, as is the case for *FGFR3* mutations. In addition, mutations in *PIK3CA* and the *RAS* genes may be of use as companion diagnostic for targeted therapies as the pathways in which these genes function will be constitutively active downstream of the mutant protein and hence upstream inhibition will be ineffective. In addition, targeted therapies with small molecule inhibitors or monoclonal antibodies are in clinical trials for tumors with an activated *FGFR3* gene. Likewise there are multiple small molecule inhibitors for the active PIK3CA protein. Finally, the high frequency with which *FGFR3* and *TERT* mutations occur makes them ideal for the identification of bladder tumor cells in DNA isolated from urinary cell pellets, both for patients under surveillance for recurrences after resection of a primary NMIBC as well as for patients presenting with hematuria to rule out that a bladder tumor is the cause of hematuria [1–3, 6, 7]. This chapter provides background information per mutation type and illustrates how mutation analysis can be carried out from voided urine or tumor tissue [8].

2 Materials

2.1 DNA Isolation from Urine

1. 50 ml centrifuge tubes.
2. Phosphate-buffered saline.
3. 1.5 ml Eppendorf vials.
4. QIAamp mini and Blood kit.
5. Ethanol (96–100%).
6. Qubit 2.0 Fluorometer device.
7. Qubit dsDNA HS Assay Kit.

2.2 DNA Isolation from Formalin-Fixed Paraffin-Embedded (FFPE) Tissue

1. Disposable 1 mm biopsy punch.
2. Xylene.
3. Ethanol 100%.
4. Ethanol 70%.
5. Lysis buffer; 10 mM Tris–HCl, pH 8.0, 100 mM EDTA, pH 8.0, 50 mM NaCl, 0.5% SDS.
6. Proteinase K, 20 mg/ml.
7. Chelex.

2.3 Mutation Analysis

2.3.1 Materials

1. KAPA2G Robust Hotstart ReadyMix.
2. Shrimp alkaline phosphatase.
3. Exonuclease-I.
4. SNaPshot Multiplex kit (Applied Biosystems, Life Technologies, UK).
5. Formamide.
6. Automatic sequencer ABI PRISM 3130 XL Genetic Analyzer or similar.
7. GeneScan Analysis Software version 2.4.2 (SoftGenetics LLC).

3 Methods

The mutations described above are good diagnostic candidates for early detection and disease surveillance. For the analysis one needs 10–100 ml of voided urine from a (potential) patient.

3.1 DNA Isolation from Urine

1. Transfer the urine sample to a 50 ml centrifuge tube.
2. Centrifuge the 50 ml tube at 1500 × *g* for 10 min.
3. Resuspend the pellet in 900 μl phosphate-buffered saline (PBS) and transfer this to a 1.5 ml Eppendorf tube.
4. Centrifuge the 1.5 ml tube at 3000 × *g* for 5 min.
5. Discard the supernatant; pellets can be kept at −80 °C until DNA isolation.
6. DNA from urine pellets is isolated using the QIAamp mini and Blood kit. Before starting, bring samples to room temperature.
7. Add 20 μl proteinase K (20 mg/ml) and 200 μl buffer AL to the sample. Mix for 15 s using the pulse-vortex and incubate for 10 min at 56 °C.
8. Centrifuge the tubes shortly to remove drops from the inside of the lid.
9. Add 200 μl ethanol (96–100%) to the sample and mix again using the pulse-vortex. Again centrifuge the tubes to remove drops from the lid.
10. Add the mixture from the 1.5 ml tube to the QIAamp Mini spin column in a 2 ml collection tube without wetting the rim.
11. Centrifuge the column at 6000 × *g* for 1 min and place the spin column in a clean 2 ml collection tube. Dispose the tube with the eluate.
12. Apply buffer AW1 to the spin column and centrifuge at 6000 × *g* for 1 min, dispose the tube with the eluate.
13. Apply buffer AW2 (500 μl) to the spin column and centrifuge at 20,000 × *g* for 3 min, discard the eluate.
14. For DNA elution transfer the spin column to a 1.5 ml Eppendorf vial and add 100 μl AE buffer to the spin column and incubate at room temperature for 5 min. Centrifuge at 6000 × *g* for 1 min. N.B. the DNA is in the eluate.
15. Measure the DNA concentration from the eluate according to manufacturer's protocol using the Qubit 2.0 Fluorometer device and corresponding Qubit dsDNA HS Assay Kit.

3.2 DNA Isolation from Formalin-Fixed Paraffin-Embedded (FFPE) Tissue

1. Use a hematoxylin-eosin-stained section of the tissue block for selection of an area with tumor cells.
2. Take a 1 mm punch from the selected region using a punch tool.

3. Transfer the sample to a 1.5 ml tube and add 800 μl xylene to remove paraffin.
4. Incubate for 10 min at room temperature.
5. Centrifuge the mixture at 16,000 × *g* for 1 min and pipet the xylene supernatant from the mixture.
6. For ethanol rehydration add 800 μl of 100% ethanol to the specimen, vortex and centrifuge at 16000 × *g* for 3 min.
7. Remove the ethanol supernatant without touching the pellet.
8. Pipet 800 μl of 70% ethanol, vortex and centrifuge at 16,000 × *g* for 3 min.
9. Remove the ethanol supernatant as much as possible.
10. Open the tube and air-dry the pellet for 10 min.
11. For the tissue dissolution add 100 μl lysis buffer, 25 μl proteinase K (20 mg/ml) and 25 μl Chelex (Bio-RAD, California, USA) to the pellet.
12. Incubate overnight in heat block at 56 °C.
13. Incubate the mixture at 95 °C for 10 min to deactivate proteinase K, and centrifuge for 1 min at 16,000 × *g*.
14. The supernatant contains the extracted DNA. Transfer into a clean tube leaving the Chelex mixture with the cell debris behind (*see* **Note 1**).
15. Measure DNA concentration as explained for urine DNA (*see* **Note 2**).

3.3 Mutation Analysis

1. For *FGFR3* mutation analysis, set up a multiplex PCR in a final volume of 10 μl containing 5 ng of DNA, 5 μl KAPA2G Robust Hotstart ReadyMix, 18 pmol of exon 7 primers and 10 pmol each of exon 10 and 15 primers (*see* Table 2 for primer sequences)(*see* **Note 3**).
2. After 3 min at 95 °C, 40 PCR cycles are carried out (15 s at 95 °C, 15 s at 55 °C and 20 s at 72 °C) followed by 10 min at 72 °C.
3. Treat the PCR product with 1.5 units of shrimp alkaline phosphatase and two units of exonuclease-I for 60 min at 37 °C to get rid of excess primers and deoxynucleotide triphosphates (ddNTPs), followed by 15 min at 85 °C to inactivate the enzymes.
4. Next, use a SNaPshot Multiplex kit for a single-nucleotide probe extension based on probes that anneal adjacent to the investigated nucleotides (probe sequences in Table 2, *see* **Note 4**).
5. The SNaPshot reaction is carried out in a total volume of 10 μl containing 1 μl of PCR product, 2.5 μl of the Snapshot ready mix, 2 μl of the 5× sequencing buffer and 1 μl of the probe mix.

Table 2
Primer and probe sequence for *FGFR3* mutation analysis

Primer	Sequence (5′- > 3′)	Product size (bp)	pmol			
FGFR3 RI Fw	AGTGGCGGTGGTGGTGAGGGAG	115	18			
FGFR3 RI Rev	GCACCGCCGTCTGGTTGG		18			
FGFR3 RII Fw	CAACGCCCATGTCTTTGCAG	138	10			
FGFR3 RII Rev	AGGCGGCAGAGCGTCACAG		10			
FGFR3 RIII Fw	GACCGAGGACAACGTGATG	160	10			
FGFR3 RIII Rev	GTGTGGGAAGGCGGTGTTG		10			
Probe	**Sequence (5′- > 3′)**	**Size (bp)**	**Strand**	**WT**	**MT**	
S373C	T19 GAGGATGCCTGCATACACAC[a]	39	sense	T[b]	A	2
K652 M/T	T20 CACAACCTCGACTACTACAAGA	42	sense	A	T/C	7
G372C	T29 GGTGGAGGCTGACGAGGCG	48	sense	G	T	2
A393E	T34 CCTGTTCATCCTGGTGGTGG	54	sense	C	A	10
R248C	T46 CGTCATCTGCCCCCACAGAG	66	sense	C	G	8
Y375C	T43 ACGAGGCGGGCAGTGTGT	61	sense	A	G	10
S249C	T36TCTGCCCCCACAGAGCGCT	55	sense	C	T	4
K652Q/E	T50 GCACAACCTCGACTACTACAAG	72	antisense	A	C/G	3
G382R	T56 GAACAGGAAGAAGCCCACACC	76	antisense	C	T	6

[a]T19 etc. indicate the length of the T-tails

[b]The color of the incorporated WT and MT nucleotides corresponds with the color of the peaks in the sequence run

6. Probe extension is for 35 cycles of 10 s at 96 °C, followed by 40 s at 58.5 °C.
7. Treat the Snapshot product with 1 U SAP for 30 min at 37 °C to remove excess ddNTPs and incubate for 15 min at 85 °C to inactivate the enzyme.
8. Add 1 μl of the reaction to 10 μl formamide and denature by incubation at 95 °C for 5 min.
9. Use this mixture for the separation of the product in a 20–25 min run on 36 cm long capillaries using the automatic sequencer. The absence or presence of a mutation is indicated by the fluorescent marker of the incorporated ddNTP.
10. Use GeneScan Analysis Software version 2.4.2 for analysis of the generated data or alternatively software provided by Applied Biosystems.

Table 3
Primer and probe sequence for *TERT* mutation analysis

Primer	Sequence (5′- > 3′)	Product size (bp)	pmol			
TERT Fw	AGCGCTGCCTGAAACTCG	155	10			
TERT Rev	CCCTTCACCTTCCAGCTC		10			
Probe	**Sequence (5′- > 3′)**	**Size (bp)**	**Strand**	**WT**	**MT**	**pmol/ reaction**
TERT; −124 C > T	T20 GGCTGGGAGGGCCCGGA[a]	37	sense	G	A/T[b]	10
TERT; −138C > T	T27 GGAGGGGGCTGGGCCGG	44	sense	G	A	5
TERT; −146 C > T	T39 CTGGGCCGGGGACCCGG	56	sense	G	A	15

[a]T20 etc. indicate the length of the T-tails
[b]The color of the incorporated WT and MT nucleotides corresponds with the color of the peaks in the sequence run

The *TERT* and *PIK3CA* mutation analyses are similar to the *FGFR3* mutation analysis. The *TERT* PCR covers the two most frequent sites for *TERT* mutations in the promoter. Primer and probe sequences for *TERT* mutation analysis are given in Table 3. Figure 2 illustrates the results of a *TERT* mutation analysis.

The *PIK3CA* PCR covers the hotspot mutation sites in the gene (E542K, E545G, E545K, and H1047R) [1]. Primer and probe sequences for PIK3CA mutation analysis are given in Table 4. Mutations in the *HRAS*, *KRAS*, and *NRAS* genes are not very common in bladder tumors. We therefore combined the most prevalent mutations in one assay as explained in Kompier et al. [1]. This assay covers 96% of the possible *RAS* mutations in bladder tumors. Details on primers and probes for the different mutations are depicted in Tables 2–5.

4 Notes

1. Take care to get rid of the Chelex beads as they may interfere with subsequent steps.
2. Do not use a spectrophotometer for determining DNA concentration. Especially with FFPE samples many proteins are still present in the DNA solution. Proteins absorb ultraviolet light in the 230 and 280 nM range and high concentrations may result in absorption at 260 nM and hence the DNA concentration may be overestimated.
3. Make up with water to 10 μl, if necessary. Optional: add a small drop of paraffin oil to prevent evaporation.
4. T-tails are added to the probe to allow separation and visualization of the different probes on the sequencer.

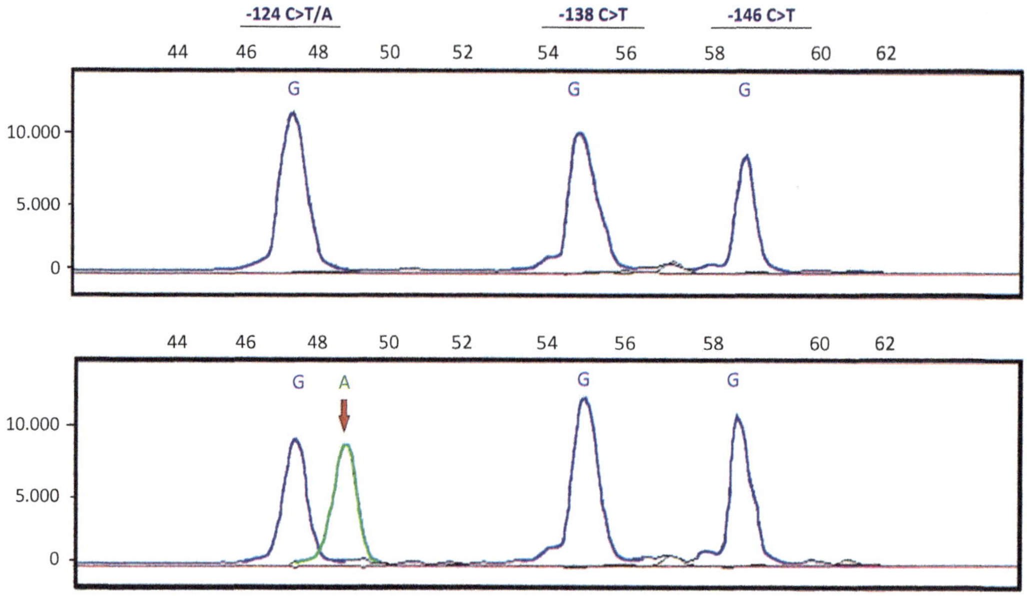

Fig. 2 Example of a wild type and mutant type (lower panel) *TERT* mutation analysis result

Table 4
Primer and probe sequence for *PIK3CA* mutation analysis

Primer	Sequence (5′- > 3′)	Product size (bp)	pmol			
PIK3CA ex9-Fw	AGTAACAGACTAGCTAGAGA	139	0.5			
PIK3CA ex9-Rev.	ATTTTAGCACTTACCTGTGAC		0.5			
PIK3CA ex20-Fw	GACCCTAGCCTTAGATAAAAC	109	1			
PIK3CA ex20-Rev	GTGGAAGATCCAATCCATTT		1			
Probe	**Sequence (5′- > 3′)**	**Size (bp)**	**Strand**	**WT**	**MT**	**pmol/ reaction**
E542K	T17 ACACGAGATCCTCCTCTCT*	35	sense	G[a]	A[b]	1.5
E545G	T21 CCTCTCTCTGAAATCACTG	40	sense	A	G	5
E545G	T25 ATCCTCTCTCTGAAATCACT	45	sense	G	A	3
H1047R	T30 GAAACAAATGAATGATGCAC	50	sense	A	G	3

[a]T17 etc. indicate the length of the T-tails
[b]The color of the incorporated WT and MT nucleotides corresponds with the color of the peaks in the sequence run

Table 5
Primer and probe sequence for *HRAS, KRAS, NRAS* mutation analysis

Primer	Sequence (5′- > 3′)	Product size (bp)	pmol
HRAS exon1 Fw	CAGGAGACCCTGTAGGAGG	139	6
HRAS exon1 Rev	TCGTCCACAAAATGGTTCTG		6
HRAS exon2 Fw	GGAGACGTGCCTGTTGGA	140	3
HRAS exon2 Rev	GGTGGATGTCCTCAAAAGAC		3
KRAS exon1 Fw	GGTCCTGCTGAAAATGACTG	163	3
KRAS exon1 Rev	GGTCCTGCACCAGTAATATG		3
KRAS exon1 Fw	CCAGACTGTGTTTCTCCCTT	155	3
KRAS exon1 Rev	CACAAAGAAAGCCCTCCCCA		3
NRAS exon1 Fw	GGTGTGAAATGACTGAGTAC	128	3
NRAS exon1 Rev	GGGCCTCACCTCTATGGTG		3
NRAS exon2 Fw	GGTGAAACCTGTTTGTTGGA	103	3
NRAS exon2 Rev	ATACACAGAGGAAGCCTTCG		3

(continued)

Table 5 (continued)

Probe	Sequence (5′- > 3′)	Size (bp)	Strand	WT	MT	pmol/ reaction
HRAS pos.34	T17 CTGGTGGTGGTGGGCGCC[a]	35	Sense	G[b]	C/T/A	5
HRAS pos.182	T18 GCATGGCGCTGTACTCCTCC	38	antisense	T	G/C/A	1.5
KRAS pos.34	T25 GGACTCTTGCCTACGCCCAC	45	antisense	C	G/A/T	5
HRAS pos.35	T31 CGCACTCTTGCCCACACCG	50	antisense	C	G/A/T	7
NRAS pos.182	T33 GACATACTGGATACAGCTGGAC	55	sense	A	G/C/T	5
KRAS pos.181	T41 CTCATTGCACTGTACTCCTCTT	63	antisense	G	T/C	2
HRAS pos.181	T46 CATCCTGGATACCGCCGGC	65	sense	C	A/G	7
KRAS pos.35	T49 AACTTGTGGTAGTTGGAGCTG	70	sense	G	C/T/A	2
HRAS pos.37	T55 CAGCGCACTCTTGCCCACAC	75	antisense	C	G/A/T	7
NRAS pos.34	T62 CTGGTGGTGGTTGGAGCA	80	sense	G	C/T/A	2

[a]T17 etc. indicate the length of the T-tails
[b]The color of the incorporated WT and MT nucleotides corresponds with the color of the peaks in the sequence

References

1. Kompier LC, Lurkin I, van der Aa M, van Rhijn BW et al (2010) FGFR3, HRAS, KRAS, NRAS and PIK3CA mutations in bladder cancer and their potential as biomarkers for surveillance and therapy. PLoS One 5:e13821
2. van Rhijn BW, Vis AN, van der Kwast TH, Kirkels WJ, Radvanyi F et al (2003) Molecular grading of urothelial cell carcinoma with fibroblast growth factor receptor 3 and MIB-1 is superior to pathologic grade for the prediction of clinical outcome. J Clin Oncol 21:1912–1921
3. Allory Y, Beukers W, Sagrera A et al (2014) Telomerase reverse transcriptase promoter mutations in bladder cancer: high frequency across stages, detection in urine, and lack of association with outcome. Eur Urol 65:360–366
4. Hurst CD, Platt FM, Knowles MA (2014) Comprehensive mutation analysis of the TERT promoter in bladder cancer and detection of mutations in voided urine. Eur Urol 65:367–369
5. Zuiverloon TC, van der Aa MN, van der Kwast TH et al (2010) Fibroblast growth factor receptor 3 mutation analysis on voided urine for surveillance of patients with low-grade non-muscle-invasive bladder cancer. Clin Cancer Res 16:3011–3018
6. van Kessel KE, van Neste L, Lurkin I et al. (2016) Evaluation of an epigenetic profile for the detection of bladder cancer in patients with hematuria. J Urol 195:601-607
7. van Kessel KE, Kompier LC, de Bekker-Grob EW, Zuiverloon TC et al (2013) FGFR3 mutation analysis in voided urine samples to decrease cystoscopies and cost in nonmuscle invasive bladder cancer surveillance: a comparison of 3 strategies. J Urol:1676–1681
8. Hurst CD, Zuiverloon TC, Hafner C et al (2009) A SNaPshot assay for the rapid and simple detection of four common hotspot codon mutations in the PIK3CA gene. BMC Res Notes 2:66

Chapter 3

A Versatile Assay for Detection of Aberrant DNA Methylation in Bladder Cancer

Stella Tommasi and Ahmad Besaratinia

Abstract

Urothelial carcinoma of the bladder is one of the most common malignancies in the industrialized world, mainly caused by smoking and occupational exposure to chemicals. The favorable prognosis of early stage bladder cancer underscores the importance of early detection for the treatment of this disease. The high recurrence rate of this malignancy also highlights the need for close post-diagnosis monitoring of bladder cancer patients. As for other malignancies, aberrant DNA methylation has been shown to play a crucial role in the initiation and progression of bladder cancer, and thus holds great promise as a diagnostic and prognostic biological marker. Here, we describe a protocol for a versatile DNA methylation enrichment method, the *M*ethylated CpG *I*sland *R*ecovery *A*ssay (MIRA), which enables analysis of the DNA methylation status in individual genes or across the entire genome. MIRA is based on the ability of the methyl-binding domain (MBD) proteins, the MBD2B/MBD3L1 complex, to specifically bind methylated CpG dinucleotides. This easy-to-perform method can be used to analyze the methylome of bladder cancer or urothelial cells shed in the urine to elucidate the evolution of bladder carcinogenesis and/or identify epigenetic signatures of chemicals known to cause this malignancy.

Key words Aromatic amines, Biomarkers, Epigenetics, Methyl-binding domain (MBD) proteins, Tobacco smoke, Urine

1 Introduction

Bladder cancer is the ninth most common cancer in the world, with an estimated 430,000 new cases and 165,000 deaths in 2012 [1–3]. In the US alone, 76,960 new cases are expected to occur in 2016, and 16,390 bladder cancer patients are expected to die from the disease in the same year [4]. The vast majority (>90%) of bladder cancer cases are urothelial carcinomas. Approximately 75% of patients are diagnosed with non-muscle-invasive bladder cancer, of which roughly 50% are of low-grade [1, 3]. The prognosis of these noninvasive tumors is usually favorable; however, up to 80% of cases will recur after complete transurethral resection, and up to 45% of cases will progress to invasive cancer within 5 years [5, 6]. Cystoscopy, followed by biopsy of suspicious lesions, remains the

Wolfgang A. Schulz et al. (eds.), *Urothelial Carcinoma: Methods and Protocols*, Methods in Molecular Biology, vol. 1655, DOI 10.1007/978-1-4939-7234-0_3, © Springer Science+Business Media LLC 2018

gold standard for the detection of both new and recurrent bladder cancer. However, this approach is highly invasive and costly and its sensitivity can be as low as 60% for the detection of carcinoma in situ [6, 7]. Noninvasive tests for bladder cancer diagnosis are available and include voided urine cytology, cytogenetic analysis by fluorescence in situ hybridization, and detection of genetic mutations in urine. Yet, these tests have limited sensitivities (54–86%), and specificities (61–90%), and often yield false positive results [3, 6, 8]. Given the high recurrence rate of bladder cancer and the costs and discomfort associated with post-diagnosis follow-ups, the quest for novel noninvasive tests to improve early detection and assist with surveillance is currently a top research priority [8, 9].

Unlike other types of human cancer with unknown or less well-defined etiologic agent(s), bladder cancer is primarily linked to exposure to aromatic amines, a family of chemicals present in tobacco smoke and various industrial products and workplace settings [10–13]. Epidemiologic studies have shown that smokers have two- to sixfold higher risk of bladder cancer relative to nonsmokers [1, 14]. Also, those who smoke black (air-cured) tobacco products are at increased risk of bladder cancer compared to those who smoke blond tobacco (flue-cured) products. The latter is consistent with the higher content of aromatic amines in smoke from black tobacco products relative to blond tobacco products [11]. Furthermore, higher incidence of bladder cancer has been observed in industrial workers exposed to aromatic amines generated during the manufacture or processing of a variety of products, including rubber, cable, textile, dye, paints, solvents, leather dust, inks, etc. [10–13, 15]. Lifestyle choices, such as the use of hair dyes containing aromatic amines, have also been suggested as a potential determinant of bladder cancer, although conclusive evidence is yet to emerge [15].

Aromatic amines are known to induce DNA damage and mutations that may cause disruption of key biological pathways that may lead to cell transformation, e.g., in normal urothelium [9, 11, 16, 17]. In addition to having a genotoxic mode of action, aromatic amines, like many other chemical carcinogens, may also exert epigenetic effects of relevance to bladder carcinogenesis [6, 18–20]. Epigenetics is a fast growing field in cancer biology with tremendous potential for environmental, clinical, and translational research [21–23]. Epigenetic effects are defined as heritable changes in gene expression that do not involve alterations in the underlying DNA sequence. Aberrant DNA methylation associated with transcriptional deregulation of cancer-related genes is the best-studied epigenetic mechanism of carcinogenesis [23–28]. Aberrancies in DNA methylation patterns commonly occur in the early stages of carcinogenesis and as such, are detectable prior to clinical diagnosis of cancer. Thus, modification of DNA methylation patterns together with alterations of gene expression may serve as predictive biomarkers for early detection of cancer [29]. Furthermore, epigenetic changes intensify as cancer progresses, and are potentially reversible through pharmacological interventions or genetic manipulation [30, 31]. Therefore, epigenetic biomarkers can also be used for both prognostic and therapeutic purposes.

Investigating the epigenetic basis of bladder carcinogenesis, especially in individuals with known history of exposure to aromatic amines, e.g., specific industry workers or smokers, holds great promise for cancer biomarker discovery [6, 8, 9, 20, 32–34]. The continuous shedding of bladder cells into the urine offers a unique opportunity for noninvasive surveillance of the epigenetic landscape both before and after clinical manifestation of bladder cancer [34–36]. The noninvasively obtainable urine specimens from, e.g., occupationally exposed individuals to aromatic amines or smokers, can be analyzed over time to evaluate alterations of the epigenome during the initiation and progression of bladder cancer. Elucidating the underlying mechanisms of bladder carcinogenesis by determining the epigenetic signature of aromatic amines in a readily available surrogate tissue (i.e., urine) will be critical to developing novel diagnostic and/or prognostic biomarkers for bladder cancer.

Over the past decades, an increasing number of methods have been developed to examine the DNA methylation profile at individual loci or on a genome-wide scale in a variety of experimental systems [37–40]. Here, we described a protocol for the *M*ethylated CpG *I*sland *R*ecovery *A*ssay (MIRA), a sensitive and versatile pull-down assay for the enrichment of methylated DNA [41, 42]. This technique is easy to perform and allows recovery of methylated DNA without relying on the use of expensive antibodies. The MIRA (outlined in Fig. 1) is based on the ability of the methyl-binding domain (MBD) proteins, the MBD2b/MBD3L1 complex, to specifically bind methylated-CpG dinucleotides [40–42]. The MIRA-enriched DNA fractions can be used in several downstream applications, including DNA methylation analysis of single loci by real-time PCR or bisulfite conversion followed by cloning and DNA sequencing [40]. MIRA is also compatible with high-throughput microarray or next-generation sequencing platforms, e.g., the Illumina Genome Analyzer (MIRA-seq). So far, several versions of MIRA-seq have been developed, all requiring ligation of specific adapters for library construction, DNA sequencing, and sequence read alignment using a reference genome [43–45]. We and others have successfully applied MIRA to detect aberrant DNA methylation in a variety of tumor types, including human melanoma, lung and breast cancer [41, 46], immortalized cell lines [47] and mice/cells treated in vivo/in vitro with prototype carcinogens [48, 49]. The MIRA technology is licensed to Active Motif (under U.S. Patent No. 7,425,415), which has developed easy-to-perform kits for MIRA (MethylCollector™ Ultra, Active Motif®) and MIRA-seq (MethylCollector™ Ultra-Seq, Active Motif®).

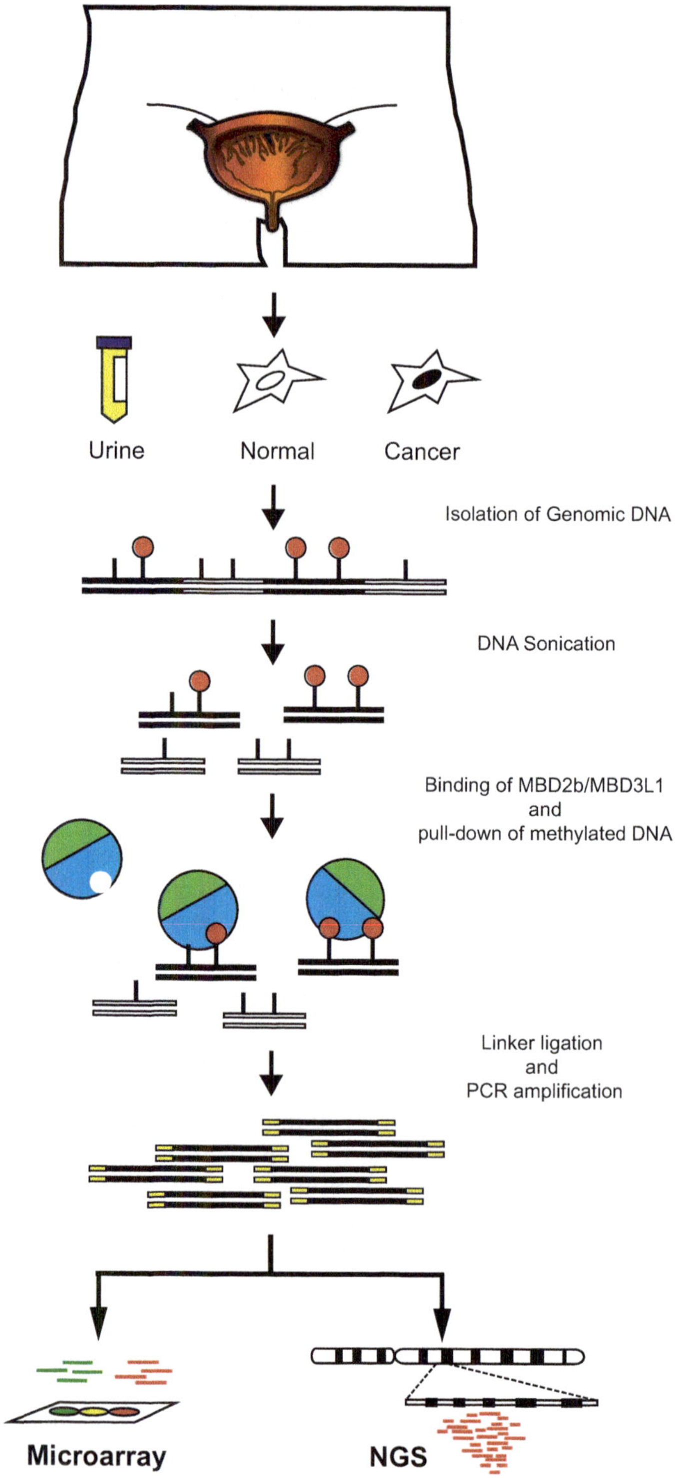

Fig. 1 Outline of MIRA. This method enables analysis of the DNA methylation status in individual genes or across the entire genome. MIRA is based on the ability of the methyl-binding domain (MBD) proteins, the MBD2B/MBD3L1 complex, to specifically bind methylated CpG dinucleotides. Enriched DNA fractions can be analyzed on high-throughput microarray or NGS platforms

2 Materials

All the reagents must be of molecular biology grade and solutions must be prepared using distilled milliQ water and then autoclaved/filter-sterilized.

2.1 Purification of GST-MBD2b and His-MBD3L1 Proteins for MIRA

1. GST-tagged MBD2b and histidine-tagged MBD3L1 expression plasmids.
2. LB broth, LB agar, and SOC medium, for bacteriological work [50].
3. BL21 (DE3) Competent Cells (Agilent Technologies, Santa Clara, CA).
4. Isopropyl-Beta-D-Thiogalatoside (IPTG). Make a 100 mM stock solution in H_2O, filter sterilize and keep at −20 °C.
5. Lysozyme. Make a 100 mg/ml stock solution in H_2O, aliquot and keep at −20 °C.
6. Sodium Chloride-Tris-EDTA (STE) buffer; 150 mM NaCl, 10 mM Tris–HCl, pH 7.8, 0.1 mM or 1 mM EDTA, pH 8.0.
7. GST-STE buffer; 150 mM NaCl, 10 mM Tris–HCl, pH 7.8, 1 mM EDTA, pH 8.0.
8. His-STE buffer; 150 mM NaCl, 10 mM Tris–HCl, pH 7.8, 0.1 mM EDTA, pH 8.0.
9. Phenylmethylsulfonylfluoride (PMSF). Make a 100 mM stock solution in isopropanol, aliquot and keep at −20 °C.
10. *N*-lauroylsarcosine. Make a 10% (w/v) stock solution in H_2O, aliquot and keep at −20 °C.
11. Glutathione Sepharose 4B beads (GE Healthcare Life Sciences, Uppsala, Sweden).
12. Ni-NTA His-Bind® Resin (MilliporeSigma, Darmstadt, Germany).
13. GST-washing buffer; 0.1% (v/v) Triton X-100 in phosphate buffered saline (PBS) buffer.
14. His-washing buffer; 50 mM $NaH_2PO_4{\cdot}H_2O$, 300 mM NaCl, 20 mM Imidazole. Adjust pH to 8.0 with 1 M NaOH.
15. GST-Elution buffer; 50 mM Tris–HCl, pH 8.5, 150 mM NaCl, 20 mM reduced glutathione, 0.1% Triton X-100.
16. His-Elution buffer: 50 mM $NaH_2PO_4{\cdot}H_2O$, 300 mM NaCl, 250 mM Imidazole. Adjust pH to 8.0 with 1 M NaOH.
17. 4-(2-hydroxyethyl)-1-piperazineethanesulfonic acid) HEPES.
18. Protein-dialysis buffer (for both GST- and His-tagged proteins): 50 mM Hepes, pH 7.4, 150 mM NaCl, 5 mM β-mercaptoethanol, 50% Glycerol.
19. Bovine Serum Albumin (BSA).

2.2 Sample Preparation for MIRA

1. Elution buffer (EB) (Qiagen, Valencia, CA).
2. TE; 10 mM Tris–HCl, 1 mM EDTA, pH 8.0.
3. Quick-DNA™ Urine kit (Zymo Research, Irvine, CA).

2.3 MIRA Enrichment and PCR Amplification

1. Purified GST-tagged MBD2b and His-tagged MBD3L1 proteins (~1 μg each).
2. Sonicated DNA from JM110 bacterial strain (*see* **Note 1**).
3. 10× MIRA-binding buffer; 100 mM Tris–HCl, pH 7.9, 500 mM NaCl, 100 mM $MgCl_2$, 10 mM DL-Dithiothreitol (DTT), 1% (v/v) Triton X-100 (*see* **Note 2**).
4. MagneGST Glutathione Particles and magnetic stand (Promega, Madison, WI).
5. Qiaquick PCR purification kit (Qiagen, Valencia, CA).
6. MIRA-washing buffer; 10 mM Tris–HCl, pH 7.5, 700 mM NaCl, 1 mM EDTA, 3 mM $MgCl_2$, 0.1% (v/v) Triton X-100.
7. T4 DNA polymerase, 10× NEB 2 buffer, T4 DNA ligase and 10× T4 DNA ligase buffer (New England Biolabs, Ipswich, MA).
8. Ligation-mediated PCR (LM-PCR) Linker is obtained by annealing a long oligo: 5′-GCGGTGACCCGGGAGATCT-GAATTC-3′ with a short complementary oligo: 5′-GAATT-CAGATCTCCCG-3′ (*see* **Note 3**).
9. Taq DNA polymerase, 10× PCR buffer, 5× Q solution (Qiagen, Valencia, CA).
10. Sybr Green I Nucleic Acid Gel Stain (Roche, Mannheim, Germany).

3 Methods

3.1 Purification of GST-MBD2b and His-MBD3L1 Proteins for MIRA

GST-MBD2b and His-MBD3L1 can be purified in parallel. Distinct buffers/reagents are usually needed.

3.1.1 Transformation

1. In two separate tubes, transform BL21 (DE3)-competent cells with:
   (a) *GST-MBD2b* protein-expressing plasmid (1 μl).
   (b) *His-MBD3L1* protein-expressing plasmid (1 μl).
2. Incubate tubes on ice for 30 min, at 42 °C for 38 s, and back on ice for 2 min.
3. Add 500 μl SOC medium and incubate at 37 °C for 1 h with shaking.

4. Following transformation, plate cells (100 μl) on:
   (a) ampicillin-containing plates for *GST-MBD2b*.
   (b) kanamycin-containing plates for *His-MBD3L1*.
5. Incubate at 37 °C overnight.

3.1.2 IPTG Induction

1. Inoculate 200 ml LB (add ampicillin for *GST-MBD2b* culture or kanamycin for *His-MBD3L1* culture) with 30–40 well-developed bacterial colonies.
2. Grow in a shaker at 37 °C until OD reaches 0.6 at a fixed wavelength of 600 nm.
3. To each flask, add 200 μl of 100 mM IPTG (0.1 mM IPTG final concentration) to induce expression of GST-tagged MBD2b or His-tagged MBD3L1 proteins.
4. Allow the cells to grow in the shaker at 37 °C for additional 4–6 h.
5. Split cell suspension in 50 ml falcon tubes (4×) and centrifuge at 3500 × *g* for 15 min at 4 °C. Discard the supernatant.
6. Cell pellets can be processed immediately or kept at −80 °C for several months.

3.1.3 Protein Purification

1. Resuspend the cell pellet (from a single falcon tube) in 10 ml of:
   (a) GST-STE buffer containing 100 μg/ml lysozyme for *GST-MBD2b*;
   (b) His-STE buffer containing 100 μg/ml lysozyme for *His-MBD3L1*.
2. To each tube, add 100 μl of 100 mM PMSF (to a final concentration of 1 mM PMSF) and incubate on ice for 10 min.
3. Lyse bacterial cells by adding 1 ml of 10% *N*-lauroylsarcosine.
4. Sonicate bacterial lysate until it clears up and loses viscosity.
5. Add 1 ml of 10% Triton-X to the lysate and vortex it for 20 s.
6. Centrifuge lysate at 3500 × *g* for 15 min (4 °C) and transfer the supernatant into a new tube (~12 ml).
7. To the cleared lysate add:
   (a) 0.1 ml 50% slurry Glutathione Sepharose 4B beads for *GST-MBD2b*;
   (b) 0.1 ml Ni-NTA Agarose beads for *His-MBD3L1*.
8. Mix gently by shaking at 4 °C for 30–45 min.
9. Pellet the beads at 1000 × *g* for 1 min.
10. Wash with:
    (a) 10 ml of GST-washing buffer for *GST-MBD2b*;
    (b) 10 ml of His-washing buffer for *His-MBD3L1*.

11. Invert tubes several times, then collect beads by centrifugation at 1000 × *g* for 1 min.
12. Repeat washes two more times.

3.1.4 Elution and Dialysis

1. Elute proteins from beads with:
   (a) 1 ml GST-Elution buffer for ~4 h at 4 °C on a rotating platform for *GST-MBD2b*;
   (b) 1 ml His-Elution buffer for 30 min at 4 °C on a rotating platform for *His-MBD3L1*.
2. Dialyze the eluted proteins against:
   (a) 1–2 l of 1× PBS (+PMSF) for 5 h at 4 °C, and then against 1–2 l of protein-dialysis buffer (+PMSF) overnight at 4 °C.
   (b) After dialysis, check protein integrity and concentration on a 10% SDS-PAGE gel using BSA as a standard.
3. Aliquots of purified MBD2b and MBD3L1 proteins can be kept at −20 °C for several months.

3.2 Sample Preparation for MIRA

3.2.1 DNA Isolation

1. High molecular weight genomic DNA can be isolated from cells and tissues using standard phenol/chloroform extraction protocols [50]. Alternatively, commercially available kits, such as the DNeasy Blood & Tissue Kit (Qiagen, Valencia, CA), can be used.
2. Genomic DNA can be extracted from urine specimens with the Quick-DNA™ Urine kit (Zymo Research, Irvine, CA).

3.2.2 Fragmentation of Genomic DNA

We routinely use a Bioruptor® sonicator (Diagenode, Denville, NJ) to shear genomic DNA to generate 200- to 600-bp fragments (*see* **Note 4**).

1. Resuspend 500–700 ng genomic DNA to a final volume of 200 μl (with EB or TE buffer).
2. Sonication is performed in apposite tubes using the medium power setting with alternating 30 s on/30 s off intervals for a total of 15 min. Avoid overheating.
3. Check an aliquot on 2% agarose gel.
4. Keep 10–20 ng sonicated DNA to use as input (non-MIRA-enriched fraction).

3.3 MIRA

3.3.1 Binding of MBD Proteins to Fragmented DNA

1. In a 1.5 ml Eppendorf tube, mix: 1× NEB buffer 2, 0.1% Triton X-100, 0.5 μg sonicated JM110 DNA, 1 μg purified GST-MBD2b, 1 μg purified His-MBD3L1, and H_2O to a final volume of 100 μl.
2. Mix by pipetting and preincubate at 4 °C for 20 min on a rotating platform. Rotate at a low speed to prevent foaming.

This step is required for MBD2b/MBD3L1 complex formation.

3. Add 500–700 ng sonicated genomic DNA to the 100 μl binding mix. Adjust final volume to 400 μl (with EB buffer).
4. Incubate at 4 °C overnight (or for at least 5 h) on a rotating platform.

3.3.2 Washing and Pre-blocking of Magne GST Beads

1. Add 2.5 μl of MagneGST Glutathione Particles into 1 ml of 1× PBS containing 0.1% Triton X-100 and invert tubes several times.
2. Capture magnetic beads using a magnetic stand and carefully decant the supernatant.
3. Add 1 ml of 1× PBS/0.1% Triton X-100 into each tube.
4. Repeat washes for two to three times.
5. To decrease nonspecific background, pre-block the washed beads with a solution of: 1× NEB buffer 2, 0.1% Triton X-100, 0.5 μg sonicated JM110 DNA, and H_2O up to 400 μl.
6. Mix by pipetting and incubate at 4 °C for 20 min on a rotating platform.
7. Remove the supernatant with the aid of a magnetic stand.
8. Add 400 μl of protein-DNA mix (Subheading 3.3.1) to the pre-blocked beads.
9. Incubate at 4 °C for ~2 h on a rotating platform.

3.3.3 Recovery of the MIRA-Enriched DNA Fraction

1. Capture the beads with the aid of a magnetic stand and carefully remove the supernatant.
2. Add 800 μl of MIRA-washing buffer into the tube and invert four to five times. Capture the beads on a magnetic stand. Discard the supernatant.
3. Wash beads (carrying the methylated CpG fraction) for two to three times with 1 ml of MIRA-washing buffer. Following beads pulldown, discard the supernatant.
4. Purify the CpG-enriched fraction from the beads with the Qiaquick PCR purification kit according to the manufacturer's instructions.
5. Elute the CpG-rich fraction from the column with 50 μl of EB buffer.

3.3.4 Generation of Blunt-Ended DNA

Following sonication, DNA fragments must undergo an end-treatment filling step for the successful ligation of the blunt-ended linker adaptor. *Remember to include the input sample (non-MIRA-enriched DNA fraction) in parallel at this point.

1. To each input and MIRA-enriched DNA sample (50 μl) add: 1× NEB buffer 2, 100 μM dNTPs, 1× BSA, 0.6 U T4 DNA polymerase, and H_2O up to a final volume of 60 μl.
2. Mix by pipetting and incubate at 12 °C for 20 min.
3. Add 300 μl PBI buffer to each tube and purify according to the Qiaquick protocol (Qiagen).
4. Elute in 50 μl EB buffer.
5. Speed vac to 5 μl.

3.3.5 Linker Ligation and PCR Amplification

1. For linker ligation, to each blunt-ended DNA sample (5 μl), add 5 μl ligation mix containing: 15 μM double-stranded LM-PCR linker, 1× T4 DNA ligase buffer, and 400 U T4 DNA ligase.
2. Incubate at 16 °C overnight.
3. For PCR amplification, add to each tube: 1× PCR Buffer, 1× Q solution, 1.2 mM $MgCl_2$, 0.35 mM dNTP, 0.375× Sybr Green, 5 U Taq Polymerase, and H_2O up to 100 μl.
4. Incubate samples in a real-time PCR machine using the following cycling conditions: 72 °C for 15 min; 95 °C for 3 min; [95 °C for 30 s, 60 °C 20 s] for 14–16 cycles; 72 °C for 3 min and 30 s (*see* **Note 5**).
5. Following PCR amplification, purify DNA by Qiaquick purification kit (Qiagen) and elute in 50 μl EB buffer.
6. Measure the concentration by a spectrophotometer or Nanodrop.
7. At this point, input and MIRA-enriched DNA from experimental and control samples can be labeled and examined by microarray analysis. Alternatively, samples can be ligated to specific adaptors followed by library construction and analysis on NGS platforms (Fig. 1).

4 Notes

1. JM110 is a bacterial strain that lacks both DNA adenine methylation (*dam*) and DNA cytosine methylation (*dcm*) activities. Purified JM110 DNA is sonicated to an average length of 400–500 bp. Sonicated JM110 DNA is used in the binding reaction to decrease nonspecific binding of DNA to MBD proteins and/or beads.
2. 10× NEB 2 buffer (New England Biolabs, Ipswich, MA) can be used as an alternative buffer. Remember to add Triton X-100 to a final concentration of 0.1%.

3. The LM-PCR linker is prepared by combining 50 μl of 100 μM long oligo with 50 μl of 100 μM short oligo. The mix (50 μM) is incubated for 3 min in a boiling water bath, and allowed to slowly cool down to room temperature. The annealed double-stranded linker is kept in small aliquots at −20 °C.
4. Alternatively, genomic DNA can be restriction digested with *MseI* (5′-TTAA-3′), which cuts outside the CpG islands. Different sets of oligos are required to make the linker adaptor. Sonication is preferable to *MseI* digestion because it does not introduce significant sequence bias.
5. The initial step at 72 °C is required to fill in the 3′ ends of the double-stranded linker adaptor. PCR cycling is monitored in a real-time thermocycler and reactions are stopped immediately before reaching the amplification plateau (14–16 cycles are usually sufficient). PCR reactions can be scaled down to 10–50 μl (final volume).

Acknowledgments

ST and AB declare no conflicts of interest.

Work of the authors is funded by grants from the National Institute of Dental and Craniofacial Research of the National Institutes of Health (1R01DE026043-01) to AB and from the University of California Tobacco-Related Disease Research Program (TRDRP-25IP-0001) to ST.

References

1. Stewart BW, Wild CP (eds) (2014) World Cancer Report 2014. International Agency for Research on Cancer (IARC), Lyon, France
2. Antoni S, Ferlay J, Soerjomataram I, Znaor A, Jemal A, Bray F (2016) Bladder cancer incidence and mortality: a global overview and recent trends. Eur Urol 71(1):96–108. doi:10.1016/j.eururo.2016.06.010
3. Kamat AM, Hahn NM, Efstathiou JA, Lerner SP, Malmstrom PU, Choi W, Guo CC, Lotan Y, Kassouf W (2016) Bladder cancer. Lancet 388(10061):2796–2810. doi:10.1016/S0140-6736(16)30512-8
4. Siegel RL, Miller KD, Jemal A (2016) Cancer statistics, 2016. CA Cancer J Clin 66(1):7–30
5. Carradori S, Cristini C, Secci D, Gulia C, Gentile V, Di Pierro GB (2012) Current and emerging strategies in bladder cancer. Anticancer Agents Med Chem 12(6):589–603
6. Besaratinia A, Cockburn M, Tommasi S (2013) Alterations of DNA methylome in human bladder cancer. Epigenetics 8(10):1013–1022
7. Griffiths TR, on behalf of Action on Bladder Cancer (2013) Current perspectives in bladder cancer management. Int J Clin Pract 67 (5):435–448
8. Miremami J, Kyprianou N (2014) The promise of novel molecular markers in bladder cancer. Int J Mol Sci 15(12):23897–23908
9. Netto GJ (2012) Molecular biomarkers in urothelial carcinoma of the bladder: are we there yet? Nat Rev Urol 9(1):41–51
10. Boffetta P (2008) Tobacco smoking and risk of bladder cancer. Scand J Urol Nephrol Suppl 218:45–54
11. Besaratinia A, Tommasi S (2013) Genotoxicity of tobacco smoke-derived aromatic amines and bladder cancer: current state of knowledge and future research directions. FASEB J 27 (6):2090–2100
12. Kiriluk KJ, Prasad SM, Patel AR, Steinberg GD, Smith ND (2012) Bladder cancer risk from occupational and environmental exposures. Urol Oncol 30(2):199–211

13. U.S. Department of Health and Human Services (2014) The health consequences of smoking – 50 years of progress. A report of the Surgeon General. U.S. Department of Health and Human Services. Public Health Service. Office of the Surgeon General. Rockville, MD
14. Freedman ND, Silverman DT, Hollenbeck AR, Schatzkin A, Abnet CC (2011) Association between smoking and risk of bladder cancer among men and women. JAMA 306 (7):737–745
15. Internationa Agency for Research on Cancer (IARC) (2010) Some aromatic amines, organic dyes, and related exposures. In: IARC monographs on the evaluation of carcinogenic risk to humans, vol 99. Lyon, France
16. Scelo G, Brennan P (2007) The epidemiology of bladder and kidney cancer. Nat Clin Pract Urol 4(4):205–217
17. Stern MC, Lin J, Figueroa JD, Kelsey KT, Kiltie AE, Yuan JM, Matullo G, Fletcher T, Benhamou S, Taylor JA, Placidi D, Zhang ZF, Steineck G, Rothman N, Kogevinas M, Silverman D, Malats N, Chanock S, Wu X, Karagas MR, Andrew AS, Nelson HH, Bishop DT, Sak SC, Choudhury A, Barrett JH, Elliot F, Corral R, Joshi AD, Gago-Dominguez M, Cortessis VK, Xiang YB, Gao YT, Vineis P, Sacerdote C, Guarrera S, Polidoro S, Allione A, Gurzau E, Koppova K, Kumar R, Rudnai P, Porru S, Carta A, Campagna M, Arici C, Park SS, Garcia-Closas M, International Consortium of Bladder C (2009) Polymorphisms in DNA repair genes, smoking, and bladder cancer risk: findings from the international consortium of bladder cancer. Cancer Res 69(17):6857–6864
18. Jirtle RL, Skinner MK (2007) Environmental epigenomics and disease susceptibility. Nat Rev Genet 8(4):253–262
19. Cortessis VK, Thomas DC, Levine AJ, Breton CV, Mack TM, Siegmund KD, Haile RW, Laird PW (2012) Environmental epigenetics: prospects for studying epigenetic mediation of exposure-response relationships. Hum Genet 131(10):1565–1589
20. Schulz WA, Goering W (2016) DNA methylation in urothelial carcinoma. Epigenomics 8 (10):1415–1428. doi:10.2217/epi-2016-0064
21. Sandoval J, Esteller M (2012) Cancer epigenomics: beyond genomics. Curr Opin Genet Dev 22(1):50–55
22. You JS, Jones PA (2012) Cancer genetics and epigenetics: two sides of the same coin? Cancer Cell 22(1):9–20
23. Feinberg AP, Koldobskiy MA, Gondor A (2016) Epigenetic modulators, modifiers and mediators in cancer aetiology and progression. Nat Rev Genet 17(5):284–299
24. Suzuki MM, Bird A (2008) DNA methylation landscapes: provocative insights from epigenomics. Nat Rev Genet 9(6):465–476
25. Kulis M, Esteller M (2010) DNA methylation and cancer. Adv Genet 70:27–56
26. Jones PA (2012) Functions of DNA methylation: islands, start sites, gene bodies and beyond. Nat Rev Genet 13(7):484–492
27. Besaratinia A, Tommasi S (2014) Epigenetics of human melanoma: promises and challenges. J Mol Cell Biol 6(5):356–367
28. Beekman R, Kulis M, Martín-Subero JI (2016) The DNA methylomes of cancer. In: Fraga M, Fernandez AF (eds) Epigenomics in health and disease Elsevier Inc, pp 183–207
29. Verma M (2015) The role of Epigenomics in the study of cancer biomarkers and in the development of diagnostic tools. Adv Exp Med Biol 867:59–80
30. Rodriguez-Paredes M, Esteller M (2011) Cancer epigenetics reaches mainstream oncology. Nat Med 17(3):330–339
31. Costa-Pinheiro P, Montezuma D, Henrique R, Jeronimo C (2015) Diagnostic and prognostic epigenetic biomarkers in cancer. Epigenomics 7(6):1003–1015
32. Chihara Y, Kanai Y, Fujimoto H, Sugano K, Kawashima K, Liang G, Jones PA, Fujimoto K, Kuniyasu H, Hirao Y (2013) Diagnostic markers of urothelial cancer based on DNA methylation analysis. BMC Cancer 13:275
33. Harb-de la Rosa A, Acker M, Kumar RA, Manoharan M (2015) Epigenetics application in the diagnosis and treatment of bladder cancer. Can J Urol 22(5):7947–7951
34. Wu P, Cao Z, Wu S (2016) New progress of epigenetic biomarkers in urological cancer. Dis Markers 2016:9864047. doi:10.1155/2016/9864047
35. Chung W, Bondaruk J, Jelinek J, Lotan Y, Liang S, Czerniak B, Issa JP (2011) Detection of bladder cancer using novel DNA methylation biomarkers in urine sediments. Cancer Epidemiol Biomarkers Prev 20(7):1483–1491
36. Sapre N, Anderson PD, Costello AJ, Hovens CM, Corcoran NM (2014) Gene-based urinary biomarkers for bladder cancer: an unfulfilled promise? Urol Oncol 32(1):48.e49–48.e17
37. Laird PW (2010) Principles and challenges of genomewide DNA methylation analysis. Nat Rev Genet 11(3):191–203
38. Fouse SD, Nagarajan RO, Costello JF (2010) Genome-scale DNA methylation analysis. Epigenomics 2(1):105–117
39. Taylor KH, Shi H, Caldwell CW (2010) Next generation sequencing: advances in characterizing the methylome. Genes 1(2):143–165

40. Olkhov-Mitsel E, Bapat B (2012) Strategies for discovery and validation of methylated and hydroxymethylated DNA biomarkers. Cancer Med 1(2):237–260
41. Tommasi S, Karm DL, Wu X, Yen Y, Pfeifer GP (2009) Methylation of homeobox genes is a frequent and early epigenetic event in breast cancer. Breast Cancer Res 11(1):R14
42. Mitchell N, Deangelis JT, Tollefsbol TO (2011) Methylated-CpG Island recovery assay. Methods Mol Biol 791:125–133
43. Choi JH, Li Y, Guo J, Pei L, Rauch TA, Kramer RS, Macmil SL, Wiley GB, Bennett LB, Schnabel JL, Taylor KH, Kim S, Xu D, Sreekumar A, Pfeifer GP, Roe BA, Caldwell CW, Bhalla KN, Shi H (2010) Genome-wide DNA methylation maps in follicular lymphoma cells determined by methylation-enriched bisulfite sequencing. PLoS One 5(9):e13020
44. Almamun M, Levinson BT, Gater ST, Schnabel RD, Arthur GL, Davis JW, Taylor KH (2014) Genome-wide DNA methylation analysis in precursor B-cells. Epigenetics 9 (12):1588–1595
45. Green BB, McKay SD, Kerr DE (2015) Age dependent changes in the LPS induced transcriptome of bovine dermal fibroblasts occurs without major changes in the methylome. BMC Genomics 16:30
46. Tommasi S, Kim SI, Zhong X, Wu X, Pfeifer GP, Besaratinia A (2010) Investigating the epigenetic effects of a prototype smoke-derived carcinogen in human cells. PLoS One 5(5): e10594
47. Tommasi S, Zheng A, Weninger A, Bates SE, Li XA, Wu X, Hollstein M, Besaratinia A (2013) Mammalian cells acquire epigenetic hallmarks of human cancer during immortalization. Nucleic Acids Res 41(1):182–195
48. Tommasi S, Zheng A, Yoon JI, Li AX, Wu X, Besaratinia A (2012) Whole DNA methylome profiling in mice exposed to secondhand smoke. Epigenetics 7(11):1302–1314
49. Tommasi S, Zheng A, Yoon JI, Besaratinia A (2014) Epigenetic targeting of the Nanog pathway and signaling networks during chemical carcinogenesis. Carcinogenesis 35 (8):1726–1736
50. Sambrook J, Fritsch EF, Maniatis T (1989) Molecular cloning: a laboratory manual. Cold Spring Harbor Laboratory Press, Cold Spring Harbor, NY

Chapter 4

Immunohistochemical Analysis of Urothelial Carcinoma Tissues for Proliferation and Differentiation Markers

Michael Rose and Nadine T. Gaisa

Abstract

Immunohistochemistry is a standard method in histopathology and enables the localized detection of proteins in histological tissue sections. Specific antibodies are bound to cellular antigens, captured by secondary antibodies or polymers, linked to enzymes and visualized by chromogenic substrates. Here, we describe an automated staining technique for larger slide batches as well as a manual protocol for only few slides using a polymer technique. We focus on differentiation markers, measures of cell proliferation, and therapeutic targets in benign and malignant urothelial tissues.

Key words Immunohistochemistry, Polymer, (Cyto)keratins, Uroplakins, Ki67

1 Introduction

Immunohistochemistry (IHC) has a long history and is still an irreplaceable method in histopathology for diagnostic, therapeutic, and prognostic purposes [1]. In the 1930s first experiments demonstrated that specificity of antibody reactions was not impaired by covalently linked molecules [2], thus laying the scientific foundation for IHC. In 1941, Albert H. Coons and colleagues performed the next step by verifying streptococcal antigens in frozen sections of rheumatic fever lesions via coupling fluorescent compounds to antibodies [3, 4]. Labeled molecules have changed over time, but linkage of enzymes [5] such as *horseradish peroxidase* (HRP) that was investigated already in the 1960s [6–8] is still used. These enzyme-linked antibodies catalyze a chromogenic substrate turnover allowing the visualization of specific antigen binding in tissue sections by light microscopy. Breaking steps toward an improved staining were the invention of monoclonal antibodies, reducing unspecific cross-reactions, in 1975 [9], and the introduction of polymer-based detection systems, enhancing the gain of chromogenic-based signals, in the 1990s. Since formalin-fixed, paraffin-embedded (FFPE) tissues were routinely applied [10],

Wolfgang A. Schulz et al. (eds.), *Urothelial Carcinoma: Methods and Protocols*, Methods in Molecular Biology, vol. 1655, DOI 10.1007/978-1-4939-7234-0_4, © Springer Science+Business Media LLC 2018

standardization in order to achieve reproducibility has become the major focus in IHC as the antigen-antibody recognition is affected by multiple working steps including sample preparation and antigen retrieval techniques [11].

In the current era of "big data" and "molecular pathology" triggered by high-throughput methods like next-generation sequencing (NGS), immunohistochemical staining remains a cost-efficient standard technique offering a wide range of applications via localized specific antigen detection. The advantages are obvious: in heterogeneous tumor tissues staining patterns, which reflect expression and stability of a distinct protein, can be quantified and assigned to different cell types such as fibroblasts, immune, muscle, or epithelial cells. On the single-cell level further information can be provided by the cellular localization distinguishing between membranous, cytoplasmic or nuclear protein expressions. In clinical use IHC has a profound impact on tumor diagnostics and, meanwhile, also on managing risk stratification and therapeutic strategies of malignant diseases [1]. Antigens such as Ki67, a nucleus-specific proliferation marker, are easy to implement into pathological evaluation and hold a clear prognostic value in urothelial cancer (UC) [12]. In combination with aberrantly expressed CK20/KRT 20 (a differentiation marker normally only expressed in umbrella cells), Ki67 is thought to predict recurrence, progression, and survival stratifying clinical important patient groups in bladder cancer [13]. Since Choi et al. and other working groups reported intrinsic subtypes of invasive UC (basal and luminal) in 2014 [14], markers such as KRT5, KRT14, CD44, or KRT 20, GATA3 and HER2 which have been previously described for breast cancer subtype classification [15], have become more important for future UC diagnostics/management. As antigens like EGFR include also information about targeted therapies, their application may also guide and improve subtype-specific UC treatment.

In the following sections, detailed instructions for reproducible immunohistochemical stains of FFPE urothelial tissue sections are provided.

2 Materials

For both, automated and manual staining procedures, various distributors offer antibodies, reagents, and machines. Thus, in the following, we describe a protocol optimized for our selected local supplier, using commercially available premade solutions. However, we keep it as general as possible in order to enable transfer to other automated systems and self-prepared staining solutions as well. For optimal performance antibodies and reagents (and also machines) should be concerted.

2.1 Antigen Retrieval

1. Low pH buffer (*see* **Note 1**); To prepare 0.01 M citrate buffer pH 6.1 weigh 2.94 g tri-sodium citrate ($Na_3C_6H_5O_7.2H_2O$) and transfer it to a cylinder or beaker. Add ultrapure water to a volume of 950 mL (*see* **Note 2**) and mix. When fully dissolved make up to 1 L with ultrapure water. Adjust pH with HCl. Store at 4 °C.
2. High pH buffer (*see* **Note 3**); To prepare 0.01 M EDTA buffer pH 9.0 weigh 0.37 g ethylendiaminetetraacetic acid disodium salt dihydrate (EDTA) and transfer it to a cylinder. Add water to a volume of 950 mL. Mix and adjust pH with NaOH/KOH (*see* **Note 4**). Make up to 1 L with ultrapure water. Again adjust pH with NaOH/KOH. Store at 4 °C.
3. Temperature-controlled water bath (alternatively microwave oven or pressure cooker).
4. Heat-resistant glass or plastic ware with cover.
5. Wet chamber.

2.2 Solutions

1. Peroxidase blocking (*see* **Note 5**); Peroxidase activity can be blocked by 3% H_2O_2 solution (in ultrapure water) (*see* **Note 6**).
2. Protein blocking; Proteins can be blocked by normal serum of species other than the used primary antibody and the used tissue source (usually the species of the secondary antibody is used). A concentration of 1–5% in PBS should be obtained (*see* **Note 7**).
3. Antibody dilution (*see* **Note 8**); Antibodies can be diluted in phosphate buffered saline (PBS).
4. Wash buffer (*see* **Note 9**); It is possible to use PBS as wash buffer. In order to reduce unspecific background staining 0.01–0.1% Tween 20 can be added (*see* **Note 10**).

2.3 Antibodies

Antibodies for proliferation and differentiation markers in urothelial tissues are listed in Table 1.

2.4 Detection Systems

There are various methods for the detection of antigen-antibody reactions. The oldest method using direct immunolabeling with enzyme-conjugated primary antibodies is (due to weak 1:1 signals) no longer used for routine immunohistochemistry, but still preferred in high resolution immunofluorescence. All current immunohistochemistry protocols apply indirect immunolabeling with a non-conjugated primary antibody and different capturing techniques with bridging secondary antibodies or polymers. In the last 10 years the polymer technique, using ten or more secondary antibodies and >70 enzymes at once for each primary-secondary antibody reaction, has proven excellent signals in tissues and is now mainly used. Therefore, this protocol is based on polymer technique (Fig. 1).

Table 1
Antibodies for proliferation and (subtype-specific) differentiation markers in urothelial tissues

Antibody/ clone	Company/order #	Dilution	Antigen retrieval	Detection system (DAKO)
Ki-67 MIB-1	DAKO M7240	1:400	pH 6.1	FLEX + M
(Cyto)keratin 5/6 D5/16 B4	DAKO M7237	1:100	pH 9.0	FLEX + M
(Cyto)keratin 5 XM26	abcam ab17130	1:50	pH 6.1	FLEX + M
(Cyto)keratin 14 LL002	abcam ab7800	1:400	pH 6.1	FLEX + M
(Cyto)keratin 20 Ks20.8	DAKO M7019	1:100	pH 6.1	FLEX + M
Uroplakin II	BIOCARE MEDICAL ACI3051C	1:100	pH 6.1	FLEX + M
Uroplakin III AU1	PROGEN 610108	1:10	pH 6.1	FLEX + M
GATA3 L50-823	BioCare Medica CM 405 B	1:250	pH 6.1	FLEX + M
HER2 (HercepTest)	DAKO K5204	1:300	pH 6.1	–
EGFR E30	DAKO M7239	1:50	–	FLEX + M

M mouse linker

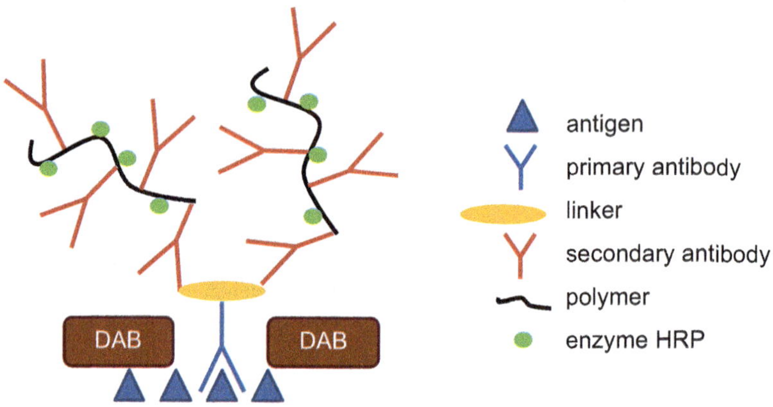

Fig. 1 Scheme of polymer-based antigen detection. A tissue antigen is captured by a primary antibody in a first step. In a facultative second step a species-specific linker molecule can be added in order to enable binding of multiple polymers. In the following step, polymers with multiple secondary antibodies and enzymes can bind to the antigen itself or the linker molecule. By addition of a chromogenic substrate (DAB) enzyme-induced color development at the targeted structures takes place

2.5 Chromogens

1. Diaminobenzidine (DAB): two component solutions of various distributors are available. These kits have to be used according to the manufacturer's instructions (e.g., mix 20 mL substrate buffer with 20 drops of DAB chromogen).
2. Fast Red: multi-component (e.g., AP substrate buffer, chromogen red 1, chromogen red 2, chromogen red 3) kit of various distributors. Depending on the total volume needed follow the protocol of the manufacturer (e.g., for ~1120 μL: 1000 μL substrate buffer, 40 μL chromogen 1, 40 μL chromogen 2, 40 μL chromogen 3) (*see* **Note 11**).
3. Others: other chromogens like nitroblue-tetrazolium (dark blue-violet) or DAB with nickel (gray-black) may be used for special purposes and chromogen kits are offered by several companies. They have to be used according to the manufacturer's protocols. It is important to select best suitable combinations of chromogen and counterstain in order to highlight the targeted structures (*see* **Note 12**).

2.6 Counterstain

Counterstaining for DAB chromogen is usually performed with premade hematoxylin solutions. According to the used automated staining system they are offered by the company. For manual staining also standard hematoxylin solutions can be used.

2.7 Mounting

Mounting of slides can either be performed by a fully automated glass/foil cover slipper or manually.

1. Cover slips.
2. Mounting medium.

3 Methods

3.1 Automated Staining Procedure

3.1.1 Pretreatment

1. Fill, switch on, and heat pretreatment device according to the manufacturer's instructions (*see* **Note 13**).
2. Place paraffin slides (*see* **Note 14**) into the racks (in the order of the programming of the stainer) and insert them into the device when starting temperature is reached.
3. Pretreatment program (our in house protocol):

Step	Action	Duration
Preheating	Heating up to 80 °C	~25 min
Insert slides		
Start heating	Heating up to 97 °C	~10 min
Demasking	Holding 97 °C	20 min
Cooling	Cooling down to 65 °C	~15 min
Take out slides		

4. Transfer slides to wash buffer and leave them for 5–10 min (*see* **Note 15**).

3.1.2 Staining Procedure

1. Program the automated slide stainer according to your requirements while pretreatment is going on.
2. Equip the stainer with the necessary reagents (*see* below).
3. Transfer slides from wash buffer to the stainer.
4. Machine staining protocol: our in-house protocol with DAKO K8002. Note that optimal dilution, antigen retrieval procedure, and detection systems are listed in Table 1.

Step	Reagent	Duration
Slide transfer/washing	Wash buffer	As required
Washing	Wash buffer	~15–20 min
Peroxidase block	Peroxidase-blocking reagent	5 min
Washing	Wash buffer	~15–20 min
Primary antibody	Primary antibody diluted in antibody diluent	30 min
Washing	Wash buffer	~2 min
Linker	Linker	15 min
Washing	Wash buffer	10 min
Secondary polymer	Polymer/HRP	20 min
Washing	Wash buffer	10 min
Washing	Wash buffer	10 min
Chromogen	DAB substrate working solution (mix)	10 min
Washing	Wash buffer	15–20 min
Counter staining	Hematoxylin	5 min
Counter staining development	Ultrapure water	20 min
Washing	Wash buffer	~2 min

According to tissue requirements 2–3 the reagent drop zones of the robot can be chosen. Volumes of peroxidase block, primary antibody, linker, and secondary polymer are 100 μL per drop zone. For chromogen and counterstaining 200 μL volume per drop zone are suggested. Washing durations are variable due to slide numbers.

3.2 Manual Staining Procedure

3.2.1 Deparaffinization

1. Keep freshly cut 1–3 μm paraffin slides overnight at 50 max. 60 °C in an oven.
2. Take the slides out of the oven and start the following dewaxing procedure (*see* **Note 16**):

Step	Reagent	Duration
Dewax	Xylene	10 min
Dewax	Xylene	10 min
Decending alcohols	100% ethanol	10 min
Decending alcohols	100% ethanol	10 min
Decending alcohols	96% ethanol	5 min
Decending alcohols	70% ethanol	5 min
Rehydration	Aqua dest	5 min

3.2.2 Antigen Retrieval

1. Place heat-resistant container filled with appropriate antigen retrieval buffer into the water bath (alternatively microwave oven or pressure cooker) and start heating.
2. When 98 °C (boiling temperature) is reached place the slides into the retrieval buffer and start demasking. Retrieval times vary among different antibodies and retrieval buffers (on average pH 6.1 citrate buffer ~15–30 min, pH 9.0 EDTA buffer ~5–15 min).
3. Stop heating, take the container out, and cool down slides by slow and continuous dilution of retrieval buffer with aqua dest. Transfer slides to wash buffer, let them cool down to room temperature, and rest for about 15 min.

3.2.3 Staining

1. Take slides out of wash buffer and transfer them to a wet chamber (plastic box with lid and wet pulp) (*see* **Note 17**).
2. Apply 200 μL peroxidase-blocking reagent per slide for 10–15 min.
3. Wash slides three times for 5 min with wash buffer/PBS.
4. For antibodies with strong background reaction protein block may be applied for 15 min. Discard protein block (do not wash).
5. Place 200 μL of diluted primary antibody (*see* Table 1) onto each slide and incubate for 30 min at room temperature.
6. Wash slides three times for 5 min with wash buffer/PBS.
7. Apply 200 μL linker for 15 min.
8. Wash slides three times for 5 min with wash buffer/PBS.
9. Incubate slides with polymer for 20 min.

10. Wash slides three times for 5 min with wash buffer/PBS.
11. Apply 200–500 μL DAB substrate working solution (mix) for 10 min.
12. Wash slides three times for 5 min with wash buffer/PBS.
13. Counterstain slides with hematoxylin for 10 min and wash briefly with tap water.
14. Differentiate staining with aqua dest. for 10 min.

3.3 Dehydration and Mounting (Automated Staining and Manual Staining)

For automated staining the following **steps 1** and **2** can be performed in any routine histology robot.

1. Dehydrate slides in an ascending alcohol series as follows:

Step	Reagent	Duration
Transfer	Aqua dest	1 min
Ascending alcohols	70% ethanol	30 s
Ascending alcohols	70% ethanol	30 s
Ascending alcohols	70% ethanol	30 s
Ascending alcohols	96% ethanol	30 s
Ascending alcohols	96% ethanol	30 s
Ascending alcohols	96% ethanol	30 s
Dehydration	100% ethanol	2 min
Dehydration	100% ethanol	2 min
Dehydration	Xylene	2–5 min
Dehydration	Xylene	2–5 min
Dehydration	Xylene	2–5 min
Dehydration	Xylene	2–5 min

2. Transfer dehydrated slides in xylene to a cover slipper machine or place 2 drops cover medium onto the slide and cover each slide with a cover slip. Apply slight pressure in order to remove air bubbles.

4 Notes

1. We use commercially available low pH buffer (pH 6.1).
2. When dissolving tri-sodium citrate the volume of the solution will increase. Therefore, start dissolving in 950 mL and fill up to nearly 1 L when the salt is fully dissolved.
3. We use commercially available high pH buffer (pH 9.0).

4. Concentrated KOH/NaOH can be used at first to approach the required pH. Close to the final pH, less concentrated bases are preferred, as the pH of EDTA buffer may suddenly rise above the required value.
5. We use commercially available peroxidase-blocking reagent.
6. Peroxidase solutions should be kept in dark plastic containers since light enhances decomposition of H_2O_2 into H_2O and O_2 reducing the effectiveness of the solution and producing gas (*cave*: glass bottles may explode). Peroxidase blocking solution is alternatively commercially available by several suppliers.
7. Protein blocking is used to reduce background staining due to hydrophobic interactions. It can be used as a blocking step prior to the incubation with the primary antibody. Blocking solution is just discarded (no washing) and then the antibody incubation follows. More elegantly the primary antibody can be diluted in antibody-diluent containing 1% bovine serum albumin (BSA) with comparable effects. Protein blocking solutions are alternatively commercially available by several suppliers.
8. We use commercially available antibody diluent.
9. We use commercially available wash buffer concentrate.
10. Adding detergent (e.g., Tween 20) reduces surface tension of the water and also dissolves membrane glycoproteins (e.g., Fc-receptors) resulting in less background staining. Pipetting of detergents may be difficult due to their viscosity; aspirate slowly.
11. Fast Red solution is not very stable. The four-component mixture should be freshly prepared maximum 10 min prior to use.
12. Optimal chromogen and counterstain combinations are the ones with best contrast: DAB (brown) & hematoxylin (light blue), DAB/DAB + Ni (brown/black) & methyl green, red chromogens & hematoxylin (light blue)/methyl green, nitroblue tetrazolium (blue) & nuclear fast red.
13. Change target retrieval solutions after three to four times of use as retrieval may be less effective afterwards.
14. 1–3 μm paraffin slides for immunohistochemistry should ideally be prepared the previous day and kept overnight at 50 °C (max. 60 °C). From 50 °C they should be directly transferred to the antigen retrieval procedure.
15. If paraffin residues are found in washing buffer or on the top of the pretreated slides, rinse slides with buffer or PBS in order to optimize antibody binding during the staining procedure.

16. Deparaffinization has to be carried out in a fume hood due to vapors. Xylene and alcohol solutions have to be checked and changed regularly. If precipitates form solutions have to be discarded.
17. For optimal staining results slides should never dry out. Place slides plane into the wet chamber, close the lid, and move the chamber as little as possible. In order to avoid spread of reagents far beyond the tissue the sections can be encircled with a wax pen.

References

1. Dabbs DJ (ed) (2014) Diagnostic immunohistochemistry: theranostic and genomic applications, 4th edn. Saunders Elsevier, Philadelphia
2. Reiner L (1930) On the chemical alteration of purified antibodies. Science 72:483
3. Coons AH, Creech HH, Jones RN (1941) Immunological properties of an antibody containing a fluorescent group. Proc Soc Exp Biol Med 47:200–202
4. Coons AH (1975) Introduction: the development of immunohistochemistry. Annals New York Acad Sci 177:5–9
5. Nakane PK, Pierce GB (1967) Enzyme-labeled antibodies for the light and electron microscopic localization of tissue antigens. J Cell Biol 33:307–318
6. Kacarai Y, Nakane PK (1970) Localization of tissue antigens on the ultrathin sections with peroxidase-labeled antibody method. J Histochem Cytochem 18:161–166
7. Leduc EH, Avrameas S, Bouteille M (1968) Ultrastracturual localization of antibody in differentiating plasma cells. J Exp Med 127:109–118
8. Ostrowski KE, Barnard A, Sawicki W, Chorzelski T, Langner A, Mikulski A (1970) Autoradiographic detection of antigens in cells using tritum-labeled antibodies. J Histochem Cytochem 22:383–392
9. McMichael AJ, Pilch JR, Galfre G, Mason DY, Fabre JW, Milstein C (1979) A human thymocyte antigen defined a hybrid myeloma monoclonal antibody. Eur J Immunol 9:205–10.7
10. Taylor CR, Burns J (1974) The demonstration of plasma cells and other immoglobulin-containing cells in formalin-fixed, paraffin-embedded tissues using peroxidase-labelled antibody. J Clin Pathol 27:14–20
11. Shi SR, Key ME, Kalra KL (1991) Antigen retrieval in formalin-fixed, paraffin-embedded tissues: a enhancement method for immunohistochemical staining based on microwave oven heating of tissue sections. J Histochem Cytochem 39:741–748
12. Asakura T, Takano Y, Iki M, Suwa Y, Noguchi S, Kubota Y, Masuda M (1997) Prognostic value of Ki-67 for recurrence and progression of superficial bladder cancer. J Urol 158:385–388
13. Bertz S, Otto W, Denzinger S, Wieland WF, Burger M, Stöhr R, Link S, Hofstädter F, Hartmann A (2014) Combination of CK20 and Ki-67 immunostaining analysis predicts recurrence, progression, and cancer-specific survival on pT1 urothelial bladder cancer. Eur Urol 65:218–226
14. Choi W, Porten S, Kim S, Willis D, Plimack ER, Hoffman-Censits J, Roth B, Cheng T, Tran M, Lee IL (2014) Identification of distinct basal and luminal subtypes of muscle-invaisve bladder cancer with different sensitivities to frontline chemotherapy. Cancer Cell 25:152–165
15. Sorlie T (2004) Molecular portraits of breast cancer: tumor subtypes as distinct disease entities. Eur J Cancer 40:2667–2675

Chapter 5

Molecular Subtype Profiling of Urothelial Carcinoma Using a Subtype-Specific Immunohistochemistry Panel

Gottfrid Sjödahl

Abstract

Molecular subtypes of bladder cancer (BC) can be determined by relatively small immunohistochemistry panels both for non-muscle invasive (NMI) and muscle invasive (MI) tumors. For analysis of NMI tumors, as few as two markers are needed, although classification is dependent also on pathological grade and histological evaluation. The result is a classification into the three tumor-cell phenotypes of NMI-BC, Urothelial-like (Uro), Genomically Unstable (GU), and Basal/SCC-like. For analysis of MI tumors, 13 markers are needed. The larger number of markers required for the classification of MI-BC reflects the inclusion of two additional phenotypes exclusively found in invasive tumors; Mesenchymal-like (Mes-like) and Small-cell/Neuroendocrine-like (Sc/NE-like). Here follows a description of how to perform and approach IHC-based subtype classification of bladder cancer.

Key words Bladder cancer, Urothelial carcinoma, Molecular subtypes, Phenotype, Classification, Urothelial-like, Genomically unstable, Basal/SCC-like, Mesenchymal-like, Small-cell/neuroendocrine-like

1 Introduction

Stratification of tumors into molecular subtypes by means of mRNA or protein profiling is becoming a prerequisite for molecular cancer research. Although unbiased mRNA expression profiling is considered the state-of-the-art method for subtype classification, some aspects of classification can only be obtained by the tissue resolution of in-situ analysis.

Here follows a description of how tissue microarray (TMA) and immunohistochemistry (IHC) techniques were combined to subtype classify urothelial carcinomas of all pathological stages from Ta to ≥T2. The method consists of three main steps: IHC staining, IHC evaluation, and data analysis and classification, which are covered separately under the methods section. The 2 × 1.0 mm TMA core format was used throughout the development of this method. In theory, however, the method should be readily

Wolfgang A. Schulz et al. (eds.), *Urothelial Carcinoma: Methods and Protocols*, Methods in Molecular Biology, vol. 1655, DOI 10.1007/978-1-4939-7234-0_5, © Springer Science+Business Media LLC 2018

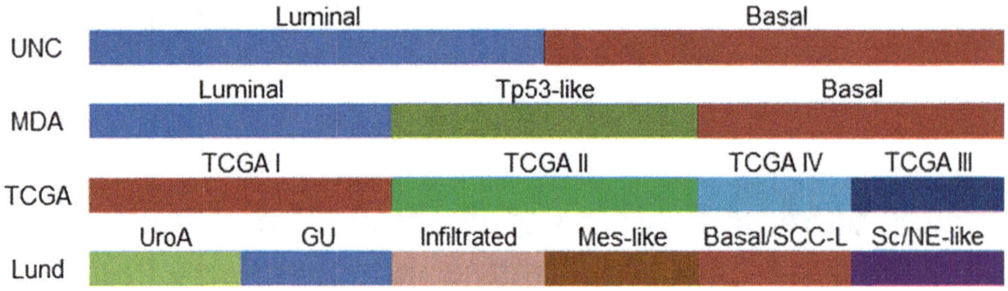

Fig. 1 Schematic approximate representation of the overlap between mRNA-based subtype classification systems of bladder cancer. UNC, University of North Carolina group [5], MDA, MD Anderson group [4], TCGA, The Cancer Genome Atlas [6]. Lund, The Lund Bladder cancer Research Group [7]. UroA. Urothelial-like A, GU, Genomically Unstable, Mes-like, mesenchymal-like, Sc/NE-like, Small-cell/Neuroendocrine-like

transferable to other TMA formats, and with some modification also to classification on full tissue-sections and cell lines/model systems. The protein markers and simple classification rules described have been applied in three TMA cohorts containing $n = 237$ [1], $N = 167$ [2], and $n = 425$ [7]. The correspondence to several mRNA subtype classification systems [3–6] was based on the parallel analysis of both IHC and mRNA data for a total of more than five hundred tumors. In comparison to subtype identification by mRNA expression profiling the main difference in IHC-based profiling is the absence of immune/stroma-rich subtypes as all the analyses are based on the phenotype of the tumor-cells alone. Such immune-enriched phenotypes are present in most classification systems (MDA Tp53-like, TCGA Cluster II, Lund Infiltrated). For a schematic guide to the different subtype classification systems of bladder cancer, *see* Fig. 1. The method detailed here is open for improvement in several ways: Although the marker profiles presented here accurately identify the existing phenotypes of bladder cancer, it is possible that even better markers exist. It is also likely that additional phenotypes of bladder cancer will be described as larger cohorts are analyzed. However, given the size of cohorts analyzed so far, novel phenotypes are not likely to comprise more than 5% of any of the stage groups Ta, T1, and ≥T2. Furthermore, additional studies are required for phenotypic classification of upper urinary tract urothelial cancer, pre-neoplastic urothelial disorders, as well as mild to severe dysplasia, and urothelial carcinoma in-situ.

2 Materials

In addition to the materials described below, standard IHC-lab equipment is required. A Dako Autostainer instrument (Dako AS, Glostrup, Denmark) was used for all stainings on which this method is based, but is not an absolute requirement. A PT link pretreatment module for tissue sections (Dako) was used for all stainings on which this method is based, but is not an absolute requirement.

1. Glass slides (Super frost plus).
2. Pertex medium for mounting and preserving of slide specimens.
3. Formalin-fixed paraffin-embedded (FFPE) cancer tissue from trans-urethral resection of the bladder (TUR-B) in TMA format. A core diameter of 1.0 mm was used in all TMAs on which this method is based.
4. Primary antibodies. For a list of antibodies including vendors and product number, *see* Table 1.
5. EnVision FLEX K8010 kit (Dako) including both low- and high-pH Target Retrieval Solutions.
6. Slide scanner with the capability of scanning TMA slides at 20× magnification.

3 Methods

Before starting the project, select which stainings to perform for subtype classification and validation. Exhaustive subtype classification requires more markers than identification of only a single subtype (e.g., identification of Basal/SCC-like cases only) or of subclassification of a subtype (e.g., classification of a cohort of luminal-type tumors into Uro and GU subtypes) (*see* **Note 1**).

3.1 Immunohistochemistry

1. Mount TMA sections of 4 μm thickness onto Super frost plus glass slides (*see* **Note 2**). Let slides dry at room temperature, and then incubate for 2 h at 60 °C.

   Step 2 is performed in a pretreatment module for tissue sections (Dako) if possible.

2. Pretreat by incubating in pH 6 or pH 9 Target Retrieval Solution (*see* **Note 3**) preheated to 65 °C. Rise the temperature to 98 °C for 20 min, and then let it cool back down to 65 °C. Remove the slides and wash them gently in Wash buffer.

   Steps 3–7 are performed in Autostainer instrument if possible. Wash the slides with Wash buffer between each step.

3. Block your slides by incubating with Peroxidase Blocking Solution for 5 min.
4. Incubate slides with primary antibody for 30 min (*see* **Note 4**). For primary antibody dilutions, *see* Table 1.
5. Incubate slides with FLEX HRP detection reagent for 25 min.
6. Incubate slides with DAB and DAB+ Chromogen solution and substrate buffer according to the kit instructions for 2 × 5 min.

Table 1
Subtype-specific primary antibodies described in this method

Marker	Catalog No.	Vendor	Dilution	Evaluation	Corr IHC-GEX (Affy)	Corr IHC-GEX (Illumina)
ACTA2	M0851	Dako	1:500	–	–	–
CCNB1	1495-1	Epitomics	1:100	Perc.	0.52	0.60
CCND1	M3635	Dako	1:100	Perc./Intensity	0.77	0.56
CDH1	M3612	Dako	1:200	Intensity	0.65	0.28
CDH3	#610228	BD Biosciences	1:200	Perc./Intensity	0.78	0.46
CHGA	M0869	Dako	1:100	Intensity	0.36	–
E2F3	MS-1063	Lab vision	1:80	Perc./Intensity	0.63	0.45
EGFR	M7239	Dako	1:25	Perc./Intensity	0.65	0.47
EPCAM	M3525	Dako	1:40	Intensity	0.64	–
ERBB2	790-2991	Ventana	RTU	Intensity	0.75	0.49
FGFR3	#4574	Cell signaling	1:40	Intensity	0.75	0.65
FOXA1 (clone 2F83)	ab40868	Abcam	1:200	Intensity	0.69	–
GATA3	#5852	Cell signaling	1:800	Perc./Intensity	0.81	–
KRT14	MS-115	Lab vision	1:200	Perc./Intensity	0.82	0.64
KRT20	M7019	Dako	1:500	Intensity	0.71	0.61
KRT5	RM-2106	Lab vision	1:200	Perc./Intensity	0.81	0.72
NCAM1	NCL-L-CD56-504	Leica	1:50	Perc./Intensity	–	–
CDKN2A (p16)	#550834	BD Biosciences	1:50	Intensity	0.57	0.56
PPARG	#2435	Cell signaling	1:400	Perc./Intensity	0.70	–
RB1	#9309	Cell signaling	1:100	Perc.	0.53	0.44
SYP	M0776	Dako	1:100	Perc./Intensity	0.42	–
TP63	IMG-80212	Imgenex	1:100	Perc.	0.83	0.73
TUBB2B	LS-B4190-50	LifeSpan	1:200	Perc./Intensity	0.61	–
UPK3	AIB-30180	Nordic Biosite	1:20	Intensity	0.44	0.19
VIM	M0725	Dako	1:200	Perc./Intensity	0.57	–
ZEB2	61095	Active Motif	1:500	Intensity	0.41	–

In addition to catalog numbers and vendors, the dilution of primary antibody in IHC and the evaluation criteria (Intensity, percentage, or both) is given for each marker. The correlation (Pearson r) between IHC (tumor-cell score) and normalized mRNA expression values was investigated using a cohort of FFPE-derived RNA samples from advanced tumors (Affymetrix ST 1.0, unpublished data), and a cohort of fresh-frozen tissue-derived RNA samples from a mixed stage cohort (Illumina HT-12 platform) [3]

7. Counterstain slides with Mayer's Hematoxylin for 2 min.
8. Dehydrate slides by serial incubation as follows: water (10 min), 96% ethanol (5 min), 99% ethanol (5 min), and xylene (10 min).
9. Apply cover slides using the Pertex medium for mounting and preserving of slide specimens.

3.2 Immunohistochemistry Evaluation

Each IHC staining is evaluated either as the intensity (0–3) of staining, or as the percentage of positive cells in bins of 10% (0–9), or both. The type of evaluation depends on the appearance of the staining. Antibodies that usually stain all tumor-cells evenly such as CDH1 are evaluated only by intensity, whereas nuclear markers with digital "on/off" type expression such as RB1 and TP63 are evaluated only by percentage positive tumor-cells. Markers that are heterogeneously expressed such as KRT5 and CDH3 are evaluated both by intensity and percentage positive tumor-cells (*see* **Note 5**). As IHC is a semiquantitative technique, the cutoffs for intensity evaluation have to be established for each project. Generally, the intensity cutoffs are set so that 0 represents no staining, 1 represents low, but detectable degree of staining, 2 represents clearly positive cases, and 3 represents strong expression.

1. For each staining, confirm that the staining patterns match those described (*see* **Note 6**) and that both low and high scoring cases can be found in the material to be evaluated.
2. Markers of the different patterns are evaluated as described in Table 1. All the cores that cannot be evaluated should be marked as "N/A," or equivalent and should be excluded from further calculations. For notes regarding individual markers' staining patterns, *see* **Note 6.**

3.3 Data Adjustments and Subtype Classification

1. Calculation of tumor-cell scores. For each marker multiply the intensity score (0–3) with the percentage score (0–9) divided by 10 (0–0.9). The resulting score is the tumor-cell score. For markers evaluated only by intensity (0–3) or percentage (now converted to 0–0.9) those values represent tumor-cell scores.
2. If cases are represented by multiple tissue cores, merging of replicate cores must be done before subtype classification. The tumor-cell score for the case is in this case equal to the mean score of all cores representing that case.
3. If the cohort contains mainly non-muscle invasive tumors, tumors should primarily be classified into "Uro-like" (Uro), "Genomically Unstable" (GU), and "Basal/SCC-like" subtypes. If the cohort contains mostly muscle invasive cases, this step can be skipped. In that case go to **step 5** below.

   For classification, count how many of the following criteria are fulfilled:

- Tumor has a urothelial-like histology. For additional information on this evaluation, *see* **Note 7.**
- Tumor is pathologically low-grade (G1-G2, and not G3) (*see* **Note 8**).
- The tumor-cell score for the proliferation marker CCNB1 is low ($\leq$0.17). For a discussion on cut-off values, *see* **Note 9.**

If two or more of the criteria delineated above are met, the tumor is classified as Uro. If none or only one of the criteria is met, the tumor is classified as GU if the tumor-cell score for KRT5 is low ($\leq$0.57) and as Basal/SCC-like if the tumor-cell score for KRT5 is high (>0.57). Examples of the relevant stainings in the three different phenotypes can be seen in Fig. 2. For a discussion on cut-off values, *see* **Note 9.**

4. Validation of non-muscle invasive (NMI) subtype classification. After subtypes have been assigned using the NMI method, it is highly recommended that the subtype classification is validated by a number of additional stainings. The most efficient markers

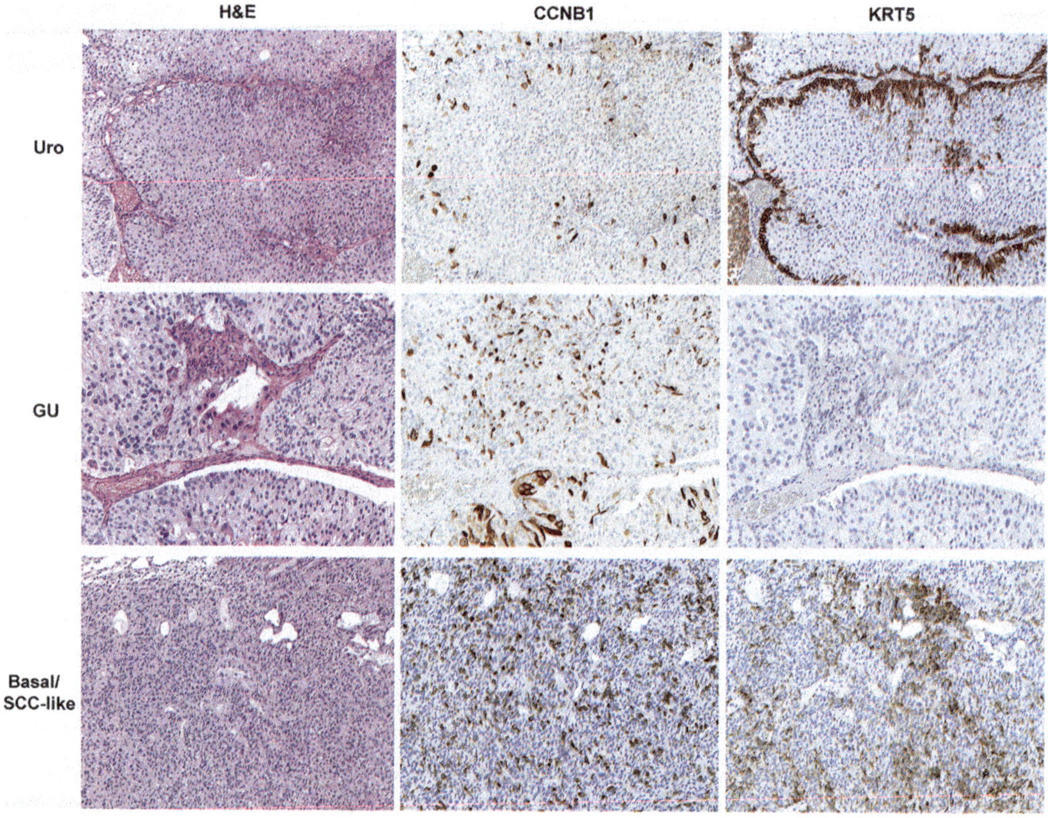

Fig. 2 Example images of Hematoxylin & Eosin (H&E), Cyclin B1 (CCNB1), and Keratin 5 (KRT5) staining in the three phenotypes of non-muscle invasive bladder cancer, Urothelial-like (Uro), Genomically Unstable (GU), and Basal/SCC-like

Table 2
Markers used to define the phenotypes of muscle invasive bladder cancer

Uro	FGFR3 +	CCND1 +	RB1 +	CDKN2A (p16) –
GU	FGFR3 –	CCND1 –	RB1 –	CDKN2A (p16) +
Basal/SCC-like	KRT5 +	KRT14 +	FOXA1 –	GATA3 –
Mes-like	VIM +	ZEB2 +	CDH1 –	EPCAM –
Sc/NE-like	TUBB2B +	EPCAM +	CDH1 –	GATA3 –

Based on the four markers shown, a definition score is calculated for each subtype. The definition score is then used to assign unclassified cases to one of the five phenotypes

for NMI subtype validation are FGFR3 and CCND1 for the Uro subtype, ERBB2 and CDKN2A (p16) for the GU subtype, and P-cadherin and DSC2/3 for the Basal/SCC-like subtype. Additionally, RB1 loss, seen as complete absence of RB1 staining, should be more frequent in GU and Basal/SCC-like cases than in Uro cases. TP63 staining should be higher in Uro cases and in Basal/SCC-like cases than in GU cases. If this relatively limited set of markers shows significant association to the corresponding group, the classification can be considered valid.

5. If the cohort contains mainly muscle invasive cases, tumors should primarily be classified into "Urothelial-like" (Uro), "Genomically Unstable" (GU), "Basal/SCC-like", "Mesenchymal-like" (Mes-like), and "Small-cell/Neuroendocrine-like" (Sc/NE-like). This classification is performed according to the samples definition scores (Table 2).

   To calculate definition scores, each marker score is divided by the range-maximum in order to normalize scores recorded as percentages versus those recorded as intensities. Definition scores are then calculated by adding/subtracting each normalized marker. If a case has a high definition score (>0.6) for the Basal/SCC-like, Mes-like, or Sc/NE-like definitions, then the case is classified according to the score that was highest of the three. If neither of these three definitions is high (>0.6), then the case is classified as Uro if the Uro definition is high (>0.6) and as GU if it is low (<0.6). The GU phenotype is thus defined as the opposite of the Uro phenotype. The examples of the relevant stainings in the five different phenotypes can be seen in Fig. 3.

6. Validation of muscle invasive (MI) subtype classification. After subtypes have been assigned using the MI method, subtype classification may be validated by additional stainings that are not allowed to affect the classification results. The validation marker results should be reported as a between groups statistical comparison.

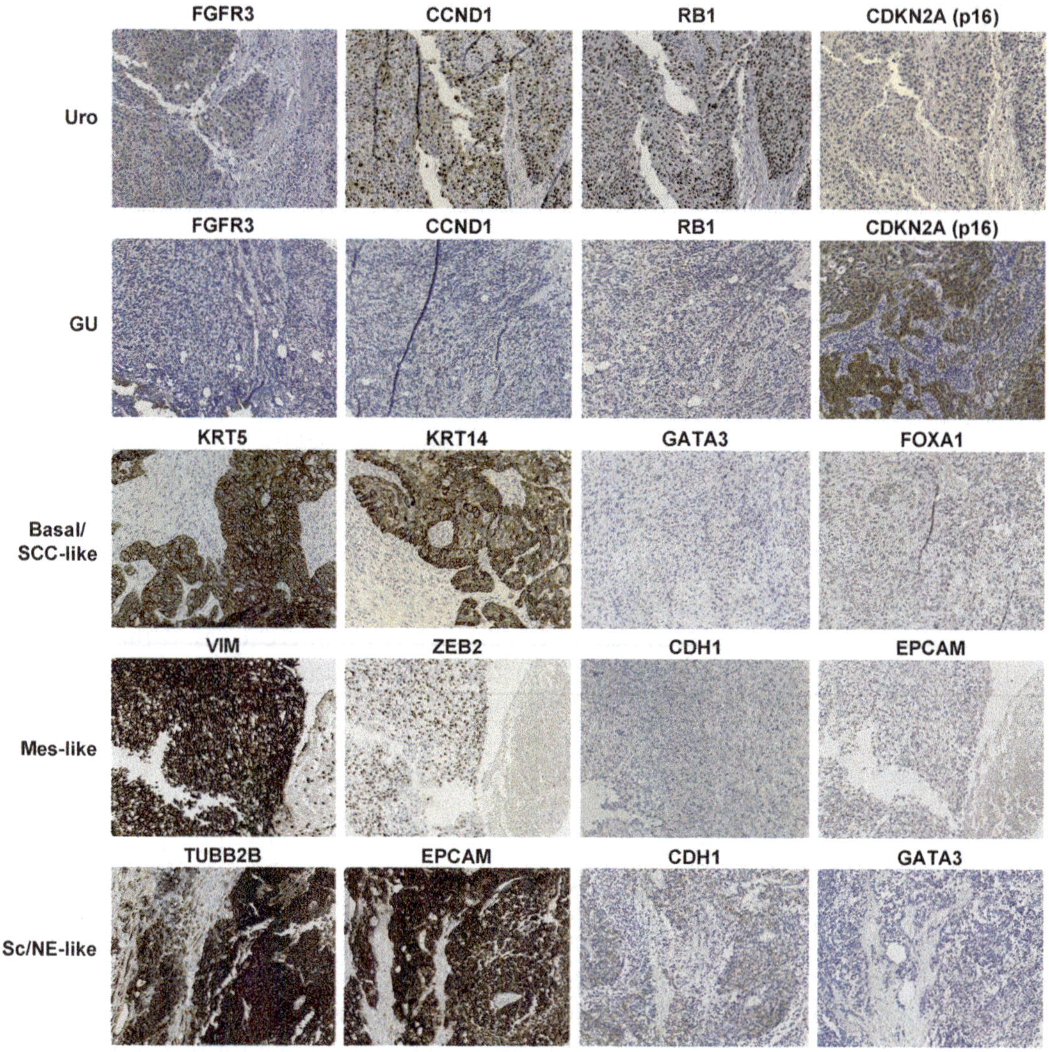

Fig. 3 Example images of markers used for subtype classification of the five phenotypes of muscle invasive bladder cancer, Urothelial-like (Uro), Genomically Unstable (GU), Basal/SCC-like, Mesenchymal-like (Mes-like), and Small-cell/Neuroendocrine-like (Sc/NE-like)

4 Notes

1. For unbiased subtype classification of NMI-based cohorts, stainings for CCNB1 and KRT5 have to be performed, as that data is used in tumor classification. Additionally, it is recommended that a number of validation markers are used in **step 4**. FGFR3, CCND1, ERBB2, CDKN2A (p16), P-Cadherin, and DSC2/3 are the ones suggested in **step 4** under Data Adjustments and Subtype Classification. For unbiased classification of MI-based cohorts the classification itself uses 13 markers. Additional validation markers in Table 1 can be used.

2. For the antibodies included in Table 1, thorough comparisons to gene expression data (Illumina HT-12 and/or Affymetrix ST 1.0 platforms) have been performed, and no staining of positive or negative control tissue needs to be performed.
3. At times, but not always, depending on the primary antibody used, switching from the standard pH 9 Target Retrieval Buffer to the pH 6 Target Retrieval Buffer can increase the contrast of the staining. Performing antigen retrieval in the more acidic buffer can thus be tried when the results using the conventional buffer need to be improved.
4. Primary antibody incubation time and dilution are the main parameters that can be changed to increase or decrease the general intensity of staining. If the results obtained using the dilutions suggested in Table 1 lead to too weak or too strong stainings, the appropriate adjustments need to be made at this step.
5. It is good practice to always include a "comments" field during evaluation. Here, it is possible to note if a marker that is normally homogeneously expressed would only be expressed in 50% of the tumor-cells. This would then be taken into account when calculating a tumor-cell score for this case even though the evaluations for this marker are done only using intensity scale (0–3).
6. This note gives a description of the staining pattern and potential usefulness of each IHC marker. For some markers, additional information can be found in the Supplementary Appendix of [1, 7]. *ACTA2*, Smooth-muscle actin. This antibody is used to visualize stroma for determining which cases are urothelial-like, *see* [1]. *CCNB1*, Cyclin B1. This is evaluated by percentage positive tumor-cells. It stains the cytoplasm and nucleus of cells in G2 and M-phases of the cell cycle. Typically, it is expressed at 10–20% in NMI-BC and 30–40% in MI-BC. *CCND1*, Cyclin D1. This is evaluated by intensity and percentage positive tumor-cells. It stains the nucleus of basal and intermediate cell layers of Uro tumors. *CDH1*, E-Cadherin. This is evaluated by intensity. It stains the plasma membrane of tumor-cells. Basal/SCC-like subtype has slightly decreased intensity, whereas Mes-like and Sc/NE-like tumors frequently lose expression entirely. *CDH3*, P-Cadherin. This is evaluated by intensity and percentage positive tumor-cells. It stains the plasma membrane of basal cells of Uro tumors and all tumor-cells of Basal/SCC-like tumors. *CHGA*, Chromogranin A. This is evaluated by intensity. It stains cells with neuroendocrine differentiation (>90% of cases are negative). Validation marker for the Sc/NE-like group. *E2F3*, this is evaluated by intensity and percentage positive tumor-cells. This is overexpressed in GU and Sc/NE-like cases due to a subtype-specific genomic amplification. It serves as a

validation marker for these subtypes. *EGFR*, Epidermal growth factor receptor. This is evaluated by intensity and percentage positive tumor-cells. It stains the cytoplasm and plasma membrane of basal cells layer of Uro tumors and all tumor-cells of Basal/SCC-like tumors. *EPCAM*, Epithelial cell adhesion molecule. This is evaluated by intensity. It stains the plasma membrane of tumor-cells. Expression is only lost in the Mes-like subtype. *ERBB2*, Epidermal growth factor receptor 2. This is evaluated by intensity. It stains the plasma membrane of tumor-cells of the Uro and, most strongly, of the GU subtype. *FGFR3*, Fibroblast growth factor receptor 3. This is evaluated by intensity. It stains the plasma membrane of tumor-cells of the Uro subtype. *FOXA1*, Forkhead-box transcription factor A1. This is evaluated by intensity. It stains the nucleus of tumor-cells of the Uro and GU subtypes. Similar expression profile to GATA3. *GATA3*, GATA binding protein 3. This is evaluated by intensity and percentage positive tumor-cells. It stains the nucleus of tumor-cells of the Uro and GU subtypes. *KRT14*, Keratin 14. This is evaluated by intensity and percentage positive tumor-cells. It stains the cytoplasm of tumor-cells of the Basal/SCC-like subtype. *KRT20*, Keratin 20. This is evaluated by intensity. It stains the cytoplasm of tumor-cells of the Uro and GU subtypes. In tumors, KRT20 is frequently strongly de-regulated and expression is not limited to morphologically differentiated cells. *KRT5*, Keratin 5. This is evaluated by intensity and percentage positive tumor-cells. It stains the cytoplasm and plasma membrane of basal cells layer of Uro tumors and all tumor-cells of Basal/SCC-like tumors. In Uro tumors usually only 10% of the cells (basal) are positive, whereas in some Uro cases and in Basal/SCC-like cases 20–100% of cells are positive. *NCAM1*, CD56, Neural cell adhesion molecule 1. This is evaluated by intensity and percentage positive tumor-cells. It stains cells with neuroendocrine differentiation (>90% of cases are negative). Validation marker for the Sc/NE-like group. *CDKN2A (p16)*, Cyclin-dependent kinase inhibitor 2A p16INK4A. This is evaluated by intensity. It stains the cytoplasm of GU tumors strongly. Normal expression represents a score of 1, and Uro tumors have frequently lost expression due to subtype-specific genomic loss, leading to complete lack of expression. *PPARG*, Peroxisome proliferator activated receptor gamma. This is evaluated by intensity and percentage positive tumor-cells. It stains the nucleus of tumor-cells of the Uro and GU subtypes. Similar expression profile to GATA3. *RB1*, Retinoblastoma 1. This is evaluated by percentage positive tumor-cells. It stains the nucleus of all tumor-cells that have not specifically lost expression. Loss of expression is least frequent in the Uro subtype, of intermediate frequency in the Basal/SCC-like subtype, and most frequent in the GU and the Sc/NE-like subtypes. *SYP*,

Synaptophysin. This is evaluated by intensity and percentage positive tumor-cells. It stains cells with neuroendocrine differentiation (>90% of cases are negative). Validation marker for the Sc/NE-like group. *TP63*, Tumor protein p63. This is evaluated by percentage positive tumor-cells. It stains the nucleus of basal and intermediate cell layers of tumor-cells of the Uro subtype. Tumors of the Basal/SCC-like subtype are positive, whereas the GU and the Sc/NE-like subtypes are negative. *TUBB2B*, Beta-tubulin class 2B. This is evaluated by intensity and percentage positive tumor-cells. It stains the cytoplasm of tumor-cells of the Sc/NE-like subtype. Skeletal muscle also stains positive. *UPK3*, Uroplakin 3. This is evaluated by intensity. It stains the plasma membrane of tumor-cells of the Uro and GU subtypes. In tumors, UPK3 is frequently strongly de-regulated and expression is not limited to morphologically differentiated cells. *VIM*, Vimentin. This is evaluated by intensity and percentage positive tumor-cells. It stains the cytoplasm of stromal cells strongly. It occasionally stains small subsets of tumor-cells at the invasive front, but stains all tumor-cells of the Mes-like subtype. *ZEB2*, Zinc Finger E-Box Binding Homeobox 2. This is evaluated by intensity. It stains the nucleus of stromal cells and tumor-cells of the Mes-like subtype.

7. To be classified as Urothelial-like histology the tumor should have a smooth, undisrupted tumor-stroma interface, nuclei of similar shape and size, and a conserved directionality of cells from basal cell layers outward [1]. This variable overlaps with low pathological grade to a quite large extent but not fully. The purpose of including the urothelial-like histology is to capture the defining aspect of the urothelial-like subtype, which is that the tumors have retained the normal stratification of cell layers seen in the urothelium.
8. WHO 1973 grade (G1-G3) or equivalent should be used. It has not been tested to what extent the use of WHO 2004 grade (High grade versus low grade) would affect classification results.
9. Due to the semiquantitative nature of the IHC analysis, the intensity cutoffs used in the evaluation step will not be defined too precisely. Thus, there will be some systematic variation between studies depending on how cut-off values are selected. A measure has been taken to minimize the effect of such a bias in the selection of markers. Most of the markers described here are easy to evaluate and naturally fall into the (0–3) intensity categories. Nevertheless, the lack of absolute correspondence between evaluation cutoffs has an effect also on the numeric cutoffs used for classification. Therefore, these numeric values are to be regarded as starting points. If validation markers give weak subtype associations or if the proportion of subtypes are skewed compared to the stage distribution of the cohort, adjustment of the numeric cutoffs for classification should be made.

Acknowledgments

The development of this method would not have been possible without the expertise of Kristina Lövgren in tissue microarray and immunohistochemistry techniques.

References

1. Sjödahl G, Lövgren K, Lauss M et al (2013) Toward a molecular pathologic classification of urothelial carcinoma. Am J Pathol 183:681–691
2. Patschan O, Sjödahl G, Chebil G (2015) A molecular pathologic framework for risk stratification of stage T1 urothelial carcinoma. Eur Urol 68:824–832
3. Sjödahl G, Lauss M, Lövgren K et al (2012) A molecular taxonomy for urothelial carcinoma. Clin Cancer Res 18:3377–3386
4. Choi W, Porten S, Kim S (2014) Identification of distinct basal and luminal subtypes of muscle-invasive bladder cancer with different sensitivities to frontline chemotherapy. Cancer Cell 25:152–165
5. Damrauer JS, Hoadley KA, Chism DD (2014) Intrinsic subtypes of high-grade bladder cancer reflect the hallmarks of breast cancer biology. Proc Natl Acad Sci U S A 111:3110–3115
6. Cancer Genome Atlas Research Network (2014) Comprehensive molecular characterization of urothelial bladder carcinoma. Nature 507: 315–322
7. Sjödahl G, Eriksson P, Liedberg F, Höglund M (2017) Molecular classification of urothelial carcinoma: global mRNA classification versus tumour-cell phenotype classification. J Pathol 242(1):113–125

Part II

Urothelial Carcinogenesis

Chapter 6

Defining the Pathways of Urogenital Schistosomiasis-Associated Urothelial Carcinogenesis through Transgenic and Bladder Wall Egg Injection Models

Evaristus C. Mbanefo and Michael H. Hsieh

Abstract

Urogenital schistosomiasis (infection with *Schistosoma haematobium*) is a major cause of bladder carcinogenesis. However, the exact mechanisms of the sequelae leading up to the development of bladder cancer are poorly understood, mainly because of a dearth of tractable mouse models. We developed a mouse model of urogenital schistosomiasis through intramural injection of parasite eggs into the bladder wall to mimic the trapping of parasite eggs in the bladder. This approach recapitulates many of the sequelae observed in infected humans. Here, we describe procedures for utilizing this surgical technique in combination with well-established transgenic mouse strains to dissect the role of cancer-related genes in the initiation and establishment of bladder carcinogenesis. The described method utilizes CRE-mediated flox activity to render mice p53 haploinsufficient before challenging them with bladder wall egg injection. These techniques are potentially amenable to studying the role of other pro-carcinogenic and cancer suppressor gene(s) in urogenital schistosomiasis-associated urothelial carcinogenesis.

Key words Bladder cancer, Urogenital schistosomiasis, Bladder wall injection, Genetic manipulation, CRE recombinase, p53

1 Introduction

Schistosoma haematobium, the etiological agent of urogenital schistosomiasis (UGS), is classified among the group 1 carcinogens by the International Agency for Research on Cancer (IARC) [1]. It is a major cause of bladder cancer in Africa and parts of the Middle-East [2]. Indeed, urogenital schistosomiasis may rival smoking, in concert with other risk factors such as diet, host genetic factors, environmental exposures, and co-infection with other uropathogens, as arguably the most important risk factors for bladder cancer globally [3] (Fig. 1). Bladder cancer is the most severe outcome of UGS, and is the product of chronic inflammation in response to

Wolfgang A. Schulz et al. (eds.), *Urothelial Carcinoma: Methods and Protocols*, Methods in Molecular Biology, vol. 1655, DOI 10.1007/978-1-4939-7234-0_6, © Springer Science+Business Media LLC 2018

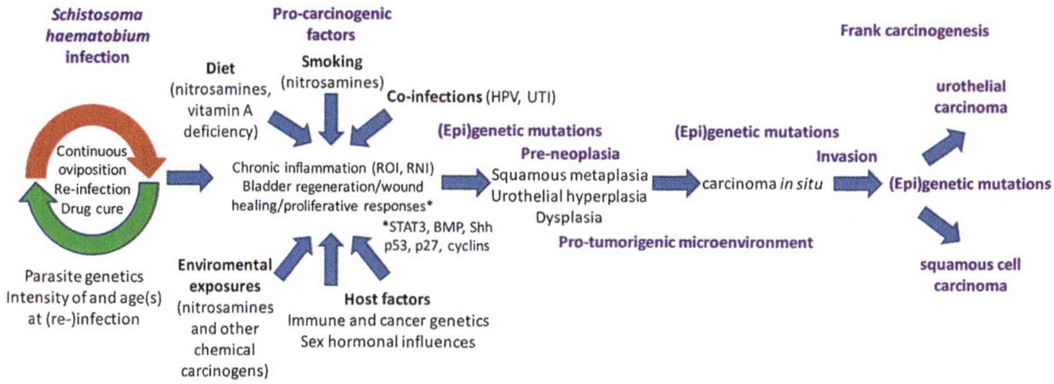

Fig. 1 Proposed mechanisms of urogenital schistosomiasis-associated bladder carcinogenesis

continuous release of antigens from parasite eggs lodged in the walls of the bladder [4, 5]. During UGS, antigens secreted from parasite eggs elicit host-induced granuloma formation around the trapped eggs [6]. The ensuing attempt at tissue repair results in fibrosis and chronic inflammation [7]. The chronic sequelae that follow lead to alterations in the urothelium, including severe ulceration and denudation, hyperplasia, dysplasia, squamous metaplasia, and sometimes bladder carcinoma [8].

Despite being a carcinogen and a major debilitating disease, the mechanisms by which urogenital schistosomiasis-associated chronic inflammation promotes bladder carcinogenesis are poorly understood, mainly because research into its basic biology is hampered by the dearth of experimental tools and tractable animal models that recapitulate the sequelae of urogenital schistosomiasis [9, 10]. For instance, natural infection of mice with *S. haematobium* cercariae, the infective larval stage for humans, results in hepatoenteric schistosomiasis rather than the pelvic form seen during human infection. Novel discoveries that fill these gaps will be the key to our understanding of the fundamental biology and associated development of preventive and therapeutic measures against urogenital schistosomiasis-associated bladder cancer. In an effort to make breakthroughs in addressing these gaps, our group has developed several mouse models of urogenital schistosomiasis [3, 9, 11–13], including tractable mouse models for urogenital schistosomiasis-associated bladder cancer [8] through a combination of use of transgenic mice and parasite egg injection into the mouse bladder wall. Here, we detail the basic procedures for effectively generating and utilizing these resources for studying the mechanisms of urogenital schistosomiasis-associated urothelial carcinogenesis. In brief, urothelial-associated, p53 haploinsufficient mice are generated by crossing Upk3a-GCE mice (featuring urothelial specific tamoxifen-inducible Cre recombinase expression) with p53-floxed mice which have the *Trp53* gene flanked by a pair of *loxP* recombination sites. The p53-haploinsufficient or intact transgenic progeny is subjected to bladder wall injection with *Schistosoma haematobium* eggs, which recapitulates the chronic pathogenic sequelae leading up to schistosomiasis-associated bladder carcinogenesis. This model can be exploited to study the effect of other bladder cancer-related gene knockouts.

2 Materials

2.1 Animals (Transgenic Mice and LVG Hamsters)

1. DBA-Tg(Upk3a-GFP/cre/ERT2)26Amc/J mice (Upk3a-GCE mice), featuring tamoxifen-inducible Cre recombinase activity in cells expressing uroplakin-3a, a urothelial-specific gene [14]. We had earlier validated the urothelial specificity of the Cre recombinase activity in this Upk3a-GCE transgenic mouse model [8].
2. p53-floxed mice with *loxP* recombination sites flanking exons 2–10 of the *Trp53* gene.
3. *Schistosoma haematobium*-infected LVG Hamsters for generating *Schistosoma haematobium* eggs.

2.2 Bladder Wall Injection of Schistosoma haematobium Eggs

1. Isoflurane general anesthesia apparatus with vaporizer system and nozzle for maintenance anesthesia of mice.
2. Dissecting microscope for magnification (optional).
3. 30-gauge needles.
4. 100 μL Hamilton syringes.
5. Sterilized surgical instruments suitable for laboratory mice (scissors, forceps, needle drivers).
6. General surgical supplies: sterile surgical drapes, gauze, and wipes.
7. Hair clippers or depilatory cream.
8. Betadine solution.
9. 4–0 Vicryl and 4–0 non-absorbable silk sutures.
10. Topical antibiotic ointment (Bacitracin 500 units/gram).
11. Buprenorphine—0.6–0.9 mg/kg (an opioid analgesic agent).
12. Bupivicaine—1 mg/kg (local anesthetic agent).
13. Electric heating pad.

2.3 Schistosoma haematobium Egg Preparation

1. *Schistosoma haematobium*-infected LVG hamsters from the NIAID Schistosomiasis Resource Center.
2. Waring blender.
3. Ice-cold 1.2% NaCl solution containing antibiotic antimycotic solution (100 units penicillin, 100 mg/mL streptomycin, and 0.25 mg/mL amphotericin B).

4. Stainless-steel sieves with pore sizes of 420 μm, 180 μm, 105 μm, and 45 μm sieve (Newark Wire Cloth).
5. Light box.
6. Flat-bottom glass Petri dishes.
7. Cell strainers.
8. Pasteur pipettes.

3 Methods

3.1 Generating Urothelial p53 Haploinsufficient Mice

1. To generate p53 haploinsufficient mice, crossbreed Upk3a-GCE mice with p53 floxed mice (Fig. 2) to generate an F1 generation (*Upk3a-GCE; p53*$^{flox/WT}$) featuring a *loxP*-flanked *Trp53* gene in one *Trp53* allele and urothelial specific Cre recombinase activity. *See* **Notes 1** and **9** for sources of these mice and other recommended alternative models.
2. Subsequently, intraperitoneally inject 3 consecutive daily doses of 0.13 g/kg tamoxifen in corn oil to the F1 progeny to induce excision of the *loxP* flanked exons (exons 2–10) of the *Trp53* gene by Cre-mediated recombinase activity, which partly truncates p53 expression and renders the F1 progeny haploinsufficient for p53 in the urothelium (Fig. 2).
3. You can now utilize the p53 haploinsufficient mice to study the implications of p53 abnormalities in schistosomiasis-associated bladder carcinogenesis. In the absence of a tractable mouse model of natural infection-induced, schistosomiasis-associated

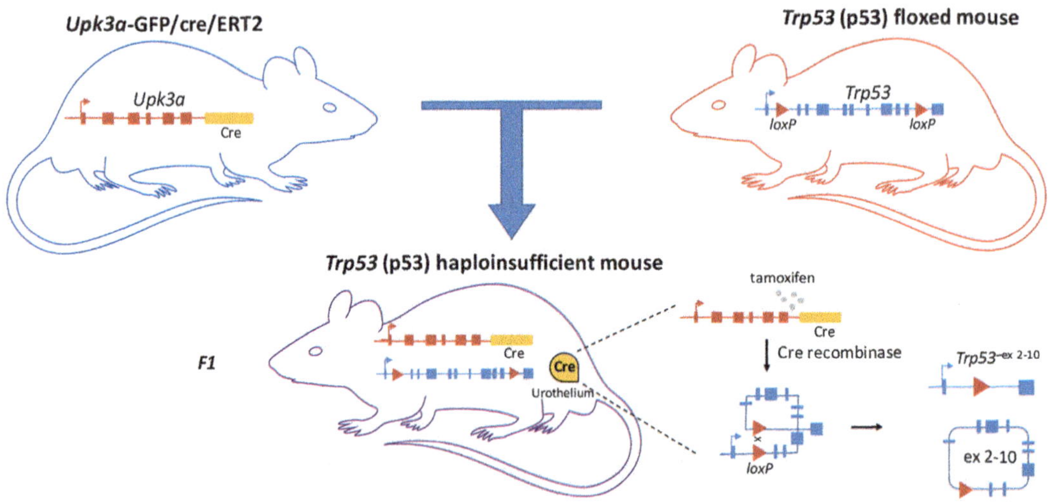

Fig. 2 Genetic crossing of Upk3a-GCE mice with p53 floxed mice and subsequent tamoxifen administration results in Cre-mediated recombinase activity at the *loxP* sites flanking exons 2–10 of the *Tpr53* gene, which renders the F1 generation p53 haploinsufficient in the urothelium

bladder carcinogenesis, our recommended alternative is to inject the parasite eggs into the walls of the bladder [11], akin to the biological lodging of parasite eggs in the host bladder walls.

3.2 Schistosoma haematobium Egg Preparation

1. Keep LVG hamsters previously infected with *Schistosoma haematobium* according to detailed procedures for infection of laboratory animals, including a wide range of schistosomiasis life cycle maintenance procedures, described at the website http://www.afbr-bri.com/schistosomiasis/ and in published protocols [15] Also *see* **Note 2**.
2. At approximately 18 weeks post infection, the peak of egg deposition in the liver and intestines [16], euthanize the infected hamsters and excise their livers and intestines. It is recommended to confirm successful infection of hamsters before this step (*see* **Note 3**).
3. Homogenize the hamster livers and intestines in ice-cold 1.2% NaCl salt solution. *See* **Notes 4** and **5** on recommendations on preparation of this solution.
4. Sequentially pass the homogenate through a series of sieves with decreasing pore sizes: 420 μm, 180 μm, and 105 μm, and then collect the eggs on a 45 μm sieve. Rinse the eggs onto a Petri dish using the salt solution.
5. To enrich for mature eggs and exclude host tissues and other extraneous debris, swirl the Petri dish on a light box in a circular motion to concentrate the eggs at the center. Carefully remove the concentrated eggs at the center using a Pasteur pipette before adding more 1.2% NaCl solution.
6. The enriched eggs may be further concentrated by transferring the content of the Pasteur pipette to a 40 μm cell strainer placed in another Petri dish half filled with the cold 1.2% NaCl solution.
7. Repeat this swirling procedure three to four times or until pure, enriched mature eggs are obtained.
8. Transfer the pure mature eggs to a 15 mL conical tube, fill with cold 1.2% NaCl, and allow eggs to settle by gravity before removing excess salt solution to concentrate eggs. Proceed with injection of eggs into the mouse bladder wall.

3.3 Bladder Wall Injection of Schistosoma haematobium Eggs

1. Ensure that the anesthesia system and all your supplies are available and in good sterile condition before starting. Also *see* **Note 6**.
2. The surgical instruments must be autoclaved beforehand. Also, prior to each use and between individual animal procedures, sterilize surgical instruments with a hot bead sterilizer.

3. Clean the surgical space with soap and water.
4. Repeatedly wipe the surgical table surface with Cide Swipes or antiseptic wipes.
5. Wash the 100 μL Hamilton syringes and 30-gauge (1/2 in. long) needles by repeatedly aspirating absolute alcohol and then phosphate buffered saline (PBS) through the channels prior to first surgery, and wash subsequently with sterile phosphate buffered saline between injections.
6. Place the subject mouse in an isoflurane induction chamber, with the isoflurane set between 2 and 5% to induce general anesthesia. *See* **Note** 7 on recommendations on general anaesthesia.
7. After general anesthesia is induced, remove the mouse from the isoflurane induction chamber and place the mouse with the ventral abdominal region facing up under a dissecting microscope on a sterile surgical space (sterile drape) set onto an electric warming pad to maintain normal body temperature. Place the snout into the anesthesia maintenance nozzle to keep the mouse anesthetized during surgery (the isoflurane flow may be adjusted to 1–3% as necessary to maintain appropriate anesthesia).
8. Using an electric clipper, shave the abdominal skin. Alternatively, apply a depilatory cream and wipe off after 1 min with sterile water.
9. Cover the anus using sterile surgical gauze to prevent contamination by fecal material when the abdomen is open during surgery.
10. Cover the surgical field (lower abdomen) with sterile surgical gauze.
11. Apply Betadine three to four times on the lower abdomen by prepping the surface with Betadine-soaked gauze.
12. Inject the local anesthetic agent (bupivicaine—1 mg/kg) subcutaneously at the site of the planned lower abdominal midline incision. Next, inject Buprenorphine (0.6–0.9 mg/kg) subcutaneously at the planned incision site.
13. Under the dissecting microscope, make a lower midline abdominal incision with scissors while holding up the skin with a pair of forceps. The incision need not be too long but should be just enough to allow exposure of the bladder.
14. Expose the bladder by gentle pressure on the sides of the incision. A full bladder will usually pop out with gentle pressure.
15. Partially decompress the bladder if too full by applying a gentle downward pressure at the dome but do not completely empty

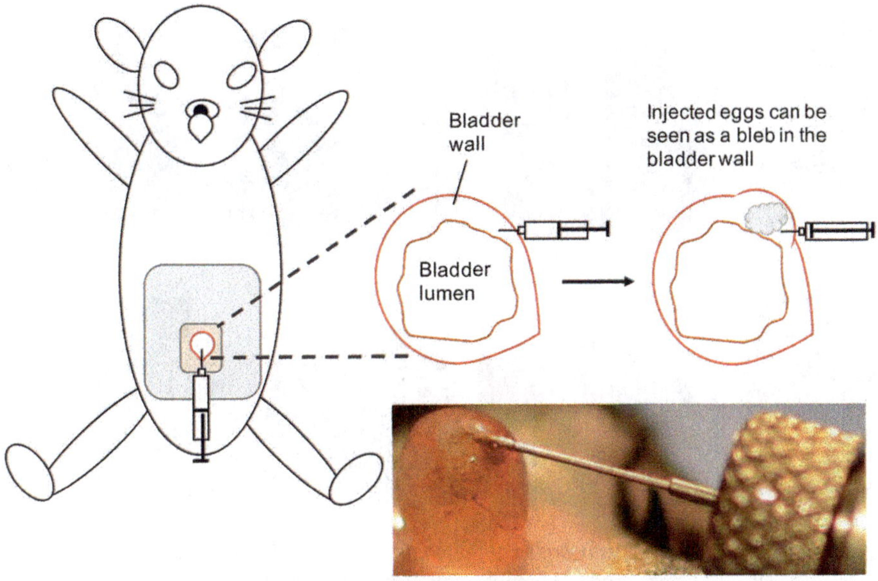

Fig. 3 Bladder wall injection of *Schistosoma haematobium* eggs. Successful injection can be confirmed as a bleb in the bladder wall

the bladder. A completely empty bladder will be more challenging to inject due to poor traction with the needle.

16. Using a 30-gauge needle and Hamilton syringe with the bevel of the needle facing upwards, slowly insert the needle into the wall of the bladder dome and gently push the plunger to inject the sample solution as shown in Fig. 3 (3000 eggs in 50 μL of PBS).
17. Confirm successful injection by verifying the presence of a well-localized bleb inside the bladder wall.
18. Once injection is complete, remove the syringe and carefully push back the exposed bladder into the abdomen with gentle pressure.
19. Close the incision with Vicryl suture for the inner layer and silk suture for the outer layer (skin). *See* **Note 8** for recommendation for injecting multiple mice in a day.
20. Apply topical antibiotic ointment (Bacitracin 500 units/gram) on the sutured incision.
21. Place the mouse on a warming pad during the recovery period before transferring to a new housing cage.
22. Inject another dose of the analgesic agent before the end of the day, and weekly thereafter, if necessary.
23. Maintain the injected mice in conventional mouse housing with an ad libitum supply of mouse chow and water for about 3 months.

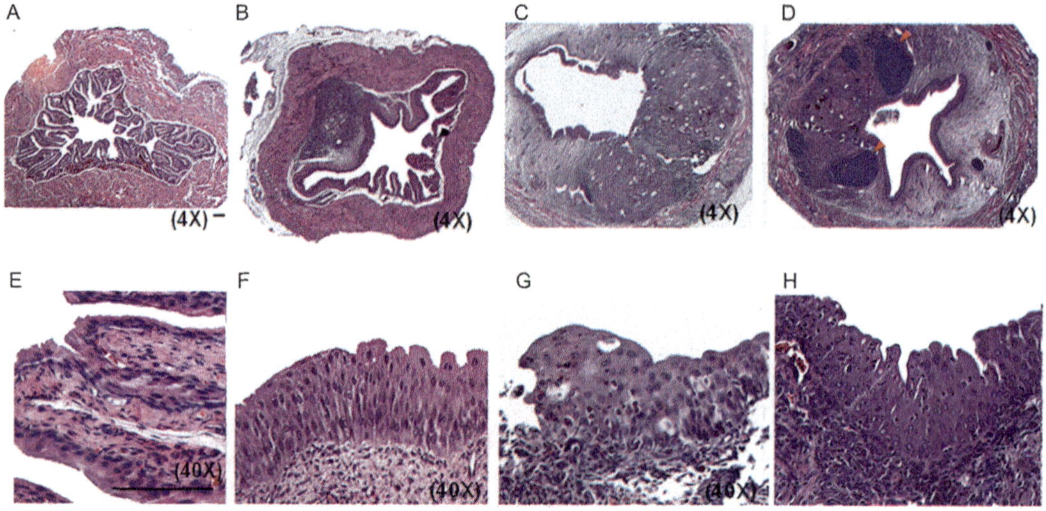

Fig. 4 Bladder wall injection of *Schistosoma haematobium* eggs results in granuloma formation, urothelial ulceration, hyperplasia, dysplasia, and squamous metaplasia. The bladder sections from control mice are shown in (**a**) and (**e**), while **b–d** and **f–h** show 4× and 40× magnification of egg-injected mice bladder sections at days 4, 28, and 99, respectively. Adapted from ref. [11]

24. Euthanize the mouse and aseptically excise the bladder.
25. Fix the bladder (in tissue cassettes) immediately in buffered 10% formalin.
26. Process the fixed bladders histologically by embedding in paraffin, sectioning, followed by hematoxylin and eosin staining.
27. Observe histopathological changes microscopically. Typical examples of histopathological changes in egg-injected bladders on days 4, 28, and 99 post-injection are depicted in Fig. 4 [11].

4 Notes

1. DBA-Tg(Upk3a-GFP/cre/ERT2)26Amc/J mice (Upk3a-GCE mice) can be purchased from Jackson Laboratories (Bar Harbor, Maine, USA), while p53-floxed mice were obtained as a gift from Zijie Sun.
2. If the generation of urothelial-specific, inducible p53 haploinsufficiency is cost- and/or time-prohibitive, one can consider the use of conventional p53 mutant transgenic mice. Another option is use of p53-floxed mice crossed with mice expressing tamoxifen-inducible Cre in all tissues, and then administer tamoxifen intravesically (through a transurethral catheter) in order to induce excision of p53 alleles in the bladder urothelium.

3. *Schistosoma haematobium*-infected LVG Hamsters for generating *Schistosoma haematobium* eggs can be ordered from the NIH Schistosomiasis Resource Center (http://afbr-bri.com/schistosomiasis).
4. Before euthanizing hamsters, it is recommended to parasitologically confirm successful infection by identification of parasite eggs in stool exam. A modified Kato Katz method for this procedure can be found in our published protocols, which also demonstrated how fulminant infection can be identified by tracking hamster weight over time [17].
5. Instead of making the 1.2% NaCl solution and storing on the long term, we find that the solution is better prepared fresh. The required amount of the NaCl salt may be weighed out and stored in 50 mL tubes, ready to be dissolved just before use.
6. An ice-cold solution of 1.2% NaCl should be used throughout the egg preparation steps to prevent premature hatching of the eggs.
7. Before starting surgery, ensure that the anesthesia system, sterile equipment, and all surgery supplies are available. We normally prepare these materials before the day of surgery. Make and use a checklist.
8. Ensure that mice are anesthetized by observing breathing patterns and responses to a gentle paw pinch.
9. When injecting many mice in a day, it is recommended to work in a team of two. The second member of the team can perform suturing and post-op care as the first operates on the next animal.

Acknowledgments

This work was supported by NIH R56AI119168. The contents are solely the responsibility of the authors and do not necessarily represent the official views of the funders. The funders had no role in the preparation of the manuscript and the decision to publish. We appreciate the significant contributions by the previous Hsieh laboratory members and collaborators in the described projects, including but not limited to Chi-Ling Fu, Jared Honeycutt, Justin Odegaard, Olfat Hamman, and De'Broski R. Herbert.

References

1. IARC (1994) Monograph on the evaluation of carcinogenic risks to humans: schistosomes, liver flukes and helicobacter pylori. WHO: International Agency for Research on Cancer 61:9–175
2. Khaled H (2013) Schistosomiasis and cancer in Egypt: review. J Adv Res 4(5):461–466. doi:10.1016/j.jare.2013.06.007

3. Conti SL, Honeycutt J, Odegaard JI et al (2015) Alterations in DNA methylation may be the key to early detection and treatment of schistosomal bladder cancer. PLoS Negl Trop Dis 9(6):e0003696. doi:10.1371/journal.pntd.0003696
4. Chung KT (2013) The etiology of bladder cancer and its prevention. J Cancer Sci Ther 5 (10):346–361. doi:10.4172/1948-5956.1000226
5. Rosin MP, Saad el Din Zaki S, Ward AJ et al (1994) Involvement of inflammatory reactions and elevated cell proliferation in the development of bladder cancer in schistosomiasis patients. Mutat Res 305(2):283–292
6. Colley DG, Secor WE (2014) Immunology of human schistosomiasis. Parasite Immunol 36 (8):347–357. doi:10.1111/pim.12087
7. Odegaard JI, Hsieh MH (2014) Immune responses to Schistosoma haematobium infection. Parasite Immunol 36(9):428–438. doi:10.1111/pim.12084
8. Honeycutt J, Hammam O, Hsieh MH (2015) Schistosoma haematobium egg-induced bladder urothelial abnormalities dependent on p53 are modulated by host sex. Exp Parasitol 158:55–60. doi:10.1016/j.exppara.2015.07.002
9. Rinaldi G, Young ND, Honeycutt JD et al (2015) New research tools for urogenital Schistosomiasis. J Infect Dis 211(6):861–869. doi:10.1093/infdis/jiu527
10. Honeycutt J, Hammam O, CL F et al (2014) Controversies and challenges in research on urogenital schistosomiasis-associated bladder cancer. Trends Parasitol 30(7):324–332. doi:10.1016/j.pt.2014.05.004
11. Fu C-L, Odegaard JI, Herbert DBR et al (2012) A novel mouse model of Schistosoma haematobium egg-induced immunopathology. PLoS Pathog 8:e1002605. doi:10.1371/journal.ppat.1002605
12. Fu CL, Apelo CA, Torres B et al (2011) Mouse bladder wall injection. J Vis Exp (53):e2523. doi:10.3791/2523
13. Richardson ML, CL F, Pennington LF et al (2014) A new mouse model for female genital schistosomiasis. PLoS Negl Trop Dis 8(5):e2825. doi:10.1371/journal.pntd.0002825
14. Harding SD, Armit C, Armstrong J et al (2011) The GUDMAP database—an online resource for genitourinary research. Development 138(13):2845–2853. doi:10.1242/dev.063594
15. Tucker MS, Karunaratne LB, Lewis FA et al (2013) Schistosomiasis. Curr Protoc Immuno 103:Unit 19.1. doi:10.1002/0471142735.im1901s103
16. Botros SS, Hammam OA, El-Lakkany NM et al (2008) Schistosoma haematobium (Egyptian strain): rate of development and effect of praziquantel treatment. J Parasitol 94:386–394. doi:10.1645/GE-1270.1
17. Le TL, Boyett DM, Hurley-Novatny A et al (2015) Hamster weight patterns predict the intensity and course of Schistosoma haematobium infection. J Parasitol 101(5):542–548. doi:10.1645/14-600

Chapter 7

Algorithm for the Automated Evaluation of *NAT2* Genotypes

Georg Michael, Ricarda Thier, Meinolf Blaszkewicz, Silvia Selinski, and Klaus Golka

Abstract

N-Acetyltransferase 2 (*NAT2*) genotyping by PCR and RFLP-based methods provides information on seven single nucleotide polymorphisms (SNPs) without deriving the chromosomal phase (haplotype). So genotyping results must be processed to get all possible *NAT2* haplotype (or allele) combinations. Here we describe the procedure for genotyping and present a program based on Microsoft® Access® which automatically generates all possible haplotype pairs for a given unphased *NAT2* genotype. *NAT2* haplotypes are important to predict the *NAT2* phenotype.

Key words *N*-Acetyltransferase 2, Alleles, Automated evaluation, Computer program, Genotyping, Haplotype

1 Introduction

N-Acetyltransferase 2 (NAT2) is a polymorphic xenobiotic metabolizing enzyme. Currently, more than 100 *NAT2* haplotypes (or alleles), mostly based on one to four single nucleotide polymorphisms (SNPs), have been identified in humans [1] with a remarkable intra- and interethnic variability [2]. Generally, presence of at least one SNP on both chromosomes leads to a decreased metabolic capacity—so-called "slow" acetylators—compared to "rapid" acetylators which have at least one copy of the gene without critical SNPs. To complicate the situation not all of the SNPs—or their combinations on the same chromosome (haplotype)—lead to a reduced NAT2 metabolism. Furthermore, recent studies indicate that different slow haplotypes also differ in their metabolic capacity, e.g., [3], also requiring haplotype information rather than simple discrimination between "rapid" and "slow" acetylators. Deriving the possible haplotype combination—and thus the

Electronic supplementary material: The online version of this chapter (doi:10.1007/978-1-4939-7234-0_7) contains supplementary material, which is available to authorized users.

Wolfgang A. Schulz et al. (eds.), *Urothelial Carcinoma: Methods and Protocols*, Methods in Molecular Biology, vol. 1655, DOI 10.1007/978-1-4939-7234-0_7, © Springer Science+Business Media LLC 2018

acetylation capacity—is important in bladder cancer studies because carcinogenic aromatic amines are substrates of this enzyme. In the past, exposure to carcinogenic aromatic amines like benzidine or 2-naphthylamine was a significant problem in occupational medicine [4], leading to more than 2000 bladder cancer cases recognized as an occupational disease in Germany [5, 6]. 2-Naphthylamine and o-toluidine, but not benzidine, are also constituents of tobacco smoke [7, 8]. In persons with a decreased metabolic capacity, an alternative oxidative pathway is increasingly used, leading to a higher proportion of the highly reactive arylnitrenium ions. These metabolites can bind directly to the DNA of the urothelial cells and thus may cause bladder cancer [9]. Therefore, it is important to determine the slow *NAT2* genotype, showing an increased risk particularly in older studies with occupational exposures [10] or in smokers [11], but also in a recently published meta-analysis [12]. However, in some more recent studies, an impact of the slow acetylation state is no more observed [13, 14]. In persons of Central European origin ("Caucasians"), *NAT2* genotyping is commonly based on seven SNPs (rs1801279, rs1041983, rs1801280, rs1799929, rs1799930, rs1208, rs1799931) [15].

The genotyping procedure consists of PCR assays yielding two amplicons of 442 and 559 base pairs, corresponding to nt −69 to 373 and 342 to 900, respectively. The application of restriction enzymes on the DNA fragments allows the identification of the 7 SNPs.

As the results of the PCR and RFLP measurements do not allow conclusion about the chromosomal phase, i.e., which SNPs are present on the same chromosome, the 'true" haplotype pair of an individual remains unclear if more than one heterozygous SNP is present [15]. In this case several different combinations of *NAT2* haplotypes can explain the measured genotype, i.e., the PCR and RFLP measurements. The program presented here matches the PCR and RFLP results to the complete set of predefined *NAT2* haplotypes as published by the Arylamine *N*-acetyltransferase Gene Nomenclature Committee [1]. For each haplotype combination a combination of DNA fragments is unique but not necessarily vice versa. The program shows for each sample ("current measurement") all haplotype combinations that match to the set of measured DNA fragments.

2 Materials

2.1 Genotyping Assay

DNA can be isolated for example by commercially available extraction kits or by phenol extraction. The assay used for *NAT2* genotyping by PCR/RFLP follows ref. [16], with modifications.

2.1.1 Reagents for PCR

1. Tenfold PCR buffer concentrate, including 15 mM $MgCl_2$, is supplied by the manufacturer of the DNA Taq polymerase; Q solution and additional $MgCl_2$ supplied with the enzyme are not required for this method.
2. Bidistilled water (autoclaved, free of DNase).
3. Deoxynucleoside triphosphates (dNTPs).
4. Restriction enzymes: *Msp*I, *Fok*I, *Dde*I, *Kpn*I, *Taq*I, *Bam*HI.
5. Restriction enzyme buffer, tenfold concentrate, supplied by the manufacturer of the restriction enzymes.
6. Bovine serum albumin (BSA), 100 μg/mL (*see* **Note 1**).
7. Sterile water for the amplification, 10 mL ampoules.
8. Thermostable DNA Taq polymerase (5 U/μL).

2.1.2 Primers

1. *NAT2*-P1: 5′-GTCACACGAGGAAATCAAATGC-3′.
2. *NAT2*-P2: 5′-ACCCAGCATCGACAATGTAATTCCTGCCC TCA-3′.
3. *NAT2*-P3: 5′-ACACAAGGGTTTATTTTGTTCC-3′.
4. *NAT2*-P4: 5′-AATTACATTGTCGATGCTGGGT-3′ (*see* **Note 2**).

2.1.3 Reagents for Agarose Gel Electrophoresis

1. Agarose.
2. NuSieve™ GTG™ Agarose.
3. Boric acid H_3BO_3.
4. Bromophenol blue, sodium salt.
5. DNA standards; 100 base pair ladder.
6. Glacial acetic acid.
7. Ethidium bromide (in solution 10 mg/mL).
8. Ficoll, Type 400 (Polysucrose).
9. Na_2-EDTA × 2 H_2O (Disodium ethylenediaminetetraacetate dihydrate) p.a.
10. TRIS (Tris(hydroxymethyl) aminomethane) p.a.

2.1.4 Solutions

The following weighed-in amounts, preparations and volumes were selected to suit the thermocycler used in this case (96 PCR analyses). These quantities must be adjusted to suit the conditions of the device in the laboratory of the user.

1. 0.5 M EDTA solution pH 8; 4.65 g ethylenediaminetetraacetic acid disodium salt dihydrate are weighed exactly in a 25 mL volumetric flask. The contents are swirled from time to time, while the volumetric flask is being filled to its nominal volume with bidistilled water. The solution is transferred into a 50 mL glass beaker and the pH value of the solution is adjusted to

pH 8 by careful dropwise addition of sodium hydroxide. The pH value is checked using a pH meter (*see* **Note 3**).

2. Fivefold TBE buffer concentrate (TRIS boric acid electrophoresis buffer).

   54 g (446 mmol) TRIS are weighed into a 1 L volumetric flask. Approx. 500 mL bidistilled water is added, and the contents of the flask are swirled around until a clear solution is obtained. Then 27.5 g (445 mmol) boric acid is added and the contents of the flask are swirled again until a clear solution is formed. 20 mL of a 0.5 M EDTA solution (pH 8) is added and the volumetric flask is subsequently filled to its nominal volume with bidistilled water. This solution is stable for several months.
3. Onefold TBE buffer concentrate.

   200 mL of the fivefold TBE buffer concentrate (*see* above) are placed in a 1 L volumetric flask. While the volumetric flask is being filled to its nominal volume with bidistilled water, the contents are swirled occasionally. This buffer is stable for 6–8 weeks.
4. Ficoll gel-loading buffer with bromophenol blue.

   7.5 g Ficoll (type 400) is weighed into a 100 mL glass beaker. 50 mL sterile bidistilled water is added and the Ficoll is dissolved while being warmed and stirred gently (magnetic stirrer). Then 125 mg bromophenol blue is added to the solution and dissolved with a gentle swirling motion. Aliquots of 1 mL of this material (sufficient for 200 analyses in each case) are pipetted into sealable reaction vessels and stored in the deep-freezer at approx. – 18 °C.
5. Calibration solutions for the DNA ladder.

   The 100 bp DNA standard (1 μg/μL) is used to check the restriction cleavage. For this purpose 100 μL of the appropriate standard is diluted with 200 μL Ficoll gel-loading buffer with bromophenol blue and 700 μL onefold TBE buffer concentrate. 10–15 μL of the dilutions is loaded into the gel wells.
6. Ethidium bromide solution.

   10 mg ethidium bromide (or 1 tablet containing 10 mg) is added to a 2 mL reaction vessel with a cover. Then 1 mL bidistilled water is added with a pipette, the vessel is closed and shaken until the solution becomes clear (*see* **Note 4**).

2.1.5 First PCR Master Mix for 100 Samples

All the solutions and chemicals needed for the first PCR are combined in the first PCR master mix. The volume of the master mix is selected so that approx. 100 DNA samples (or one plate with 96 wells) can be measured. Such a master mix must be freshly prepared on the day of analysis.

Table 1
First PCR master mix batch

Reagents	Volume of reagents (μL)	Final concentration[a]
Tenfold PCR buffer (incl. $MgCl_2$)	500	Onefold PCR buffer (1.5 mM $MgCl_2$)
10 mM dNTPs	100	200 μM per dNTP
10 μM primer *NAT2* P1	160	0.32 μM
10 μM primer *NAT2* P2	160	0.32 μM
DNA *Taq* polymerase (5 U/μL)	25	1.25 U
Bidistilled H_2O (sterile!)	3555	–

[a]The final concentration given here is calculated on the basis of the volume after addition of 5 μL DNA sample to 45 μL master mix in each individual sample

For this purpose the reagent volumes given in Table 1 are pipetted into a 10 mL screw-capped jar. Then the contents are thoroughly mixed by intensive shaking.

2.1.6 Second PCR Master Mix for 100 Samples

All the solutions and chemicals needed for the second PCR are combined in the second PCR master mix. The volume of the master mix is selected so that approx. 100 DNA samples (or one plate with 96 wells) can be measured. Such a master mix must be freshly prepared on the day of analysis. It differs from the master mix for the first PCR in the type of primer added.

For this purpose the reagent volumes given in Table 2 are pipetted into a 10 mL screw-capped jar. Then the contents are thoroughly mixed by intensive shaking.

The volume of the following compositions of the master mix for the restriction enzymes is selected so that approx. 100 samples (for a plate with 96 wells) can be processed.

2.1.7 Master Mix for Restriction Enzyme MspI (First PCR)

50 μL *Msp*I, 200 μL tenfold restriction enzyme buffer and 750 μL sterile bidistilled water are pipetted into a 2 mL reaction vessel with a cover. The vessel is closed and shaken intensively. This master mix must be freshly prepared on the day of analysis (*see* also Table 3).

2.1.8 Master Mix for Restriction Enzyme FokI (First PCR)

100 μL *Fok*I, 200 μL tenfold restriction enzyme buffer and 700 μL sterile bidistilled water are pipetted into a 2 mL reaction vessel with a cover. The vessel is closed and shaken intensively. This master mix must be freshly prepared on the day of analysis (*see* also Table 3).

2.1.9 Master Mix for Restriction Enzyme DdeI (First PCR)

50 μL *Dde*I, 200 μL tenfold restriction enzyme buffer and 750 μL sterile bidistilled water are pipetted into a 2 mL reaction vessel with a cover. The vessel is closed and shaken intensively. This master mix must be freshly prepared on the day of analysis (*see* also Table 3).

Table 2
Master mix batch for second PCR

Reagents	Volume of reagents (μL)	Final concentration[a]
Tenfold PCR buffer (incl. $MgCl_2$)	500	Onefold PCR buffer (1.5 mM $MgCl_2$)
10 mM dNTPs	100	200 μM per dNTP
10 μM primer *NAT2* P3	160	0.32 μM
10 μM primer *NAT2* P4	160	0.32 μM
DNA *Taq* polymerase (5 U/μL)	25	1.25 U
Bidistilled H_2O (sterile!)	3555	–

[a]The final concentration given here is calculated on the basis of the volume after addition of 5 μL DNA sample to 45 μL master mix in each individual sample

Table 3
Pipetting scheme of the master mixes for the restriction enzymes

	Volumes for 100 samples						
	***Msp*I**	***Fok*I**	***Dde*I**	***Kpn*I**	***Taq*I**	***Dde*I**	***Bam*HI**
Restriction enzyme	50 μL 1000 U	100 μL 400 U	50 μL 500 U	100 μL 1000 U	50 μL 1000 U	50 μL 500 U	50 μL 1000 U
Tenfold restriction enzyme buffer (incl. $MgCl_2$)	200 μL	200 μL	200 μL	200 μL	200 μL	200 μL	200 μL
BSA	–	–	–	20 μL	20 μL	–	20 μL
Bidistilled H_2O (sterile!)	750 μL	700 μL	750 μL	680 μL	730 μL	750 μL	730 μL

2.1.10 Master Mix for Restriction Enzyme KpnI (Second PCR)

100 μL *Kpn*I, 200 μL tenfold restriction enzyme buffer, 20 μL bovine serum albumin (BSA) and 680 μL sterile bidistilled water are pipetted into a 2 mL reaction vessel with a cover. The vessel is closed and shaken intensively. This master mix must be freshly prepared on the day of analysis (*see* also Table 3).

2.1.11 Master Mix for Restriction Enzyme TaqI (Second PCR)

50 μL *Taq*I, 200 μL tenfold restriction enzyme buffer, 20 μL bovine serum albumin (BSA), and 730 μL sterile bidistilled water are pipetted into a 2 mL reaction vessel with a cover. The vessel is closed and shaken intensively. This master mix must be freshly prepared on the day of analysis (*see* also Table 3).

2.1.12 Master Mix for Restriction Enzyme DdeI (Second PCR)

50 μL *Dde*I, 200 μL tenfold restriction enzyme buffer and 750 μL sterile bidistilled water are pipetted into a 2 mL reaction vessel with a cover. The vessel is closed and shaken intensively. This master mix must be freshly prepared on the day of analysis (*see* also Table 3).

2.1.13 Master Mix for Restriction Enzyme BamHI (Second PCR)

50 μL *Bam*HI, 200 μL tenfold restriction enzyme buffer, 20 μL bovine serum albumin (BSA) and 730 μL sterile bidistilled water are pipetted into a 2 mL reaction vessel with a cover. The vessel is closed and shaken intensively. This master mix must be freshly prepared on the day of analysis (*see* also Table 3).

2.2 Program for Evaluation of NAT2 Genotypes

An IBM® compatible computer with the operating system Microsoft® Windows® XP, 2000, 7 or higher is needed. The application runs under Microsoft® Access® 2003 or higher. The format of the data is *.mdb.

The program comprises a library of subroutines of 32 alleles and is available on the Springer Link and on the homepage of the Leibniz Research Centre for Working Environment and Human Factors at TU Dortmund (www.ifado.de/SourcecodeNAT2GenotypingProgram/).

3 Methods

3.1 Genotyping Assay

The procedure to retrieve the information needed for the computer program is given in Fig. 1 and the text below (according to Blaszkewicz et al., 2004 [16], modified).

3.1.1 Gels

3.1.1.1 Agarose Gel (1.5%)

1. Dissolve 1.5 g agarose in 100 mL onefold TBE buffer by heating to the boiling point (microwave oven 600 W, 500 mL screw-capped flask made of e.g., Duran glass) and swirl around from time to time to avoid delayed boiling.
2. Add 2 μL (10 mg/mL) ethidium bromide solution per 100 mL total volume and cool the prepared agarose solution to about 60–80 °C while being stirred gently (*see* **Note 4**).
3. Pour the prepared agarose solution into the previously prepared gel-pouring stand (insert the gel tray and the gel cutters) and allow the gel to stand for 2 h at RT to set. A gel of 25 cm width and 7.5 cm height with 50 wells can be prepared from the amount given here.
4. Pack the gel in Clingfilm for food storage and keep it in the refrigerator for up to 5 days.

3.1.1.2 NuSieve Agarose: Agarose 3:1 (3.2%)

1. Dissolve 2.4 g NuSieve agarose and 0.8 g agarose as described above in 100 mL onefold TBE buffer by intensive shaking and repeated boiling.

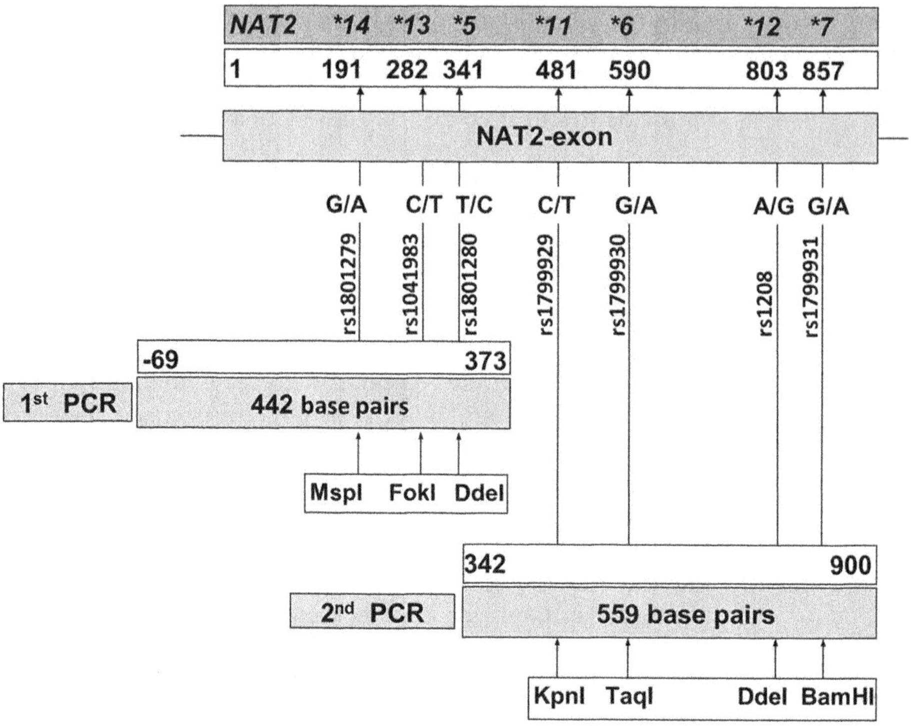

Fig. 1 Amplicon and restriction cleavage sites

2. Add 2 μL (10 mg/mL) ethidium bromide solution and cool the solution to about 60–80 °C while being stirred gently (*see* **Note 4**).
3. Pour the prepared NuSieve agarose solution into the gel-pouring stand and allow the gel to stand for 2 h at RT to set. The gel size and storage are identical to those described for the agarose gel (1.5%).

3.1.2 First PCR (nt −69 to 373)

1. Add 45 μL of the master mix per reaction in a well of a 96 well-plate inserted in a cooling block for well plates.
2. Add 5 μL DNA sample (100 ng DNA/μL) each and mix thoroughly by sucking up and ejecting the samples repeatedly with a pipette (*see* **Note 5**).
3. After all the reagents have been pipetted and mixed, cover the plate with a rubber full plate cover and centrifuge briefly (100 × *g*) to remove any air bubbles and to collect the liquid in the bottom of the wells.
4. Place the plate in the PCR device, which is programmed as shown in Table 5 and start the reaction. In the last step the amplicon is kept cooled in the device until the success of the reaction has been checked.

Table 4
Thermocycler program for the first PCR

Denaturation	94 °C	3 min	
Denaturation	94 °C	0.5 min	35 cycles
Annealing	58 °C	1 min	
Extension	72 °C	1 min	
Concluding extension	72 °C	10 min	
Cooling	4 °C	∞	

Table 5
Restriction cleavage for the amplicons of the first PCR

	Volumes for one sample		
	***Msp*I**	***Fok*I**	***Dde*I**
Product of first PCR	10 μL	10 μL	10 μL
Master mix			
Restriction enzyme	0.50 μL (10 U)	1.0 μL (4 U)	0.50 μL (5 U)
Tenfold restriction enzyme buffer	2 μL	2 μL	2 μL
H_2O sterile	7.50 μL	7.0 μL	7.50 μL
Incubation time	2 h	2 h	4 h
Incubation temp.	37 °C	37 °C	37 °C
Agarose gel	3.2% NuSieve 3: 1	1.5% agarose	3.2% NuSieve 3: 1

3.1.3 Electrophoresis 1 (Check of the Success of the First Amplification)

Check the PCR product by means of electrophoresis on 1.5% agarose gel.

1. Mix 5 μL of the amplicon, 5 μL onefold TBE buffer and 1 μL gel-loading buffer (incl. bromophenol blue).
2. Transfer the mixture to the gel wells. The heavy loading buffer ensures that the samples stay in the application wells.
3. Perform all the subsequent electrophoreses at 160 V (constant) for approx. 60–80 min (migration path approx. 5 cm).
4. Terminate the separation when the bromophenol blue front has almost reached the edge of the gel.

3.1.4 Restriction Cleavage of the First PCR

After successful amplification (positive amplification control) process a total of three 10 μL aliquots of the PCR products of the first amplification per sample separately (according to Table 5) and cleave the PCR products by restriction enzymes as follows:

1. Add 10 μL of the appropriate restriction enzyme master mix to each separate 10 μL aliquot of the product of the first PCR.
2. Incubate the samples at 37 °C in a thermostatically controlled water bath for the incubation times shown in Table 4. These times are based on the information given by the manufacturer of the enzymes and on the experience of the authors.

3.1.5 Electrophoresis 2

1. Transfer the products of restriction cleavage immediately to gel electrophoresis. Use agarose gels given in Table 5.
2. Place the gel with the gel tray in the electrophoresis unit filled with onefold TBE buffer. Cover the gel with buffer.
3. Add 2 μL Ficoll gel-loading buffer each and 20 μL of the product of restriction cleavage and mix thoroughly by sucking up and ejecting the samples repeatedly with a pipette.
4. After all the reagents have been pipetted and mixed, add approx. 15 μL into the gel wells of a 96-well plate.

3.1.6 Second PCR (nt 342 to 900)

1. Add 45 μL of the master mix for the second PCR in the well of a plate inserted in a cooling block for well plates.
2. Add 5 μL DNA sample (100 ng DNA/μL) each and mix thoroughly by sucking up and ejecting the samples repeatedly with a pipette.
3. After all the reagents have been pipetted and mixed, cover the plate with a rubber full plate cover and centrifuge briefly (100 × *g*) to remove any air bubbles and to collect the liquid in the bottom of the wells.
4. Place the plate in the PCR device, which is programmed as shown in Table 6 and start the reaction. The composition and

Table 6
Thermocycler program for the second PCR

Denaturation	94 °C	3 min	
Denaturation	94 °C	0.5 min	35 cycles
Annealing	53 °C	1 min	
Extension	72 °C	1 min	
Concluding extension	72 °C	10 min	
Cooling	4 °C	∞	

Table 7
Restriction cleavage for the amplicons of the second PCR

	Volumes for one sample			
	KpnI	*TaqI*	*DdeI*	*BamHI*
Product 2nd PCR	10 μL	10 μL	10 μL	10 μL
Master mix				
Restriction enzyme	1.00 μL (10 U)	0.50 μL (10 U)	0.50 μL (5 U)	0.50 μL (10 U)
Tenfold restriction enzyme buffer	2 μL	2 μL	2 μL	2 μL
BSA	0.20 μL	0.20 μL	Without BSA	0.20 μL
H_2O sterile	6.80 μL	7.30 μL	7.50 μL	7.30 μL
Incubation time	2 h	18 h (overnight)	4 h	2.0 h
Incubation temp.	37 °C	65 °C	37 °C	37 °C
Agarose gel	1.5% agarose	3.2% NuSieve	3.2% NuSieve	1.5% agarose

the temperature program for the second PCR are shown in the following tables. In the last step the amplicon is kept cooled in the device until the success of the reaction has been checked.

3.1.7 Electrophoresis 3 (Check of the Success of the Second Amplification)

Check the PCR product by means of electrophoresis on 1.5% agarose gel.

1. Add 5 μL of the amplicon, 5 μL onefold TBE buffer and 1 μL gel loading buffer (incl. bromophenol blue) and mix thoroughly by sucking up and ejecting the samples repeatedly with a pipette.
2. After all the reagents have been pipetted and mixed, load the reagents into the gel wells.

3.1.8 Restriction Cleavage of the Second PCR

1. Control for successful amplification.
2. Provide a total of three 10 μL aliquots of the PCR products of the second amplification per sample for further processing (according to Table 7) and restriction cleavage.
3. Add 10 μL of the appropriate restriction enzyme master mix to each separate 10 μL aliquot of the product of the second PCR and incubate the samples at 37 °C (65 °C in the case of *TaqI*) in a thermostatically controlled water bath for the incubation times shown in Table 7. These times are based on the information given by the manufacturer of the enzymes and on the experience of the authors.

3.1.9 Electrophoresis 4

1. Transfer the products of restriction cleavage as quickly as possible to the gel electrophoresis device, as the DNA fragments obtained cannot be stored.
2. Use the agarose gels given in Table 7.
3. Place the gel with the gel tray in the electrophoresis unit filled with onefold TBE buffer. The gel must be covered with buffer.
4. Thoroughly mix 2 μL Ficoll gel-loading buffer with 20 μL product of restriction cleavage by sucking up and ejecting the samples repeatedly with a pipette.
5. After all the reagents have been pipetted and mixed, pipette 15 μL of the reagents in the gel wells of a 96-well plate.

3.1.10 Calibration

1. Use the 100 bp DNA ladder to calibrate the samples after restriction cleavage and analyse these standards in each gel electrophoresis in the outermost wells of each row.

3.1.11 Evaluation

1. Place the wet gel on the UV transilluminator. The ethidium bromide intercalated in the DNA is excited to cause fluorescence emission at 312 nm (*see* **Note 6**).
2. Photograph the band pattern with the camera of the evaluation device and print out.
3. Use the computer program for the results of the investigated sample (Table 8) and determine the allele combination in the samples by the presented algorithm for automated evaluation of *NAT2* genotypes.

3.2 Application of the Program

3.2.1 Mathematical Principles

A DNA fragment in a RFLP measurement is either present (=1) or not (=0). Because of this the binary counting method is used for the evaluation of the mutation, as this allows an unequivocal identification of the actual variations at this position (Table 9).

The decimal sum 4 for example can only be presented by the binary combination "1 0 0". This is also valid for all binary values and can be used to identify variations that consist of 14 digits.

3.2.2 How to Use the Program

Before an evaluation can take place the different haplotypes (or alleles) have to be defined by the user. This is performed in the table "Alleles" (Fig. 2).

The input of the measurement result has to be done in the form "Auswertung (Evaluation)". The SNP-information is assigned to the cells f1 to f14 representing the seven SNPs in each haplotype (*see* Fig. 2, Tab. 10, 11). Each SNP is represented by two cells: the first one for the wild-type (or major) allele, the second one for the variant (or minor) allele. The cells f1 (*wildtype*) and f2 (*minor allele*) correspond to the SNP rs1801279 G/A (*Msp*I 191), f3 and f4 to the SNP rs1041983 C/T (*Fok*I 282) etc. (*see* Fig. 1). If a haplotype shows the wildtype allele at a particular locus—rs1801279[G], for

Table 8
DNA fragment lengths from the restriction cleavage

Restriction cleavage	Mutation site	Sequence	Fragment lengths (bp)				
*Msp*I (from first PCR)		Reference sequence		181	168	93	
	191	Sequence variation	274		168		
*Fok*I (from first PCR)		Reference sequence	337	105			
	282	Sequence variation	442				
*Dde*I (from first PCR)		Reference sequence	221		163	58	
	341	Sequence variation		189	163	58	32
*Kpn*I (from second PCR)		Reference sequence		424	135		
	481	Sequence variation	559				
*Taq*I (from second PCR)		Reference sequence		226	170	142	21
	590	Sequence variation	396			142	21
*Dde*I (from second PCR)		Reference sequence	345	124		90	
	803	Sequence variation	345		97	90	27
*Bam*HI (from second PCR)		Reference sequence		515	44		
	857	Sequence variation	559				
First PCR = 442 bp		Second PCR = 559 bp					

Table 9
Binary counting method

Decimal sum	Binary value (decimal)	2^2 (4)	2^1 (2)	2^0 (1)
0		0	0	0
1		0	0	1
2		0	1	0
3		0	1	1
4		1	0	0
5		1	0	1
6		1	1	0
7		1	1	1

instance—the first f-cell is marked. If there is a base pair exchange at the locus the second f-cell is marked. This procedure is repeated for the other six SNPs of the haplotype. Then a binary code is created for each haplotype by the program from the designations of the cells f1 to f14. A marked cell is designated figure "1", an empty cell

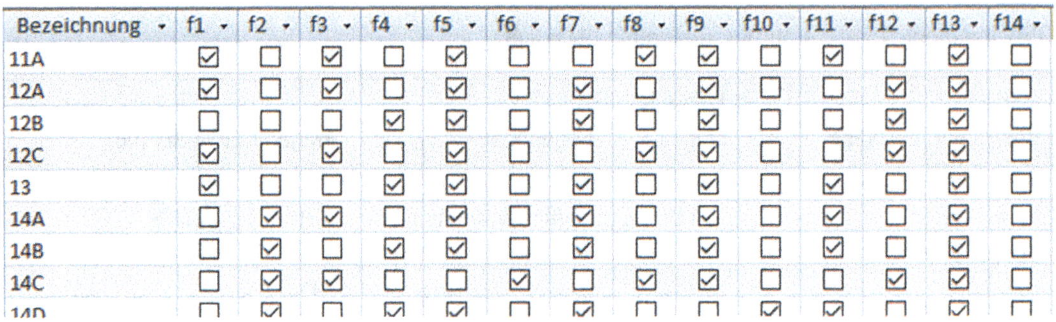

Bezeichnung	f1	f2	f3	f4	f5	f6	f7	f8	f9	f10	f11	f12	f13	f14
11A	☑	☐	☑	☐	☑	☐	☐	☑	☑	☐	☑	☐	☑	☐
12A	☑	☐	☑	☐	☑	☐	☑	☐	☑	☐	☐	☑	☑	☐
12B	☐	☐	☐	☑	☑	☐	☑	☐	☑	☐	☐	☑	☑	☐
12C	☑	☐	☑	☐	☑	☐	☐	☑	☑	☐	☐	☑	☑	☐
13	☑	☐	☐	☑	☑	☐	☑	☐	☑	☐	☑	☐	☑	☐
14A	☐	☑	☑	☐	☑	☐	☑	☐	☑	☐	☑	☐	☑	☐
14B	☐	☑	☐	☑	☑	☐	☑	☐	☑	☐	☑	☐	☑	☐
14C	☐	☑	☑	☐	☐	☑	☐	☑	☑	☐	☐	☑	☑	☐
14D	☐	☑	☐	☑	☑	☐	☑	☐	☐	☑	☑	☐	☑	☐

Fig. 2 Screenshot table "Alleles"

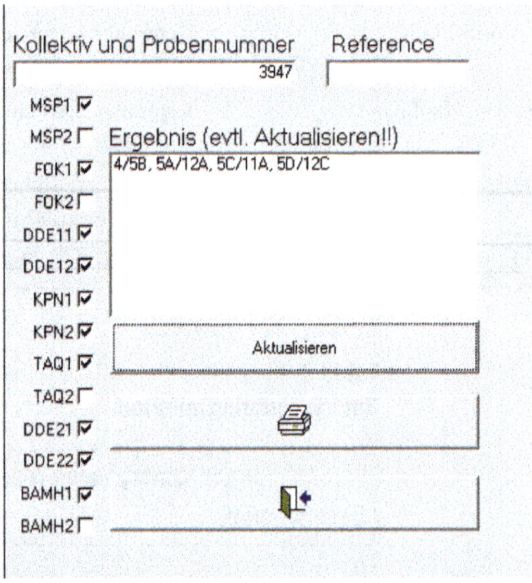

Fig. 3 Screenshot form "Evaluation (Auswertung)" after evaluation is done

gets the figure "0". The generated 14 digit binary code is then converted into a decimal, e.g., the binary code for *NAT2**4 is 1 0 1 0 1 0 1 0 1 0 1 0 1 0, corresponding to 10922, and the binary code for *5B is 1 0 1 0 0 1 0 1 1 0 0 1 1 0, corresponding to 10598. Current measurements and predefined haplotype pairs are coded respectively as presence or absence of a particular allele at the particular locus, e.g., the binary code 1 0 1 0 1 1 1 1 1 0 1 1 1 0 (= haplotype pairs *NAT2**4/5B, *5A/*12A, *5C/*11A, *5D/*12C) becomes 11246 (Fig. 3).

By pressing the button "Aktualisieren (Update)" you will get the result of the evaluation: All possible haplotype combinations are listed.

3.2.3 The Evaluation

For the identification of the different variants in the current measurement (or sample) the binary structures will be compared with those of the predefined haplotypes. If all DNA fragments of a predefined haplotype are present in the current measurement the program will identify it as a possible combination candidate and shows this on the screen. The identification is hereby based on an "OR" comparison. If a DNA fragment is part of the predefined haplotype or part of the current measurement the result is "1". If both DNA fragments are not present the result is "0". The result of this comparison will again be compared with the current measurement. If the result is the same then the haplotype is part of the current measurement (*see* examples below).

There are three options for each of the seven SNPs. Either the band pattern matches the homozygous major allele or the homozygous minor allele or the heterozygous type. These results are filled in the input template (*see* Fig. 2) of the program. If the band pattern reveals the homozygous major allele, e.g., G/G at *Msp*I 191, f1 is marked, if the pattern shows the homozygous minor allele A/A at *Msp*I 191, cell f2 is marked. If the analysis of the pattern indicates both options G/A at *Msp*I 191, the cells f1 as well as f2 are marked. This procedure is repeated for the other six SNPs. Then the binary code is created by the program from the designations of the cells f1 to f14 (*see* above) and then converted into a decimal.

To determine all possible haplotype pairs matching to the genotype of a person the program merges all possible haplotype pairs (i.e., all combinations of two equal or unequal haplotypes) of the 32 predefined library haplotypes, generates the binary code and converts it into a decimal. Next all library decimals are compared with the decimal of the sample. If the decimals are in coincidence, the program outputs the corresponding haplotype pair. Note, that the decimal of a haplotype pair is not unique, i.e., it is possible that different haplotype pairs have the same decimal. For instance, *4/*6A and *6B/*13 both have the code 1 0 1 1 1 0 1 0 1 1 1 0 1 0 with the decimal 11962 and are listed as possible haplotype pairs for all sample with this decimal 11962 (Table 12).

All DNA fragments of the library haplotype *11A are part of the current measurement. Therefore the result of the comparison and of the current measurement is identical and haplotype *11A is consistent with the current measurement. Note, that consistency with the current measurement requires that *5C is the second haplotype in the pair (Table 10).

The DNA fragment *Fok*I2 of the haplotype *12B is not part of the current measurement. Measurement and result of the comparison are incompatible, the library haplotype *12B is therefore not part of this measurement (Table 11).

Some results of an evaluation performed with this program are shown in Table 12, 13 (*see* **Note 7**).

Table 10
Example A (the allele is part of the current measurement)

SNP	rs1801279[G]	rs1801279[A]	rs1041983[C]	rs1041983[T]	rs1801280[T]	rs1801280[C]	rs1799929[C]	rs1799929[T]	rs1799930[G]	rs1799930[A]	rs1208[A]	rs1208[G]	rs1799931[G]	rs1799931[A]
DNA Fragment	*MspI1*	*MspI2*	*FokI1*	*FokI2*	*DdeI11*	*DdeI12*	*KpnI1*	*KpnI2*	*TaqI1*	*TaqI2*	*DdeI21*	*DdeI22*	*BamHI1*	*BamHI2*
Current Measurement	1	0	1	0	1	1	1	1	1	0	1	1	1	0
Allele *11A	1	0	1	0	1	0	0	1	1	0	1	0	1	0
Result	1	0	1	0	1	1	1	1	1	0	1	1	1	0

The Arabic numerals of the names of the restriction enzymes are indices. Index 1 = reference sequence (wild type), index 2 = sequence variation (mutation). In the case of a double-digit index, the first digit codes for the first or second PCR and the second digit codes for reference sequence and sequence variation, resp.

Table 11
Example B (the allele is not part of the current measurement)

SNP	rs1801279[G]	rs1801279[A]	rs1041983[C]	rs1041983[T]	rs1801280[T]	rs1801280[C]	rs1799929[C]	rs1799929[T]	rs1799930[G]	rs1799930[A]	rs1208[A]	rs1208[G]	rs1799931[G]	rs1799931[A]
DNA Fragment	*MspI1*	*MspI2*	*FokI1*	*FokI2*	*DdeI11*	*DdeI12*	*KpnI1*	*KpnI2*	*TaqI1*	*TaqI2*	*DdeI21*	*DdeI22*	*BamHI1*	*BamHI2*
Current Measurement	1	0	1	0	1	1	1	1	1	0	1	1	1	0
Allele *12B	0	0	0	1	1	0	1	0	1	0	0	1	1	0
Result	1	0	1	1	1	1	1	1	1	0	1	1	1	0

The Arabic numerals of the names of the restriction enzymes are indices. Index 1 = reference sequence (wild type), index 2 = sequence variation (mutation). In the case of a double-digit index, the first digit codes for the first or second PCR and the second digit codes for reference sequence and sequence variation, resp.

4 Notes

1. Bovine serum albumin (BSA), 100 μg/mL, is supplied by the manufacturer of the restriction enzymes if required.
2. The primers are dissolved in sterile water so that concentrations of 100 pmol/μL are available. They are stored at −20 °C. The primers are stable for approx. 1–2 years under these conditions.

Table 12
Calculation principle for an example resulting in the two possible allele combinations *NAT24/*6A, *NAT2**6B/*13**

Input template	f1	f2	f3	f4	f5	f6	f7	f8	f9	f10	f11	f12	f13	f14	Decimal
Code of two alleles (sample)	1	0	1	1	1	0	1	0	1	1	1	0	1	0	11962
*The decimal 11962 refers to the allele pair: *4/*6A*															
Single allele code *NAT2**4	1	0	1	0	1	0	1	0	1	0	1	0	1	0	
Single allele code *NAT2**6A	1	0	0	1	1	0	1	0	0	1	1	0	1	0	
Merged code of two alleles	1	0	1	1	1	0	1	0	1	1	1	0	1	0	11962
*This decimal also refers to the allele pair: *6B/*13*															
Single allele code *NAT2**6B	1	0	1	0	1	0	1	0	0	1	1	0	1	0	
Single allele code *NAT2**13	1	0	0	1	1	0	1	0	1	0	1	0	1	0	
Merged code of two alleles	1	0	1	1	1	0	1	0	1	1	1	0	1	0	11962
Input template	f1	f2	f3	f4	f5	f6	f7	f8	f9	f10	f11	f12	f13	f14	
Restriction enzyme	*Msp*I		*Fok*I		*Dde*I		*Kpn*I		*Taq*I		*Dde*I		*Bam*HI		
Base exchange	G/A		C/T		T/C		C/T		G/A		A/G		G/A		

3. This solution can be stored in the refrigerator at approx. 6 °C for several months.
4. Extreme care must be taken when handling ethidium bromide, vinyl gloves must be worn. Ethidium bromide is mutagenic! These solutions must be freshly prepared on the day of analysis. Ethidium bromide is sensitive to light.
5. Necessary amounts are thawed before use in the PCR and kept in the cooling block for PCR reagents until pipetting is carried out. Gloves must be worn when preparing the PCR in order to avoid contamination of the sample with extraneous DNA and DNases, which cause degradation of DNA.
6. Suitable gloves must be worn to protect the skin against UV irradiation!
7. If more than one allele pair is found and you would like to know how likely a haplotype combination is, you have to use highly sophisticated haplotyping programs like PHASE [17–19].

Table 13
Possible haplotype combinations after application of this program, based on 32 *NAT2* haplotypes (alleles)

Sample	Results after DNA restriction cleavage																
	*Msp*I 1	*Msp*I 2	*Fok*I 1	*Fok*I 2	*Dde*I 11	*Dde*I 12	*Kpn*I 1	*Kpn*I 2	*Taq*I 1	*Taq*I 2	*Dde*I 21	*Dde*I 22	*Bam*HI 1	*Bam*HI 2	Possible allele combinations	Most likely alleles acc. to PHASE calculations[1]	Acetylator type
Individual 1	yes	no	yes	no	yes	no	yes	no	yes	no	yes	no	yes	no	*4/*4	*4/*4 = 1	R
Individual 2	yes	no	yes	no	yes	yes	yes	yes	yes	no	yes	no	yes	no	*4/*5A, *5D/ *11A	*4/*5A >0.999	R/S
Individual 3	yes	no	yes	no	yes	yes	yes	yes	yes	no	yes	yes	yes	no	*4/*5B, *5A/ *12A, 5*C/*5C *11A, *5D/ *12C	*4/*5B >0.999	R/S
Individual 4	yes	no	yes	no	yes	yes	yes	no	yes	no	yes	yes	yes	no	*4/*5C, *5D/ *12A	*4/*5C >0.999	R/S
Individual 5	yes	no	yes	yes	yes	no	yes	no	yes	yes	yes	no	yes	no	*4/*6A, *6B/*13	*4/*6A >0.999	R/S
Individual 6	yes	no	yes	no	yes	yes	yes	yes	yes	no	no	yes	yes	no	*5B/*12A, *5C/ *12C	*5B/*12A >0.995	R/S

Individual 7	yes	no	yes	no	no	yes	no	yes	yes	no	no	yes	yes	no	*5B/*5B	*5B/*5B =1	S
Individual 8	yes	no	yes	yes	yes	yes	yes	yes	yes	yes	yes	yes	yes	no	*4/*5P, *5A/*6C, *5B/*6A, *5G/*6B, *5 J/*12C	*5B/*6A >0.999	S
Individual 9	yes	no	yes	yes	yes	no	yes	no	yes	yes	yes	yes	yes	no	*4/*6C, *6A/*12A, *6B/*12B, *6F/*13	*6A/*12A >0.995	S/R
Individual 10	yes	no	yes	yes	yes	no	yes	yes	yes	yes	yes	yes	yes	no	*6A/*12C, *6C/*11A, *6E/*12B	*6A/*12C >0.999	S/R
Individual 11	yes	no	no	yes	yes	no	yes	no	no	yes	yes	no	yes	no	*6A/*6A	*6A/*6A =1	S
Individual 12	yes	no	no	yes	yes	no	yes	no	yes	yes	yes	no	yes	yes	*6A/*7B, *6I/*13	*6A/*7B >0.999	S

Acetylator: S = slow, S/R (R/S) = intermediate, R = rapid. The Arabic numerals of the names of the restriction enzymes are indices. Index 1 = wild type, index 2 = mutation. In the case of a double-digit index, the second digit codes for wild type and mutation, resp. These calculations were performed with the program PHASE [17–19]

Likelihood > or = 1

References

1. Arylamine N-Acetyltransferase Nomenclature Committee. http://nat.mbg.duth.gr/
2. Golka K, Wiese A, Assennato G, Bolt HM (2004) Occupational exposure and urological cancer. World J Urol 21:382–391
3. Patillon B, Luisi P, Poloni ES, Boukouvala S, Darlu P, Genin E, Sabbagh A (2014) A homogenizing process of selection has maintained an "ultra-slow" acetylation NAT2 variant in humans. Hum Biol 86:185–214
4. Selinski S, Blaszkewicz M, Ickstadt K, Hengstler JG, Golka K (2013) Refinement of the prediction of N-acetyltransferase 2 (NAT2) phenotypes with respect to enzyme activity and urinary bladder cancer risk. Arch Toxicol 87:2129–2139
5. Schöps W, Jungmann O, Zumbe J, Zellner M, Hengstler JG, Golka K (2013) Assessment criteria for compensation of occupational bladder cancer. Front Biosci (Elite Ed) 5:653–661
6. Schöps W, Jungmann OP, Zellner M, Zumbé J, Golka K (2016) Tumoren der ableitenden Harnwege Erkrankt durch berufliche Exposition. URO-NEWS 20(1):23–29
7. Luceri F, Moneti G, Pieraccini G (1994) Bestimmung des Amingehaltes im Zigarettenrauch. HP Peak 1:2–4
8. Hoffmann D, Hoffmann I (1997) The changing cigarette, 1950-1995. J Toxicol Environ Health 50:307–364
9. Lang NP, Kadlubar FF (1991) Aromatic and heterocyclic amine metabolism and phenotyping in humans. Prog Clin Biol Res 372:33–47
10. Golka K, Prior V, Blaszkewicz M, Bolt HM (2002) The enhanced bladder cancer susceptibility of NAT2 slow acetylators towards aromatic amines: a review considering ethnic differences. Toxicol Lett 128:229–241
11. Vineis P, Marinelli D, Autrup H, Brockmoller J, Cascorbi I, Daly AJ et al (2001) Smoking, occupation, N-acetyltransferase-2 and bladder cancer: a pooled analysis of genotyped studies. Cancer Epidemiol Biomark Prev 10:1249–1252
12. Zhu Z, Zhang J, Jiang W, Zhang X, Li Y, Xu X (2015) Risks on N-acetyltransferase 2 and bladder cancer: a meta-analysis. Onco Targets Ther 8:3715–3720
13. Ovsiannikov D, Selinski S, Lehmann ML, Blaszkewicz M, Moormann O, Haenel MW et al (2012) Polymorphic enzymes, urinary bladder cancer risk, and structural change in the local industry. J Toxicol Environ Health A 75:557–565
14. Krech E, Selinski S, Blaszkewicz M, Bürger H, Kadhum T, Hengstler JG, Truß MC, Golka K (2017) Urinary bladder cancer risk factors in an area of former coal, iron and steel industries in Germany. J Toxicol Environ Health A. in press. DOI: 10.1080/10937404.2017.1304719
15. Selinski S, Blaszkewicz M, Ickstadt K, Hengstler JG, Golka K (2014) Improvements in algorithms for phenotype inference: the NAT2 example. Curr Drug Metab 15:233–249
16. Blaszkewicz M, Dannappel D, Thier R, Lewalter J (2004) N-Acetyltransferase 2 (genotyping). In: Angerer J, Müller M (eds) Analyses of hazardous substances in biological materials, Special issue: Marker of susceptibility, vol 9. Wiley-VCH, Weinheim, pp 135–163. http://onlinelibrary.wiley.com/doi/10.1002/3527600418.bi0nat2gene0009/pdf
17. Stephens M, Smith NJ, Donnelly P (2001) A new statistical method for haplotype reconstruction from population data. Am J Hum Genet 68:978–998
18. Stephens M, Donnelly P (2003) A comparison of Bayesian methods for haplotype reconstruction. Am J Hum Genet 73:1162–1169
19. Li N, Stephens M (2003) Modelling linkage disequilibrium, and identifying recombination hotspots using SNP data. Genetics 165:2213–2233

Chapter 8

Detection of APOBEC3 Proteins and Catalytic Activity in Urothelial Carcinoma

Ananda Ayyappan Jaguva Vasudevan, Wolfgang Goering, Dieter Häussinger, and Carsten Münk

Abstract

Members of the APOBEC3 (A3) family of enzymes were shown to act in an oncogenic manner in several cancer types. Immunodetection of APOBEC3A (A3A), APOBEC3B (A3B), and APOBEC3G (A3G) proteins is particularly challenging due to the large sequence homology of these proteins and limited availability of antibodies. Here we combine independent immunoblotting with an in vitro activity assay technique, to detect and categorize specific A3s expressed in urothelial bladder cancer and other cancer cells.

Key words APOBEC3, Cytidine deaminase, Urothelial bladder cancer, Mutation, Deamination assay, Cancer cell

1 Introduction

APOBEC3G (apolipoprotein B mRNA-editing, enzyme-catalytic, polypeptide-like 3G; referred to as A3G), one of the cellular polynucleotide cytidine deaminases of the APOBEC3 (A3) family, is extensively studied as a retroviral (HIV-1) restriction factor [1–3]. On infection, A3 proteins encapsidated into the virus catalyze the deamination of cytidines to uridines in single-stranded viral cDNA generated during reverse transcription in the target cells, thereby hypermutating the viral genome and subsequently inhibiting productive infection (for reviews on the antiviral role of A3s and their protein features, *see* [4–6]). The preferred dinucleotides of A3G and other A3s are C<u>C</u> and T<u>C</u> in the DNA substrate, respectively [7–10]. A3 act only on single-stranded DNA and can deaminate the cytosines on the substrate molecule in a processive manner in $3' \rightarrow 5'$ direction [11, 12]. To counter A3-mediated mutagenesis, lentiviruses acquired the accessory protein Vif (viral infectivity

Wolfgang A. Schulz et al. (eds.), *Urothelial Carcinoma: Methods and Protocols*, Methods in Molecular Biology, vol. 1655, DOI 10.1007/978-1-4939-7234-0_8, © Springer Science+Business Media LLC 2018

factor) that anchors A3s to target them for polyubiquitylation and proteasomal degradation [13, 14].

Recently, mutation signatures resulting from the catalytic activity of A3s (especially A3A and A3B) were reported in several cancer types, including bladder, cervical, head and neck, breast and lung cancers [8, 15–18]. Specifically, mRNA levels of A3B were found to be elevated in breast, urothelial and several other cancer tissues [8, 19] positively correlating with overall mutation loads in the respective tumor genomes [8, 17]. Even though the mRNA levels of A3B appear to be much higher [20], the mutation spectrum in the bladder tumor patient cohort was found to be two times more A3A specific (YTCA) than A3B specific (RTCA) [20, 21]. Interestingly, an A3B deletion polymorphism was reported to increase the risk of breast cancers [22, 23] and further analysis revealed that the fusion form of protein A3A_B (A3A coding sequence with A3B 3′ UTR) tends to be more mutagenic [24, 25]. In addition, the haplotype I of APOBEC3H (A3H) was recently linked to breast and lung cancer mutagenesis [26].

In experimental research, A3 proteins are often fused to an epitope tag (such as hemagglutinin (HA), V5, or FLAG), which is then used for detection of the particular proteins from the cell and virus lysates using tag- specific antibodies. Although antibodies raised against A3G and A3B are available, they broadly detect A3A, A3B, and A3G due to their high sequence homology (for example A3A and A3B C-terminal domains share >90% identity at nucleotide and amino acid level). This makes it difficult to quantitatively determine the endogenous A3(s) as well as to study the localization of A3s by immunohistochemistry [9, 10]. However, the approximate molecular weight of A3A, A3B and A3G are 23, 45.9 and 46.4 kDa, respectively. Because of this difficulty in assessing A3 family members using mRNA expression profile and available antibodies, an additional independent method to validate endogenous enzymatic activity of A3s in cancer research is crucial. This validation is important to understand whether A3 borne mutations in the genome are a consequence of malignancy and whether this mutation load drives tumor development [9].

Our method involves immunodetection of A3s and determining deamination activity of the A3s using different substrate nucleotides from cell lysates (Fig. 1). We adapted the PCR-based in vitro deamination assay described by Nowarski et al. [12] which depends on a cytidine to uridine conversion in an 80 nt ssDNA by A3. A subsequent PCR generates a double-stranded DNA, replaces the uridine with thymidine, and thus generates a new restriction site (Fig. 1). The efficiency of the restriction enzyme digestion is monitored using a similar 80 nt ssDNA containing uridine instead of a cytidine in the hotspot. This method was shown to be effective in determining specific A3 activity from various samples [27, 28]. Here we used two different bladder cancer cell lines (UMUC-3

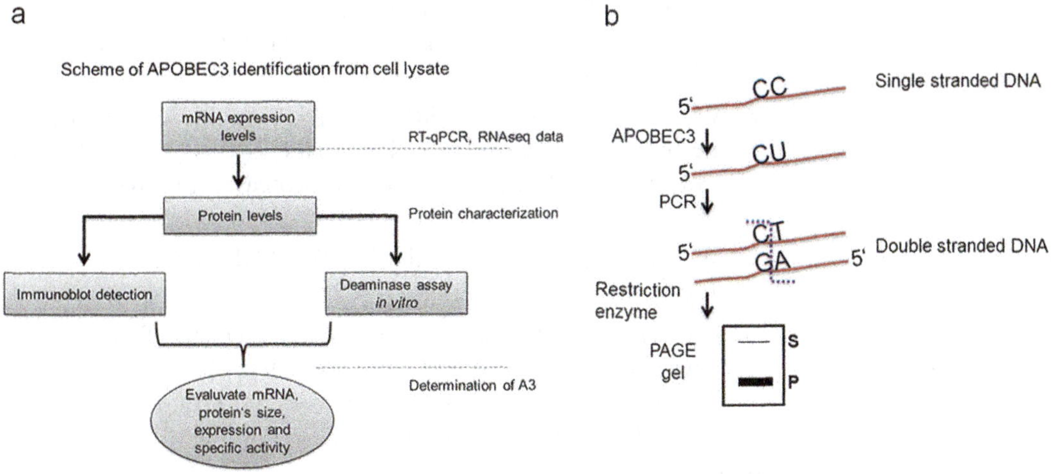

Fig. 1 (**a**) Flow chart representing the combination of techniques used for the characterization of endogenous APOBEC3 from bladder cancer cell lines. (**b**) Principle of DNA deamination assay adapted from Nowarski et al. [12] Incubation of ssDNA with A3 results in deamination of cytidine to uridine in the target motif (CC→CU), generating a specific restriction site following PCR. S-substrate; P-product; RE-restriction enzyme

and VMCUB-1) to demonstrate our method. As a source of defined cell-derived A3s, 293T cells transiently transfected with A3-encoding plasmids were used.

2 Materials

Prepare all buffers using ultrapure water and analytical grade reagents. Prepare and store all reagents at room temperature (unless indicated otherwise). Diligently follow all waste disposal regulations when disposing waste materials (*see* **Note 1**). Note that we did not include the operating procedure for SDS-PAGE and immunoblotting in this chapter, as it follows commonly used standard protocols.

2.1 Cells and Immunoblotting

1. Cell culture: Bladder cancer cell lines of interest and HEK293T cells for transient transfection (*see* **Note 2**).
2. Complete Dulbecco's Modified Eagle Medium (DMEM). For 293T: Dulbecco's high-glucose modified Eagle's medium (DMEM), supplemented with 10% fetal bovine serum (FBS), 2 mM L-glutamine, 50 units/ml penicillin, and 50 μg/ml streptomycin. For bladder cancer cell lines: DMEM plus 10% FBS and 2 mM L-glutamine.
3. Phosphate buffered saline (PBS).
4. Trypsin-EDTA.
5. Transfection reagent such as Lipofectamine.

6. Human APOBEC3 expression plasmids for A3B or A3G can be obtained from the NIH AIDS reagent program (www.aidsreagent.org/).
7. Mild lysis buffer (1×): 50 mM Tris, pH 8, 1 mM phenylmethylsulfonyl fluoride (PMSF), 10% glycerol, 0.8% NP-40, 150 mM NaCl and 1× complete protease inhibitor cocktail. Store at 4 °C (*see* **Note 3**).
8. Materials needed for standard SDS-PAGE and immunoblotting (semi-dry or wet blotting).

   The data presented here was obtained using Mini PROTEAN® three System glass plates and semi-dry blotting procedure (Biorad). It is also expected to work in a similar way with other glass plates and wet blotting.
9. PVDF membrane (*see* **Note 4**)
10. TBST (1×): 10 mM Tris, pH 8, 150 mM NaCl and 0.05% Tween-20, adjust the pH to 8 using 1 M hydrochloric acid. TBST can be prepared as 10× stock, store at room temperature.
11. Blocking solution: 5% skimmed-milk powder in 1× TBST (*see* **Note 5**). Store at 4 °C.
12. A plastic container to handle blot.
13. Anti-HA antibody (1:7500 dilution, MMS-101P, Covance) and anti-APOBEC3G antiserum (NIH catalog number 9906) (*see* **Note 6**).
14. Appropriate anti-mouse and anti-rabbit secondary antibodies (*see* **Note 7**).
15. Chemiluminescent reagent (*see* **Note 8**).

2.2 In Vitro DNA Deamination Assay

1. Single-stranded oligonucleotide DNA substrates (ss DNA), and control oligonucleotides as given in Table 1 (*see* **Note 9**).
2. 250 mM Tris buffer; adjust the pH to 7.0 using 1 M hydrochloric acid, store at room temperature.
3. RNAse A.
4. Thermoblock.
5. Standard thermocycler
6. PCR reaction tubes.
7. PCR components: Taq DNA polymerase and its buffer, 10 mM dNTPs, 10 μM forward and reverse primers (Table 1).
8. Restriction enzymes: Eco147I and MseI

2.3 Native-PAGE Electrophoresis of DNA

1. In-house, native-PAGE gel: 10× TBE buffer: 890 mM Tris (pH 8), 890 mM borate and 20 mM EDTA (can be diluted from 0.5 M EDTA, pH 8), store at room temperature (*see* **Note 10**).

Table 1
Oligonucleotides used in the deamination assay (substrate DNA and PCR primers) are listed. Note that the underlined cytosine is the target base for deamination by A3. A3G and A3B prefer CC and TC motif in the ssDNA, respectively. Uracil-containing modified DNA (CU and TU) oligonucleotides were used as a control to denote the restriction enzyme digestion

Designation	Oligonucleotide sequence
CC	5′- GGATTGGTTGGTTATTTGTTTAAGGAAGGTGGATTAAAGGCCCAAGAA GGTGATGGAAGTTATGTTTGGTAGATTGATGG
CU	5′- GGATTGGTTGGTTATTTGTTTAAGGAAGGTGGATTAAAGGCCUAAGA AGGTGATGGAAGTTATGTTTGGTA GATTGATGG
TC	5′-GGATTGGTTGGTTATTTGTATAAGGAAGGTGGATTGAAGGTTCAAGAA GGTGATGGAAGTTATGTTTGGTAGATTGATGG
TU	5′-GGATTGGTTGGTTATTTGTATAAGGAAGGTGGATTGAAGGTTUAAGAA GGTGATGGAAGTTATGTTTGGTAGATTGATGG
CC-forward	5′-GGATTGGTTGGTTATTTGTTTAAGGA
Common reverse	5′-CCATCAATCTACCAAACATAACTTCCA
TC-forward	5′-GGATTGGTTGGTTATTTGTATAAGGA

2. Aqueous 30% acrylamide and bisacrylamide stock solution at a ratio of 37.5:1, store at 4 °C (*see* **Note 11**).
3. Ammonium persulfate (APS): 10% solution in water
4. N,N,N′,N′-tetramethylethylenediamine, 1,2-bis(dimethylamino)-ethane (TEMED), store at 4 °C.
5. Ethidium bromide staining solution in water, 7.5 μg/ml final concentration (*see* **Note 12**).
6. UV-detection and documentation system

3 Methods

Perform the following procedures at room temperature unless otherwise specified.

3.1 Cell Lysis and Immunoblotting

1. Maintain HEK293T cells and bladder cancer cell lines at 37 °C in a humidified atmosphere of 5% CO_2 in complete DMEM as specified in 2.1. Treat the cancer cell line of interest as required.
2. Seed 6 × 10^5 293T cells per well in a 6-well plate. Next day, transfect 293T cells with 1 μg of A3B or A3G expression plasmids using a suitable transfection reagent. Incubate the cells for 2 days.

3. Lyse with 250–300 μl mild lysis buffer, incubate on ice for at least 15 min and clarify the lysate at 21000 × *g* for 20 min at 4 °C, transfer the soluble fraction into a new tube (*see* **Note 13**).
4. Determine the protein concentration in the cell lysate using BCA assay.
5. Load 20 μg of total protein on the 12% SDS-PAGE gel after heating the protein at 95 °C for 5 min with loading dye containing denaturing agent.
6. Run the gel at a constant 40 mA/gel until the bromophenol blue dye front has reached the bottom of the gel.
7. Transfer the protein onto a PVDF membrane using blotting technique.
8. Block the membrane with 5% milk in TBST for 30 min (in a blot shaker).
9. Incubate the blot with the primary antibody (anti-HA or anti-A3G antiserum) for overnight at 4 °C or in a cold room with slight shaking.
10. Next day, wash 3× with TBST, 10 min each time.
11. Probe the blot with appropriate secondary antibody and incubate it for 1 h at room temperature.
12. Wash 3× with TBST, 10 min each time.
13. Detect the signals using appropriate chemiluminescent reagent, image on the X-ray film or direct imaging system (Fig. 2a).

3.2 In Vitro DNA Cytidine Deamination Assay

1. Set up the deamination reaction as follows: 100 fmol ssDNA, 1 μl of 250 mM Tris, pH 7, 2 μl of cell lysate, make up to 10 μl volume with water and mix gently (*see* **Note 14**).
2. Split the reaction mixture into two halves; to one tube add 50 μg/ml RNAse A (final concentration) (*see* **Note 15**).
3. Incubate the reaction mixture at 37 °C for at least 1 h and then terminate by boiling at 95 °C for 5 min (*see* **Note 16**).
4. Dilute the reaction mixture to 1/10 with water, in order to get the substrate concentration to1 fmol/μl. Use 1 μl of this as template DNA in the subsequent PCR reaction.
5. Set the PCR reaction (to a total volume 25 μl) with 1 μl of template, 1 μl of each appropriate forward and reverse primers (stock 10 μM) (Table 1), 1 μl of dNTPs (10 mM), 2.5 μl Taq polymerase buffer containing $MgCl_2$ (10×), 1.5 units Taq DNA polymerase (*see* **Note 17**). The PCR parameters are 95 °C for 3 min, followed by 30 cycles of 61 °C for 30 s and 94 °C for 30 s (*see* **Note 18**).

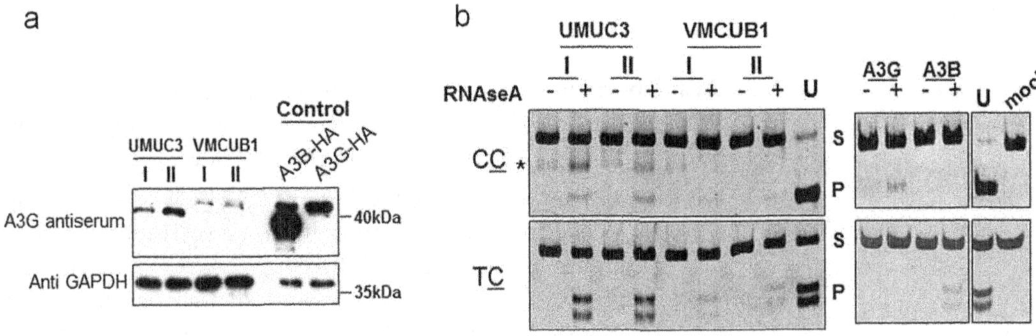

Fig. 2 (**a**) Immunodetection of endogenous A3 from bladder cancer cell lines UMUC-3 and VMCUB-1 lysates and detection of ectopically expressed HA-tagged A3B and A3G from 293 T cells. Blot was stained with anti A3G antiserum, where GAPDH served as a loading control. I and II represent two independent samples. (**b**) Deamination activity of endogenous A3 proteins was tested on two different oligonucleotide substrates containing either CC or TC. RNase A treatment was performed to derive physiologically active A3 proteins from higher mass RNA complexes. Deamination substrate band (S) and product band (P) were marked. "U" specifies the cleavage of CU or TU substrate by its respective restriction enzyme to be used as a marker to denote deaminated product. "*" indicates an unspecific band. In a separate panel, activity assay gel image representing A3G and A3B protein derived from 293 T cells was included

6. As a control for restriction enzyme digestion, include parallel PCR reactions with CU and TU oligos (1 fmol) together.
7. Add 10 units of the respective restriction enzyme Eco147I or MseI to the PCR reactions, mix thoroughly and incubate for at least 1 h at 37 °C (*see* **Note 19**).

3.3 Native Page and Visualization of DNA

1. Prepare a 15% NATIVE-PAGE gel as follows: Add 10 ml of 30% acrylamide-bisacrylamide solution, 8 ml water, 2 ml 10× TBE, 165 μl APS and add finally 16.6 μl TEMED. Quickly mix the casting solution by swirling the container and pour between the glass plates placed in the casting frame. Insert a comb immediately without introducing air bubbles (*see* **Note 20**).
2. When polymerization is complete, immediately transfer the gel to a running container, fill with 1× TBE buffer, and pre-run the gel in 1× TBE for 30 min at 100 V before adding any sample (*see* **Note 21**).
3. To avoid heat formation in the gel tank and buffer, running the native gel in a cold room or on ice is recommended. Load the digested PCR products with 6× loading dye.
4. Following electrophoresis, pry the gel plates open using a gel releaser, stain with ethidium bromide solution in water for 5 min at room temperature.
5. Detect the DNA signal using a 320 nm UV-lamp and appropriate documentation system (Fig. 2b).

4 Notes

1. Wear laboratory safety equipment such as goggles, nitrile gloves, mask, and lab coat, follow the safety instructions suggested by the manufacturer of chemicals and the local legal regulations.
2. We used UMUC-3 and VMCUB-1 bladder cancer cell lines as a model in this chapter. Our method can be used for any other cancer cell line as required. Cell lines can also be subjected to drug treatment, ectopic co-expression of another factor or downregulation by siRNA. Maintain the cells with appropriate medium and conditions as required. HEK293T cells were used for transient transfection of A3 since these cells are easily transfectable using Lipofectamine reagent.
3. Prepare mild lysis buffer without adding the PMSF and 1× protease inhibitor cocktail. It is suggested to make an aliquot of the buffer and freshly add the above components for cell lysis.
4. We obtained optimum results using Immobilon-P Membrane, 0.45 μm from Millipore.
5. We routinely use 5% milk in TBST for blocking and diluting primary and secondary antibodies. It doesn't mean that you must not use 5% BSA in TBST. Empirically determine the better one suits for your antibody and detection method.
6. The NIH antibody was obtained through the NIH AIDS reagent program. Researchers can request reagents through their website (www.aidsreagent.org/).
7. We used anti-mouse, anti-rabbit antibody from GE healthcare at dilution of 1: 10,000 as final concentration.
8. Our immunoblot was developed using ECL prime reagent and X-ray film (both from GE healthcare). It should also work in a similar manner with other reagents or imaging systems. Note that different cell lines may have higher or lower A3 protein levels; hence the detection reagent must be chosen accordingly to avoid capturing saturated signal.
9. We recommend HPLC-purified standard oligonucleotides for this assay. Salt-purified oligonucleotides may result in unspecific DNA amplification.
10. 10× TBE buffer on long storage often tends to precipitate. This complication can be resolved by warming up the buffer for a while prior to use or by using a 5× TBE stock.
11. Due to the neurotoxicity of acrylamide, we prefer buying this reagent rather than preparing it ourselves. Handle this solution inside the hood while making gels.

12. Alternatively, SYBR gold (1:1000 dilution) nucleic acid gel stain from Thermo Fischer Scientific can be used, which better stains weak signals. Note that the number of PCR cycles then needs to be reduced to 18 (instead of 30) for optimal amplification and staining.
13. We use mild lysis buffer for keeping the protein content native for activity assay, but it is also good to try using other harsh buffers such as RIPA if required for the cell lysis. Choose the same buffer and conditions throughout for all the cell lines.
14. If required, for convenient sample handling, the 15 μl reaction volume can be made up with the same substrate concentration.
15. It is easy to dilute the RNAse A to a concentration ten times higher than the final working concentration required in 25 mM Tris buffer, pH 7. RNAse treatment is important to release the A3 protein from the higher mass RNA complexes.
16. Spin the tube shortly to settle down the contents immediately after boiling.
17. Archaeal DNA polymerases such as the Pfu enzyme bind tightly to template-strand uracil and stall replication [29] unless a point mutation V93Q is introduced [30]).
18. The PCR reaction volume was kept within 20–25 μl, because it facilitates loading the complete products on the gel after restriction digestion.
19. Following PCR, add the restriction enzyme directly to the PCR product. PCR purification is not suggested (and not needed) because the columns may not be able to bind the 80 bp ds DNA fragments. Specific restriction enzyme buffers may not be required as well. We do this incubation in a PCR machine, by setting 1 h at 37 °C and then 4 °C indefinitely.
20. Given here is a composition to make a mini-gel with 1.5 mm thick glass plates from Biorad. The volumes can be scaled according to the need. Note that here we have only one layer of gel to cast, unlike stacking and separating gels of SDS-PAGE.
21. It is suggested to wash each well of the gel before and after pre-run with a syringe (to remove unwanted gel fragments). This ensures the convenient loading of samples.

Acknowledgments

We would like to thank Klaus Strebel and the NIH AIDS Research and Reference Reagent Program for anti-ApoC17 (A3G) antibody. We are grateful to W. A. Schulz for his constant support. CM is supported by the Heinz Ansmann foundation.

References

1. Sheehy AM, Gaddis NC, Choi JD, Malim MH (2002) Isolation of a human gene that inhibits HIV-1 infection and is suppressed by the viral Vif protein. Nature 418(6898):646–650. doi:10.1038/nature00939
2. Bishop KN, Holmes RK, Sheehy AM, Davidson NO, Cho SJ, Malim MH (2004) Cytidine deamination of retroviral DNA by diverse APOBEC proteins. Curr Biol 14 (15):1392–1396. doi:10.1016/j.cub.2004.06.057
3. Zhang H, Yang B, Pomerantz RJ, Zhang C, Arunachalam SC, Gao L (2003) The cytidine deaminase CEM15 induces hypermutation in newly synthesized HIV-1 DNA. Nature 424 (6944):94–98. doi:10.1038/nature01707
4. Harris RS, Dudley JP (2015) APOBECs and virus restriction. Virology 479-480:131–145. doi:10.1016/j.virol.2015.03.012
5. Chiu YL, Greene WC (2008) The APOBEC3 cytidine deaminases: an innate defensive network opposing exogenous retroviruses and endogenous retroelements. Annu Rev Immunol 26:317–353. doi:10.1146/annurev.immunol.26.021607.090350
6. Vasudevan AA, Smits SH, Hoppner A, Häussinger D, Koenig BW, Münk C (2013) Structural features of antiviral DNA cytidine deaminases. Biol Chem 394(11):1357–1370. doi:10.1515/hsz-2013-0165
7. Yu Q, Konig R, Pillai S, Chiles K, Kearney M, Palmer S et al (2004) Single-strand specificity of APOBEC3G accounts for minus-strand deamination of the HIV genome. Nat Struct Mol Biol 11(5):435–442. doi:10.1038/nsmb758
8. Burns MB, Lackey L, Carpenter MA, Rathore A, Land AM, Leonard B et al (2013) APOBEC3B is an enzymatic source of mutation in breast cancer. Nature 494(7437):366–370. doi:10.1038/nature11881
9. Henderson S, Fenton T (2015) APOBEC3 genes: retroviral restriction factors to cancer drivers. Trends Mol Med 21(5):274–284. doi:10.1016/j.molmed.2015.02.007
10. Burns MB, Leonard B, Harris RS (2015) APOBEC3B: pathological consequences of an innate immune DNA mutator. Biom J 38 (2):102–110. doi:10.4103/2319-4170.148904
11. Chelico L, Pham P, Calabrese P, Goodman MF (2006) APOBEC3G DNA deaminase acts processively 3′ –> 5′ on single-stranded DNA. Nat Struct Mol Biol 13(5):392–399. doi:10.1038/nsmb1086
12. Nowarski R, Britan-Rosich E, Shiloach T, Kotler M (2008) Hypermutation by intersegmental transfer of APOBEC3G cytidine deaminase. Nat Struct Mol Biol 15(10):1059–1066. doi:10.1038/nsmb.1495
13. Sheehy AM, Gaddis NC, Malim MH (2003) The antiretroviral enzyme APOBEC3G is degraded by the proteasome in response to HIV-1 Vif. Nat Med 9(11):1404–1407. doi:10.1038/nm945
14. Yu X, Yu Y, Liu B, Luo K, Kong W, Mao P et al (2003) Induction of APOBEC3G ubiquitination and degradation by an HIV-1 Vif-Cul5-SCF complex. Science 302(5647):1056–1060. doi:10.1126/science.1089591
15. Roberts SA, Sterling J, Thompson C, Harris S, Mav D, Shah R et al (2012) Clustered mutations in yeast and in human cancers can arise from damaged long single-strand DNA regions. Mol Cell 46(4):424–435. doi:10.1016/j.molcel.2012.03.030
16. Nik-Zainal S, Alexandrov LB, Wedge DC, Van Loo P, Greenman CD, Raine K et al (2012) Mutational processes molding the genomes of 21 breast cancers. Cell 149(5):979–993. doi:10.1016/j.cell.2012.04.024
17. Roberts SA, Lawrence MS, Klimczak LJ, Grimm SA, Fargo D, Stojanov P et al (2013) An APOBEC cytidine deaminase mutagenesis pattern is widespread in human cancers. Nat Genet 45(9):970–976. doi:10.1038/ng.2702
18. Cancer Genome Atlas Research N (2014) Comprehensive molecular characterization of urothelial bladder carcinoma. Nature 507 (7492):315–322. doi:10.1038/nature12965
19. Hedegaard J, Lamy P, Nordentoft I, Algaba F, Hoyer S, Ulhoi BP et al (2016) Comprehensive transcriptional analysis of early-stage urothelial carcinoma. Cancer Cell 30(1):27–42. doi:10.1016/j.ccell.2016.05.004
20. Lamy P, Nordentoft I, Birkenkamp-Demtroder K, Thomsen MB, Villesen P, Vang S et al (2016) Paired exome analysis reveals clonal evolution and potential therapeutic targets in urothelial carcinoma. Cancer Res 76 (19):5894–5906. doi:10.1158/0008-5472.CAN-16-0436
21. Chan K, Roberts SA, Klimczak LJ, Sterling JF, Saini N, Malc EP et al (2015) An APOBEC3A hypermutation signature is distinguishable from the signature of background mutagenesis by APOBEC3B in human cancers. Nat Genet 47(9):1067–1072. doi:10.1038/ng.3378
22. Long J, Delahanty RJ, Li G, Gao YT, Lu W, Cai Q et al (2013) A common deletion in the

APOBEC3 genes and breast cancer risk. J Natl Cancer Inst 105(8):573–579. doi:10.1093/jnci/djt018

23. Xuan D, Li G, Cai Q, Deming-Halverson S, Shrubsole MJ, Shu XO et al (2013) APOBEC3 deletion polymorphism is associated with breast cancer risk among women of European ancestry. Carcinogenesis 34(10):2240–2243. doi:10.1093/carcin/bgt185
24. Caval V, Suspene R, Shapira M, Vartanian JP, Wain-Hobson S (2014) A prevalent cancer susceptibility APOBEC3A hybrid allele bearing APOBEC3B 3'UTR enhances chromosomal DNA damage. Nat Commun 5:5129. doi:10.1038/ncomms6129
25. Nik-Zainal S, Wedge DC, Alexandrov LB, Petljak M, Butler AP, Bolli N et al (2014) Association of a germline copy number polymorphism of APOBEC3A and APOBEC3B with burden of putative APOBEC-dependent mutations in breast cancer. Nat Genet 46(5):487–491. doi:10.1038/ng.2955
26. Starrett GJ, Luengas EM, McCann JL, Ebrahimi D, Temiz NA, Love RP et al (2016) The DNA cytosine deaminase APOBEC3H haplotype I likely contributes to breast and lung cancer mutagenesis. Nat Commun 7:12918. doi:10.1038/ncomms12918
27. Jaguva Vasudevan AA, Perkovic M, Bulliard Y, Cichutek K, Trono D, Häussinger D, Münk C (2013) Prototype foamy virus bet impairs the dimerization and cytosolic solubility of human APOBEC3G. J Virol 87(16):9030–9040. doi:10.1128/JVI.03385-12
28. Marino D, Perkovic M, Hain A, Jaguva Vasudevan AA, Hofmann H, Hanschmann KM et al (2016) APOBEC4 enhances the replication of HIV-1. PLoS One 11(6):e0155422. doi:10.1371/journal.pone.0155422
29. Fogg MJ, Pearl LH, Connolly BA (2002) Structural basis for uracil recognition by archaeal family B DNA polymerases. Nat Struct Biol 9(12):922–927. doi:10.1038/nsb867
30. Firbank SJ, Wardle J, Heslop P, Lewis RJ, Connolly BA (2008) Uracil recognition in archaeal DNA polymerases captured by X-ray crystallography. J Mol Biol 381(3):529–539. doi:10.1016/j.jmb.2008.06.004

Chapter 9

Oxidative Stress in Urothelial Carcinogenesis: Measurements of Protein Carbonylation and Intracellular Production of Reactive Oxygen Species

Patcharawalai Whongsiri, Suchittra Phoyen, and Chanchai Boonla

Abstract

Oxidative stress contributes substantially to urothelial carcinogenesis. Its extent can be assessed by measurements of reactive species (mainly reactive oxygen species (ROS)), oxidatively modified damage products, and levels of various antioxidants. We presented herein the methods for the measurement of protein carbonyl content and intracellular production of ROS. Protein carbonyl is the most commonly used indicator of protein oxidation because it is early formed and relatively stable under oxidative stress. Determination of protein carbonyl relies on the derivatization of carbonyl groups (aldehydes: R-CHO and ketones: R-CO-R) with 2,4-dinitrophenylhydrazine (DNPH) under strongly acidic conditions to yield stable dinitrophenyl (DNP) hydrazones. Absorbance of the DNP hydrazones at 370–375 nm is proportional to the content of carbonyl groups. To report the protein carbonyl content, it is usually normalized by total proteins. Detection of intracellular ROS production is based on oxidation of 2′,7′-dichlorofluorescein-diacetate (DCFH-DA) by ROS to produce the highly fluorescent 2′,7′-dichlorofluorescein (DCF). Fluorescent intensity measured at 480 nm excitation and 535 nm emission is directly proportional to the amount of ROS generated.

Key words Bladder cancer, Oxidative stress, Protein carbonyl, DNPH, ROS, DCFH

1 Introduction

Oxidative stress was first conceptualized by H. Sies as an imbalance between reactive oxidant species and antioxidants leading to potential oxidative damage. Due to aerobic metabolism and environment, reactive oxygen species (ROS) is principally produced in the cells, and it is a main cause of oxidative stress. ROS directly attacks biomolecules yielding oxidatively modified damage products, which leads to cell injury and death. It is well documented in both animal models [1–3] and human studies [4–8] that oxidative stress critically contribute to the development of urothelial cancer. Although oxidative stress has been shown to accelerate both genetic mutations and epigenetic alterations, mechanistic

Wolfgang A. Schulz et al. (eds.), *Urothelial Carcinoma: Methods and Protocols*, Methods in Molecular Biology, vol. 1655, DOI 10.1007/978-1-4939-7234-0_9, © Springer Science+Business Media LLC 2018

insight into how ROS promotes carcinogenesis and progression of bladder cancer is largely unknown. We recently demonstrated that ROS induce hypomethylation of LINE-1 element via depletion of methyl donor S-adenosylmethionine [9, 10]. Measurement of oxidative stress level is required in experiments dealing with ROS. To define the level of oxidative stress, direct measurement of ROS is the best means. However, since ROS have a short half-life and very low concentration in the cells, an indirect measure is more practical by detecting the products oxidatively modified by ROS. In this chapter, we present our experience in measurements of protein carbonyl and intracellular ROS production in a cell culture model.

The carbonyl groups (aldehydes and ketones) are formed directly by oxidation of amino acid side chains (Lys, Arg, Pro, and Thr) and indirectly through reaction of nucleophilic side chains (Cys, His, and Lys) with aldehyde substances (malondialdehyde, 4-hydroxynonenal, acrolein) generated during lipid peroxidation [11, 12]. It should be kept in mind that carbonylated proteins are not solely generated from the oxidation reaction, but can also be produced from glycation and glycoxidation reactions [13]. However, protein carbonyl is still the most commonly used marker of ROS-mediated protein oxidation. Determination of protein carbonyl depends on a classic reaction of carbonyl groups with 2,4-dinitrophenylhydrazine (DNPH) pioneered by Levine and colleagues [14]. The dinitrophenyl (DNP) hydrazone products are detected and quantified either by means of spectrophotometry or immunodetection [15].

A variety of probes have been developed for detection and quantification of ROS [16]. Among them, 2′,7′-dichlorofluorescein-diacetate (DCFH-DA), developed in 1965, is the most widely used ROS sensing probe for motoring total ROS production in cells [17, 18]. DCFH-DA is oxidized, not exclusively, by ROS to yield a fluorescent product, 2′,7′-dichlorofluorescein (DCF). Similar to protein carbonyls, this is not the only source as it can also be oxidized by reactive nitrogen species. Therefore, DCFH-DA is rather a fluorescent sensor of total reactive species [18]. However, it is generally accepted that the majority of reactive species produced in the cells are ROS, and the detected DCF fluorescent signal reflects mainly ROS in cells.

2 Materials

We use purified water based on type II water purification system (resistance of 15 MΩ-cm at 25 °C, TKA-Pacific) for preparing all solutions.

2.1 Protein Carbonyl Measurement

1. Phosphate buffer saline (1× PBS), pH 7.4 for cell culture.
2. RIPA buffer; 50 mM Tris, 150 mM NaCl, 0.1% sodium dodecyl sulfate (SDS), 1% Tritron X-100, pH 7.4. Dissolve 0.6 g Tris base, 0.87 g NaCl, 0.1 g SDS, add 1 mL Triton-X-100, adjust pH to 7.4 and volume to 100 mL.
3. 100× Protease inhibitor cocktail (Cell signaling technology, USA).
4. Bradford reagent.
5. Bovine serum albumin (BSA) (100× Purified BSA).
6. 10 mM 2,4-dinitrophenylhydrazine in 2 N HCl; Dissolve 0.991 g DNPH (TCI) in 500 mL of 2 N HCl.
7. 2 N HCl.
8. 20% (w/v) Trichloroacetic acid (TCA), keep it at 4 °C to be used as cold TCA.
9. Ethanol:ethyl acetate (1:1, v/v).
10. 6 M Guanidine hydrochloride (GdmCl) in 0.5 M potassium phosphate monobasic (KH_2PO_4), pH 2.5. Dissolve 286.6 g GdmCl, 34.023 g KH_2PO_4, adjust pH to 2.5 with HCl, and add water up to 500 mL (*see* **Note 1**).
11. Cell scrapers.
12. 1.5 mL microcentrifuge tubes.
13. Centrifuge.
14. Microplate reader.
15. 96-well ELISA plates and UV plates.
16. Water bath.

2.2 Intracellular ROS Measurement

1. 0.25% Trypsin-EDTA.
2. Fetal bovine serum (FBS).
3. Dulbecco's Modified Eagle Medium (DMEM).
4. 2′,7′-Dichlorofluorescin diacetate; Prepare stock solution of 50 mM DCFH-DA by dissolving 0.122 g of DCFH-DA in 5 mL of dimethyl sulfoxide. Wrap tube with aluminum foil and keep at −20 °C. To prepare a working DCFH-DA solution (0.5 mM), add 100 μL of stock solution in 9.9 mL serum-free DMEM medium (1:100 dilution).
5. 96-well clear-bottom black microplate.
6. Trypan blue.
7. Neubauer chamber.
8. CO_2 incubator.
9. Microplate reader.

3 Methods

3.1 Protein Carbonyl Measurement (DNPH Assay)

3.1.1 Protein Extraction from Cells: Cell Lysate Sample Preparation

1. After finishing cell treatment, discard media, place cells on ice, and wash twice with cold 1× PBS (2 mL each for 6-well plate).
2. Add RIPA buffer containing 1× Protease inhibitor cocktail (*see* **Note 2**) to the cells and incubate for 10 min on ice.
3. Thoroughly scrape the cells by cell scraper, transfer the cell lysate to a 1.5 mL microcentrifuge tube; incubate for 30 min on ice (mix well every 10 min interval).
4. Centrifuge the cell lysate at 12,000 × *g* at 4 °C for 10 min.
5. Discard pellet, carefully collect the supernatant as a cell lysate sample, put the lysate sample into a new 1.5 mL microcentrifuge.
6. Cell lysate sample is ready for analysis or it can be stored at −70 °C until testing.

3.1.2 Determination of Protein Concentration by Bradford Assay

1. Prepare BSA standard at concentrations of 0.25, 0.5, and 1 mg/mL. Water is used as blank control (0 mg/mL).
2. Add 5 μL of each BSA standard or blank or samples in triplicates to 250 μL of Bradford reagent in a 96-well microplate, and then mix well.
3. Incubate at room temperature for 5 min.
4. Measure absorbance (**A**) at 595 nm using Microplate reader. Absorbance of each standard or sample is calculated from: **A**standard or sample − **A**blank.
5. Create BSA standard curve (Absorbance, *Y*-axis vs. BSA concentrations, *X*-axis) and calculate linear equation (y = mx + c). We do not use the option pass origin. A good standard curve should have R^2 over 0.99.
6. Protein concentration in each sample is calculated from: $\frac{(\text{Asample}-\text{Ablank})-\text{c}}{\text{m}}$ mg/mL.

3.1.3 Spectrophotometric DNPH Method for Protein Carbonyl

1. Basically, protein concentration for DNPH assay should not exceed 5 mg/mL. In our experience, protein concentration in cell lysate samples ranges between 1 and 2 mg/mL. Cell lysate sample with very high protein concentration should be diluted to 1–5 mg/mL with lysis buffer.
2. Each sample is divided into two tubes, derivatization or DNPH reagent blank and test (Fig. 1).
3. Add 62.5 μL of cell lysate sample to each tube.
4. Add 250 μL of 10 mM DNPH into the test tube and 250 μL of 2 N HCl into the blank (*see* **Note 3**). Fundamentally, concentration of DNPH should be maintained at least at 2 M during

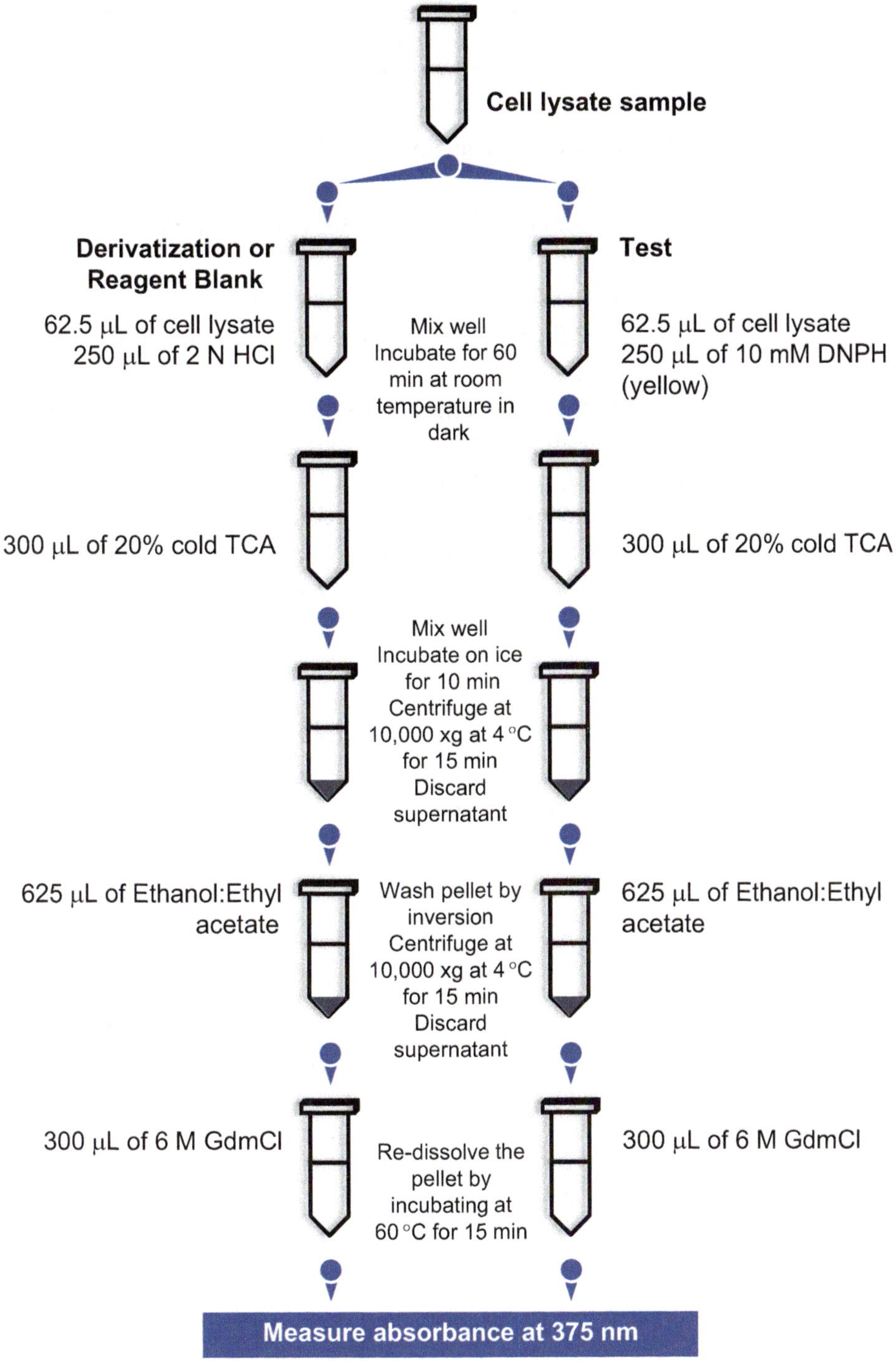

Fig. 1 Procedure of DNPH assay

the derivatization reaction [14]. In our case, we perform the reaction at a final DNPH concentration of 8 M. We do the assay in triplicate (3 tubes for blank and 3 tubes for test in each sample).

5. Mix well and incubate in the dark at room temperature for 60 min.
6. Add 300 μL of 20% cold TCA, mix well, and incubate on ice for 10 min.
7. Centrifuge at 10,000 × *g* at 4 °C for 15 min.
8. Carefully discard the supernatant without disturbing the pellet, keep pellet.
9. Add 625 μL of ethanol:ethyl acetate mixture (*see* **Note 4**) to the pellet and mix by inversion to wash the pellet.
10. Centrifuge at 10,000 × *g* at 4 °C for 15 min (up to 30 min to obtain a more densely packed pellet).
11. Discard the supernatant, collect the pellet.
12. Add 300 μL of 6 M GdmCl and incubate at 60 °C for 15–30 min to dissolve the pellet (*see* **Note 5**).
13. Transfer 250 μL of the mixture to a 96-well UV microplate (*see* **Note 6**) and measure the absorbance at 375 nm. Absorbance (A) of each sample is calculated from: **Atest** – **Ablank**.
14. Protein carbonyl content is calculated based on the obtained absorbance and absorption coefficient of DNP (22,000 M^{-1} cm^{-1}) as follows:

$$\text{Protein carbonyl}\left(\frac{\text{nmol}}{\text{mL}}\right) = \frac{A}{22,000}\,x\frac{10^9}{10^3} = A\,x\,45.45$$

15. Protein carbonyl is normalized to total protein content in the sample: Protein carbonyl $\left(\frac{\text{nmol}}{\text{mL}}\right)$/total proteins $\left(\frac{\text{mg}}{\text{mL}}\right)$. Therefore, the unit of protein carbonyl content in samples is nmol per mg proteins (nmol/mg proteins).

3.2 Intracellular ROS Measurement (DCFH-DA Assay)

3.2.1 Cell Preparation (Seeding)

1. Remove the medium from the confluent cells and wash the cells twice with 1× PBS.
2. Add 0.25% Trypsin-EDTA and incubate at 37 °C, 5% CO_2, 95% humidity in a CO_2 incubator for 3–5 min.
3. Add DMEM (about 3 volume of the added volume of 0.25% Trypsin-EDTA) to inactivate activity of trypsin, mix well by pipetting.
4. Count the number of cells by trypan blue staining in Neubauer chamber.
5. Dilute the cells to 25,000 cells/mL in DMEM.

6. Add 200 μL of cell suspension to each well (5,000 cells/well) in a 96-well black plate.
7. Incubate at 37 °C, 5% CO_2, 95% humidity for 16–18 h for cell adherence.

3.2.2 DCFH-DA Procedure (See Note 7)

1. After overnight incubation, remove the medium from each well.
2. Add 100 μL of working DCFH-DA and incubate for 30 min at 37 °C, 5% CO_2, 95% humidity.
3. Remove the working DCFH-DA and immediately wash with 100 μL of 1× PBS.
4. Add 100 μL of conditioned medium for each treatment. We perform the cell treatment in serum-free DMEM.
5. Measure the initial fluorescent intensity (480 nm excitation and 535 nm emission) (0 min time point, T_0).
6. Place the plate back in the CO_2 incubator again, incubate for 60 min at 37 °C, 5% CO_2, 95% humidity.
7. Measure the fluorescent intensity again at the end (60 min time point, T_{60}).
8. Increment of ROS generation is calculated as the ratio of fluorescent intensity (T_{60}-to-T_0 ratio). An example of our result in bladder cancer cells exposed to H_2O_2 is shown in Fig. 2.

$$\text{Intracellular ROS generation (arbitrary fluorescent unit, AFU)} \\ = \text{Fluorescent intensity of T60/Fluorescent intensity of T0}$$

4 Notes

1. Usually, 6 M GdmCL dissolves with difficulty. We gradually add GdmCl to water and heat up to 37 °C to facilitate the dissolution.
2. Working RIPA buffer containing protease inhibitors has to be freshly prepared. Just prior to use, add 100× protease inhibitor cocktail (10 μL) into RIPA buffer (1 mL). It is necessary to perform all the steps on ice and keep the working lysis buffer on ice.
3. DNPH is light sensitive. The DNPH solution should be stored in an amber or brown glass bottle for light protection. All the steps involving DNPH should be performed in the dark or dimmed light.
4. Caution: Ethyl acetate possibly causes the irritation of the respiratory system. Beware of inhalation.

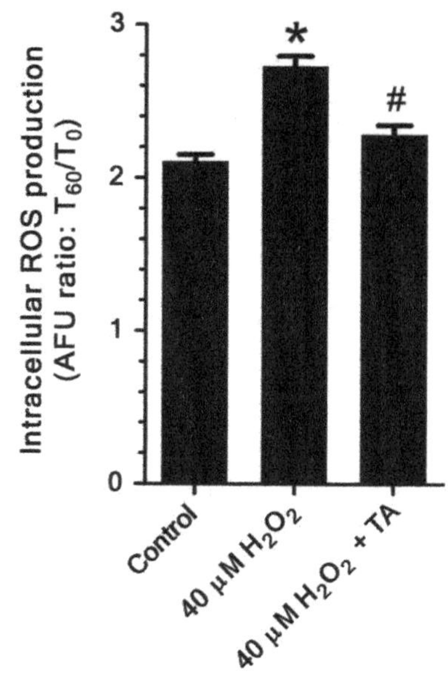

Fig. 2 Example of our result from DCFH-DA assay. Intracellular ROS production in bladder cancer cells (TCCSUP) exposed to 40 μM H_2O_2 (72 h) was significantly higher than that in the untreated control cells. Co-treatment with 300 μM tocopheryl acetate (TA) caused significantly decreased ROS generation in the H_2O_2-treated cells. $^*P < 0.05$ vs. control. $\#P < 0.05$ vs. H_2O_2. AFU: arbitrary fluorescent unit

5. In some cases, the pellet is hard to redissolve. If the pellet cannot be completely dissolved by heating at 60 °C, sonication is additionally needed.
6. Alternatively, a quartz cuvette may be used. In this case, derivatization blank is used to set zero.
7. As DCFH-DA is a fluorescent probe, all the steps handling with this probe need to avoid exposure to light.

Acknowledgment

This work was supported by Thailand Research Fund and Chulalongkorn University (RSA5680019), and Ratchadapiseksompotch Fund, Faculty of Medicine, Chulalongkorn University (RA57/118).

References

1. Kawai K, Yamamoto M, Kameyama S, Kawamata H, Rademaker A, Oyasu R (1993) Enhancement of rat urinary bladder tumorigenesis by lipopolysaccharide-induced inflammation. Cancer Res 53(21):5172–5175
2. Wei M, Wanibuchi H, Morimura K et al (2002) Carcinogenicity of dimethylarsinic acid in male F344 rats and genetic alterations in induced urinary bladder tumors. Carcinogenesis 23 (8):1387–1397

3. Brown NS, Streeter EH, Jones A, Harris AL, Bicknell R (2005) Cooperative stimulation of vascular endothelial growth factor expression by hypoxia and reactive oxygen species: the effect of targeting vascular endothelial growth factor and oxidative stress in an orthotopic xenograft model of bladder carcinoma. Br J Cancer 92(9):1696–1701
4. Akcay T, Saygili I, Andican G, Yalcin V (2003) Increased formation of 8-hydroxy-2′-deoxyguanosine in peripheral blood leukocytes in bladder cancer. Urol Int 71(3):271–274
5. Badjatia N, Satyam A, Singh P, Seth A, Sharma A (2010) Altered antioxidant status and lipid peroxidation in Indian patients with urothelial bladder carcinoma. Urol Oncol 28 (4):360–367
6. Opanuraks J, Boonla C, Saelim C et al (2010) Elevated urinary total sialic acid and increased oxidative stress in patients with bladder cancer. Asian Biomed 4(5):703–710
7. Soini Y, Haapasaari KM, Vaarala MH, Turpeenniemi-Hujanen T, Karja V, Karihtala P (2011) 8-hydroxydeguanosine and nitrotyrosine are prognostic factors in urinary bladder carcinoma. Int J Clin Exp Pathol 4 (3):267–275
8. Patchsung M, Boonla C, Amnattrakul P, Dissayabutra T, Mutirangura A, Tosukhowong P (2012) Long interspersed nuclear element-1 hypomethylation and oxidative stress: correlation and bladder cancer diagnostic potential. PLoS One 7(5):e37009
9. Wongpaiboonwattana W, Tosukhowong P, Dissayabutra T, Mutirangura A, Boonla C (2013) Oxidative stress induces hypomethylation of LINE-1 and hypermethylation of the RUNX3 promoter in a bladder cancer cell line. Asian Pac J Cancer Prev 14(6):3773–3778
10. Kloypan C, Srisa-art M, Mutirangura A, Boonla C (2015) LINE-1 hypomethylation induced by reactive oxygen species is mediated via depletion of S-adenosylmethionine. Cell Biochem Funct 33(6):375–385
11. Berlett BS, Stadtman ER (1997) Protein oxidation in aging, disease, and oxidative stress. J Biol Chem 272(33):20313–20316
12. Suzuki YJ, Carini M, Butterfield DA (2010) Protein carbonylation. Antioxid Redox Signal 12(3):323–325
13. Levine RL, Wehr N, Williams JA, Stadtman ER, Shacter E (2000) Determination of carbonyl groups in oxidized proteins. Methods Mol Biol 99:15–24
14. Levine RL, Garland D, Oliver CN et al (1990) Determination of carbonyl content in oxidatively modified proteins. Methods Enzymol 186:464–478
15. Dalle-Donne I, Rossi R, Giustarini D, Milzani A, Colombo R (2003) Protein carbonyl groups as biomarkers of oxidative stress. Clin Chim Acta 329(1–2):23–38
16. Bartosz G (2006) Use of spectroscopic probes for detection of reactive oxygen species. Clin Chim Acta 368(1–2):53–76
17. Gomes A, Fernandes E, Lima JL (2005) Fluorescence probes used for detection of reactive oxygen species. J Biochem Biophys Methods 65(2–3):45–80
18. Chen X, Zhong Z, Xu Z, Chen L, Wang Y (2010) 2′,7′-Dichlorodihydrofluorescein as a fluorescent probe for reactive oxygen species measurement: forty years of application and controversy. Free Radic Res 44(6):587–604

Part III

Cellular and Animal Models

Chapter 10

Urothelial Carcinoma Stem Cells: Current Concepts, Controversies, and Methods

Jiri Hatina, Hamendra Singh Parmar, Michaela Kripnerova, Anastasia Hepburn, and Rakesh Heer

Abstract

Cancer stem cells are defined as a self-renewing and self-protecting subpopulation of cancer cells able to differentiate into morphologically and functionally diverse cancer cells with a limited lifespan. To purify cancer stem cells, two basic approaches can be applied, the marker-based approach employing various more of less-specific cell surface marker molecules and a marker-free approach largely based on various self-protection mechanisms. Within the context of urothelial carcinoma, both methods could find use. The cell surface markers have been mainly derived from the urothelial basal cell, a probable cell of origin of muscle-invasive urothelial carcinoma, with CD14, CD44, CD90, and 67LR representing successful examples of this strategy. The marker-free approaches involve side population sorting, for which a detailed protocol is provided, as well as the Aldefluor assay, which rely on a specific overexpression of efflux pumps or the detoxification enzyme aldehyde dehydrogenase, respectively, in stem cells. These assays have been applied to both non-muscle-invasive and muscle-invasive bladder cancer samples and cell lines. Urothelial carcinoma stem cells feature a pronounced heterogeneity as to their molecular stemness mechanisms. Several aspects of urothelial cancer stem cell biology could enter translational development rather soon, e.g., a specific $CD44^{+}$-derived gene expression signature able to identify non-muscle-invasive bladder cancer patients with a high risk of progression, or deciphering a mechanism responsible for repopulating activity of urothelial carcinoma stem cells within the context of therapeutic resistance.

Key words Cancer stem cells, Urothelial regeneration, Urothelium stem cells, Urothelial carcinoma, Urothelial carcinoma cells of origin, Urothelial carcinoma stem cell markers, Side population, Drug resistance

1 Introduction

1.1 Cancer Stem Cell Concept

The cancer stem cell (CSC) model is a relatively new concept in cancer biology. Unlike the more traditional theories of clonal selection, where tumors are thought to develop genetic and phenotypic heterogeneity following repeated rounds of mutation and selection, the CSC concept relies on a notion of an intrinsic hierarchy among tumor cells. The most primitive cancer cell population—the CSCs—is endowed with several unique properties fairly similar to

Wolfgang A. Schulz et al. (eds.), *Urothelial Carcinoma: Methods and Protocols*, Methods in Molecular Biology, vol. 1655, DOI 10.1007/978-1-4939-7234-0_10, © Springer Science+Business Media LLC 2018

normal (especially adult) stem cells, first and foremost with the ability to self-renew. Accordingly, the tumor cell heterogeneity develops via CSC differentiation, conceptually similar to normal tissue differentiation; implicit in this concept is the idea that differentiated cells, both normal and cancerous, have limited lifespan and tend to be gradually eliminated. In addition to self-renewal and differentiation abilities, both normal and cancer stem cells display multiple self-protection mechanisms, making them long-lived and self-perpetuating cell populations. The CSC concept thus tends to view cancer as a sort of aberrant organ, by and large governed by the same principles of cell turnover and replenishment as any other organ in the body. Nevertheless, distinct differences are still seen between cancer and normal tissue and several explanations have been put forward to elucidate the loss of homeostatic regulation in transformed cells. In this regard, it is worth noting that the clonal evolution theory and the CSC concept are not mutually exclusive and both appear to play a role in combination to account for tumor heterogeneity and underpinning mechanisms of disease progression. In this view, tumors would be composed of multiple genetically distinct cell clones, each or at least some of them being organized in a hierarchical manner, with its own CSC population. In addition, cancer cells have been shown to manifest considerable plasticity, which in some instances have been shown to undermine the conventional model of a strict hierarchical arrangement of stemness within tumors. Within this context, CSCs might represent more an operational term and some prefer to use the term "tumor initiating cell." The same is true for cancerous differentiation, which should be interpreted as a functional diversification [1, 2]. Despite the facultative nature of plasticity, in many cancers it has now been shown that only a very small fraction of the total cell population have the ability to regenerate the tumor and targeting these cells may well be the way to kill the roots of the cancer "weed" and not just the leaves.

1.2 Stem Cells in Normal Urothelium

Urothelium represents a rather complicated and specialized multilayered epithelium. Based on both morphology and specific marker expression, three cell types can be distinguished. Basal cells are small cuboidal cells (~ 10 μm) sitting on the basement membrane. They express basal type cytokeratins (CK-5, -14, and -17), Sonic Hedgehog (Shh) and p63, and they are negative for uroplakins. The uppermost layer of urothelium is occupied by large (70–100 μm) umbrella cells that are, frequently, bi- or multinucleated. These cells are central to maintaining the blood-urine barrier through a specialized structure in their apical pole composed of uroplakins (Upk). Additional umbrella cell markers are two low-molecular weight cytokeratins, CK-18 and CK-20. The middle part of the urothelium is represented by multiple layers of intermediate cells (10–40 μm), some of them also in contact with the basement membrane and expressing a specific marker mixture (Shh$^+$, CK-5$^-$, CK-14$^-$, p63 heterogenous, Upk$^+$). The urothelium, under homeostatic conditions, displays a slow turnover (3–6 months), but it is able to react to damage with a rapid regenerative response culminating in full repair within days [3, 4].

The traditional view of the stem cell biology of urothelial homeostasis and regeneration works on the assumption that urothelial stem cells are located in the basal cell layer; according to the label-retention experiment performed in rat, ~9% of basal cells are slowly cycling and thus good candidates for urothelial stem cells [5]. The intermediate cells would in this notion represent so-called transit amplifying cells, i.e., mitotically active precursors able to differentiate into postmitotic umbrella cells, but not of self-renewing [3, 4]. During the last years, this traditional model has been challenged by several lineage-tracing experiments accomplished in mouse. Studies of CK-5-driven fluorescent marking of the basal layer showed that these cells failed to differentiate into umbrella cells, whereas lineage tracing under the Uroplakin-2 gene control resulted in a patch of urothelium involving both intermediate and umbrella cells. This lead to the formulation of a new model proposing a coexistence of two separate stem cell populations in the normal urothelium, the basal urothelial stem cells on the one hand, being solely responsible for the preservation of the basal cell layer, and the intermediate urothelial stem cells on the other hand, both self-renewing and differentiating into umbrella cells [6]. Conceptually similar lineage tracing, with longer term readouts performed in human urothelium, based on shared inactivated X-chromosome or shared mitochondrial DNA mutations, are more in keeping with the traditional view, nevertheless, revealing patches of clonally related cells spanning the entire urothelial thickness (i.e., from basal cells to umbrella cells) [7]. Thus the debate about the lineage origins in the urothelium remains active. If there are two independent stem cell populations in the mouse urothelium, then the biological function of basal cells remains an open question—are these cells providing a niche for intermediate stem cells? Or is their function to signal to and thereby preserve the suburothelial stroma? Alternative explanations, as shown with the long-term lineage tracing in human, are that a rare common multipotent stem cell ancestor exists beyond the resolution of present assays or that homeostatic mechanisms differ between mouse and human urothelium.

1.3 Urothelial Carcinoma Initiating Cell

Irrespective of the identity of normal urothelial stem cells(s), there is a fairly good consensus as to the origin of urothelial carcinoma, especially regarding the muscle invasive subtype. The dual track model of urothelial carcinoma, build on typical mutational spectra for both non-muscle invasive bladder cancer (NMIBC) and muscle invasive bladder cancer (MIBC) does not directly account for a possible difference in the respective cell of origin. Two independent mouse models, both combining lineage tracing and bladder-specific chemical mutagenesis, have convincingly shown that the cell of origin for MIBC is a basal cell [8, 9], whereas a conceptually very similar approach identified an intermediate cell as a probable cell of origin for non-muscle invasive papillary tumors [8]. Moreover, the notion of independent cells of origin for both urothelial carcinoma types in humans has been corroborated by a genome-wide gene expression analysis [10].

Interestingly, Sonic Hedgehog seems to play a crucial and, from a certain point of view, antithetical role in both urothelial regeneration and muscle invasive tumor initiation, respectively, in both cases involving tumor-stroma interaction. Expressed preferentially by basal cells, this signaling molecule initiates a remarkable epithelial-stromal interplay within the context of urothelial regenerative response. Acceptors of this signal are suburothelial stromal fibroblasts, the Shh signal resulting in coordinated expression of both mitogenic (Wnt 2, Wnt 4, and Fgf 16) and differentiation promoting (Bmp 4, Bmp 5) factors, which signal back to the urothelium, collectively promoting the very rapid regenerative response [11, 12]. This differentiation promoting activity of stromal fibroblasts is at the same time a break to cancer development, nevertheless, and within the context of MIBC development, the initiated basal cells switch off the Shh expression to allow for mutation-driven cell proliferation [13].

1.4 Urothelial Carcinoma Stem Cells and Their Clinical Impact

Apart from the label retention assay mentioned above, which makes use of one particular biological aspect of both normal and cancer stem cells, namely their relative quiescence, and which is only able to identify stem cells retrospectively, there are two basic approaches to prospectively isolate normal or cancer stem cells by fluorescent-activated cells sorting (FACS). The first one exploits convenient cell surface marker molecules, the second one another general biological property of stem cells, namely their self-protection. Because of the widespread consensus that MIBC has its origin in a basal urothelial cell, it comes as little surprise that specific markers of basal urothelial cells provided good candidates to purify stem-like cells from muscle invasive tumors. Successful examples of this strategy are CD44 [14] and the 67 kDa high affinity laminin receptor (67LR) [15]. Even the basal cell cytokeratins turned out to be very useful. Of course, being intracellular proteins, they are not apt as target proteins in FACS purification protocols. They could be used in two other ways, nevertheless. First, high specificity of basal cytokeratins gene promoters can be used to drive the expression of a convenient fluorescent marker protein, like destabilized green fluorescent protein (dGFP) [16]. Second, a specific algorithm has been created to correlate the expression of basal type cytokeratins with cell surface marker molecules, which lead to the discovery of additional cell surface markers, especially CD14 [17] and CD90 [18]. Another new urothelial cancer stem cell surface marker molecule is CD47, which has been identified based on a high correlation between its expression with that of CD44 [14].

There are two possibilities of using specific self-protection strategies of (cancer) stem cells to allow for their prospective isolation. The term "side population" (SP) describes cells, which protect themselves from small toxic compounds by constitutively overexpressing ABC-efflux pumps; as several small fluorophores, like Hoechst 33342 or Dye Cycle Violet belong to the substrates of the ABC efflux pumps as well, their use in staining protocols (*see* below) enables to sort out populations of dim cells corresponding to stem cells. The Aldefluor assay is based on another self-protection mechanism, namely on the constitutive expression of the detoxification enzyme aldehyde dehydrogenase ALDH1A1. It modifies a specific fluorescent dye Bodipy-aminoacetaldehyde in such a way that it becomes very hydrophilic and thus unable to leave the cell yielding a specific fluorescent signal in stem cells [1]. Both these approaches have been used for both NMIBC and MIBC samples and respective cell lines.

The $CD44^+$ cells have been analyzed as to the expression of generally accepted stem cell factors that could be responsible for their stemness [14]. This analysis revealed a significant heterogeneity; about 5% of cancer samples had activated β-catenin in their $CD44^+$ cells, 20% expressed nuclear Bmi-1, 40% activated nuclear STAT-3 and 80% GLI-1, a transcription factor downstream of SHH. How does this relate to the abrupt and widespread shutdown of the Shh expression immediately after MIBC initiation discussed above? It is possible that tumor stroma takes over the SHH expression, or even that tumor cells reexpress it at some point during tumor development [19]. Alternatively, the GLI-1 activity might become imposed by environmental carcinogens [20]. As for the activated nuclear STAT-3, its activation might directly result from a stromal influence. It has been reported that urothelial cancer stem cells (defined as $CD14^+$ cells in that case) are able to actively recruit myeloid cells and promote their differentiation into tumor-associated macrophages (TAMs), which signal back to cancer cells by multiple mechanisms including the secretion of inflammatory cytokines like Interleukin-6 [17], a known activator of STAT-3.

Interestingly, in the analysis above no $CD44^+$ urothelial carcinoma stem cell samples expressed basic stem cell factors OCT-4 and NANOG. Two other factors ranked into the basic stem cell circuitry have been rather thoroughly analyzed in context of urothelial CSCs, nevertheless, namely SOX-2 and SOX-4. The first has been found as specifically overexpressed in Aldefluor positive populations of invasive bladder cancer cell lines, and has been proposed to form, together with the aldehyde dehydrogenase itself (ALDH2 in this case, however), a simple diagnostic signature able to discriminate NMIBC from MIBC with accuracy exceeding 90% [21].

SOX-4 has been analyzed in at least two independent studies, each involving different cell lines and different patient sample collections, and the results of both studies are completely contradictory. While Aaboe et al. identified SOX-4 as a tumor suppressor gene, whose high expression imparted a more favorable prognosis [22], an exact opposite has been found by Shen et al., who associated SOX-4 expression with the acquisition of several stemness-related traits and a clear poor prognostic significance [23]. The reasons for such a flagrant discrepancy are entirely unclear. The story becomes even more complicated with the realization that SOX-4 is an upstream transcription activator of SOX-2 [24]. Finally, another member of the SOX family calls for attention, namely SOX-9. Within the context of urothelial regeneration, SOX-9 has been found to be a downstream transcription factor of the mitogen-activated protein kinase (MAPK) cascade, triggered by the autocrine epidermal growth factor (EGF) signaling [25]. This finding could be relevant for urothelial CSCs in so far as a constitutively active MAPK cascade, revealed by constitutively phosphorylated ERK2, seems to be typical for NMIBC SP-cells [26].

In addition to the SOX-2–ALDH2 bigenic profile mentioned above, at least three other complex genomewide urothelial cancer stem cell expression signatures have been published: $CD44^+$ vs. $CD44^-$ cells isolated from primary tumor (both NMIBC and MIBC) samples [14], $67LR^{high}$ vs. $67LR^{low}$ cells isolated from xenografted MIBC cell line SW780 [15], and normal urothelium derived signature based on comparing gene expression profiles of basal vs. umbrella cells [10]. From the clinical point of view, the first one could be of a special value. Not only that the $CD44^+$-specific gene expression signature was able to correctly discriminate between the majority of NMIBC and MIBC samples, but it also turned out to harbor an important prognostic value for NMIBC tumors. It is well established that a small but meaningful fraction of NMIBC cases (~15%) eventually progresses to the muscle invasive stage, with a corresponding significant drop in the overall prognosis. And exactly these cases seem to have reactivated the $CD44^+$ gene expression signature. Obviously, a timely identification of these patients would be crucial to appropriately adopt their therapy, and vice versa, the other group of NMIBC patients with inactive $CD44^+$ gene expression signature could be spared of unnecessary therapy with all its side effects and costs. As noted independently previously [4], this finding bears striking similarity to currently clinically exploited complex gene expression profiles MammaPrint® and Onco*type* DX® serving principally the same purpose in breast cancer. This aspect seems thus to be ready for translational development.

How to explain that originally NMIBC, derived probably from an intermediate cell, adopts a basal cell-derived stem cell signature? An important role in this respect could be attributed to stromal cancer elements. Indeed, it has been clearly shown that xenografted

CD44^{+}-derived [14] or 67LR^{high} SW780-derived tumors [15] adopt a strikingly similar stem—non-stem cell distribution, with stem cells occupying the outermost cell layer of the resulting tumor nodules, i.e., in direct contact with the mouse stromal cells, and differentiated tumor cells extending towards the nodule center. In addition to the tumor-associated macrophages mentioned above, carcinoma-associated fibroblasts (CAFs) seem to play a very important role as a niche-providing and stemness-promoting tumor cell population. Using a novel coculture model of carcinoma cells and CAFs established as pure cell lines from a single urothelial carcinoma, we have previously shown that the coculture markedly increased the expression of the stem cell-specific CK-17 in tumor cells [3]. Within the context of antitumor therapy this stemness-promoting role of CAFs can achieve another significance; as stem cells feature various self-protection mechanisms, stroma-promoted stemness could at the same time translate into a stroma-promoted therapeutic resistance (Fig. 1).

The notion that CSCs, due to their relative quiescence and numerous self-protection mechanisms, can survive chemotherapy and after a latency period of variable length initiate renewed tumor

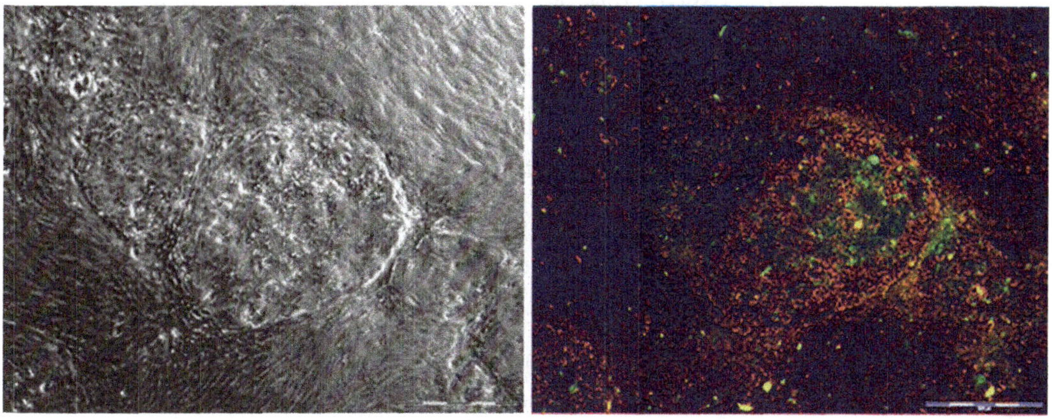

Fig. 1 Cancer-associated fibroblasts impart stemness and chemoresistance to carcinoma cells. Bladder carcinoma cell line BC44 and cell line of carcinoma-associated fibroblasts BC44Fibr, both established from the same tumor [27], were cocultured and subsequently treated with cisplatin (0.5 μg/ml) for 48 h. Mitochondrial apoptosis detection staining was carried out by the Mitochondrial apoptosis detection kit (Mitocapture™ from BioVision Incorporation, CA, USA). The kit utilizes a cationic dye that fluoresces differently in healthy vs. apoptotic cells. Disruption of mitochondrial transmembrane potential is one of the earliest events of apoptosis, preventing accumulation and aggregation of the mitocapture dye in mitochondria, resulting in solely cytoplasmic localization of monomeric mitocapture dye and *green* fluorescence. In healthy cells, mitocapture dye accumulates into mitochondria and aggregates into an oligomeric form, resulting in *bright red* fluorescence. *Left*: Phase contrast image, with a large central colony of BC44 surrounded by BC44Fibr cells. *Right*: The same colony stained with the Mitochondrial apoptosis detection kit. Apoptotic cells are concentrated towards the colony center (*green* fluorescent signal), whereas cancer cells situated at the adjunct of fibroblast cells (in peripheral region) show cisplatin resistance (*red* fluorescence-healthy cells). Cell imaging was performed by Olympus IX 81-Cell-R microscopy system. Bar = 500 μm

growth does not give the complete picture, nevertheless. Being spared of a direct chemotherapeutic attack, CSCs seem to be rapidly and transiently mobilized to enter active proliferation by mediators released from dying differentiated tumor cells. As a result, tumors might clinically behave as primary chemoresistant, as their repopulation capacity ensures that the differentiated tumor cells being killed by chemotherapy are immediately replaced by expanding and differentiating CSCs. A particular role for this CSCs mobilization could be attributed to the prostaglandin E_2 (PGE_2), and indeed, pharmacological inhibition of Cyclooxygenase 2 (COX2), which is responsible for PGE_2 synthesis), has been able to prevent this rapid CSCs mobilization and resulting tumor repopulation and restore chemosensitivity [16]—another field ready for translational development.

1.5 Methodological Approaches to Identify Urothelial Carcinoma Stem Cells

As already discussed above, cancer stem cells can be identified and isolated either by virtue of the expression of surface molecular markers (such as CD44, CD90, CD47, or 67LR) using antibody-based flow cytometry or immunomagnetic-based selections, or by marker-free approaches as side population or as Aldefluor-bright cells. In any case, a purified tentative stem cell population has to be subject to one or more bioassays to verify their stemness. Some of the basic methodologies are described in detail herein.

1.5.1 Side Population

The method for identification of side population cells was first described in 1996 by Goodell et al. [28] for murine bone marrow hemopoietic stem cells and has since been adapted for numerous tissues [29] and cancers [30]. The SP assay is based on the differential capacity of cells to efflux the fluorescent DNA binding dye Hoechst 33342 (4). Hoechst 33342 dye binds to AT-rich regions of DNA and when excited with UV laser at 350 nm its fluorescence can be detected in the "Hoechst Blue" (450 nm filter) and "Hoechst Red" (675 nm filter) channels on a flow cytometer. Simultaneous collection of the two fluorescence signals enables the observation of a tail-shaped low fluorescent population extending from the main high fluorescent bulk. This "tail" population is the SP (Fig. 2). SP cells display high levels of expression of multidrug resistance membrane pumps belonging to the superfamily of ATP-Binding Cassette (ABC) transporters, such as P-glycoprotein/ABC superfamily B member 1 (ABCB1) and breast cancer resistance protein (BCRP)/ABC superfamily G member 2 (ABCG2), which they use to actively pump out Hoechst 33342 dye. SP cells are sensitive to ABC transporter inhibitors which reverse their phenotype and are used as a control to confirm SP identification. A number of ABC transporter inhibitors with different specificities for ABC family members are available, including ABCB1 inhibitor Verapamil and ABCG2 inhibitor Fumitremorgin C, or a broad-range inhibitor Reserpine, and their use can further determine the identity of the transporter mediating SP (Fig. 3). SP has been shown to identify populations

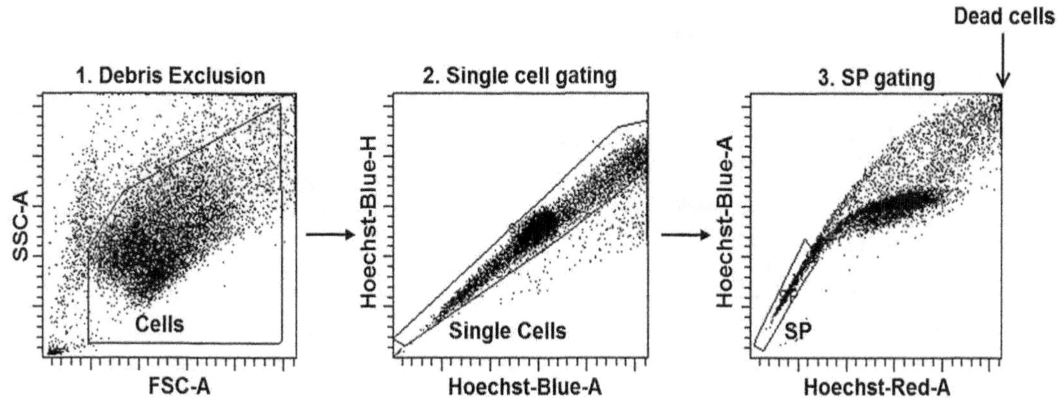

Fig. 2 Gating strategy for SP assay. An example of the step-by-step gating strategy. Cells are distinguished from debris on the flow cytometric profile based on Forward Scatter (FSC) and Side Scatter (SSC) (*1*). Hoechst 33342 dye is excited with UV laser at 350 nm and its fluorescence is measured through the "*Hoechst Blue*" and "*Hoechst Red*" channels. Doublets and aggregates are gated out based on *Hoechst Blue* area versus height to ensure that a detected signal arises from single cells (*2*). SP cells are recognized as a distinct tail extending from the main population with the characteristic low fluorescent profile based on *Hoechst Red* versus *Hoechst Blue* area. PI, having been excited at 350 nm, is also measured through the "*Hoechst Red*" channel but is much brighter than the *Hoechst red* signal so the dead cells line up on a vertical line to the far right (*3*)

enriched for stem cell markers and endowed with long-term repopulating capacity. Malignant SP cells have been shown to display higher clonogenic and tumorigenic potential as well as higher resistance to chemotherapy than non-SP cells [31–33].

1.5.2 Biological Assays to Verify Stemness of Purified Putative Cancer Stem Cells

Irrespective of whether purified on the basis of a specific marker expression, or as SP or Aldefluor-positive cells, stemness of the purified cell population must be verified by a series of widely acceptable biological assays. The two most extensively used bioassay types for cancer stem cells are in-vitro-clonogenicity and in-vivo-tumorigenicity assays.

The clonogenic ability can be defined as an ability to initiate productive growth of a cell colony out of a single sorted cell in vitro. There are several versions of clonogenic assay. The most simple one is based on the mere ability of self-renewing cells to found a colony in a standard two-dimensional cell culture; in low-grade cancer samples or cell lines established from low-grade tumors, which keep epithelial character, the stemness of the colony founding cell can be in addition deduced from a specific colony morphology of small densely packed cells (holoclones), whereas differentiated cells are either devoid of any clonogenic activity, or they only form small colonies of enlarged and loosely packed cells (paraclones or meroclones) [34]. Three-dimensional clonogenic assays are usually carried out either as anchorage-independent clonogenic assays in semisolid media (agar, agarose, methylcellulose) [35], or a specific sphere assay is applied. The latter consists in culturing cells on ultra-low-attachment plastic in serum-free specifically supplemented media, most

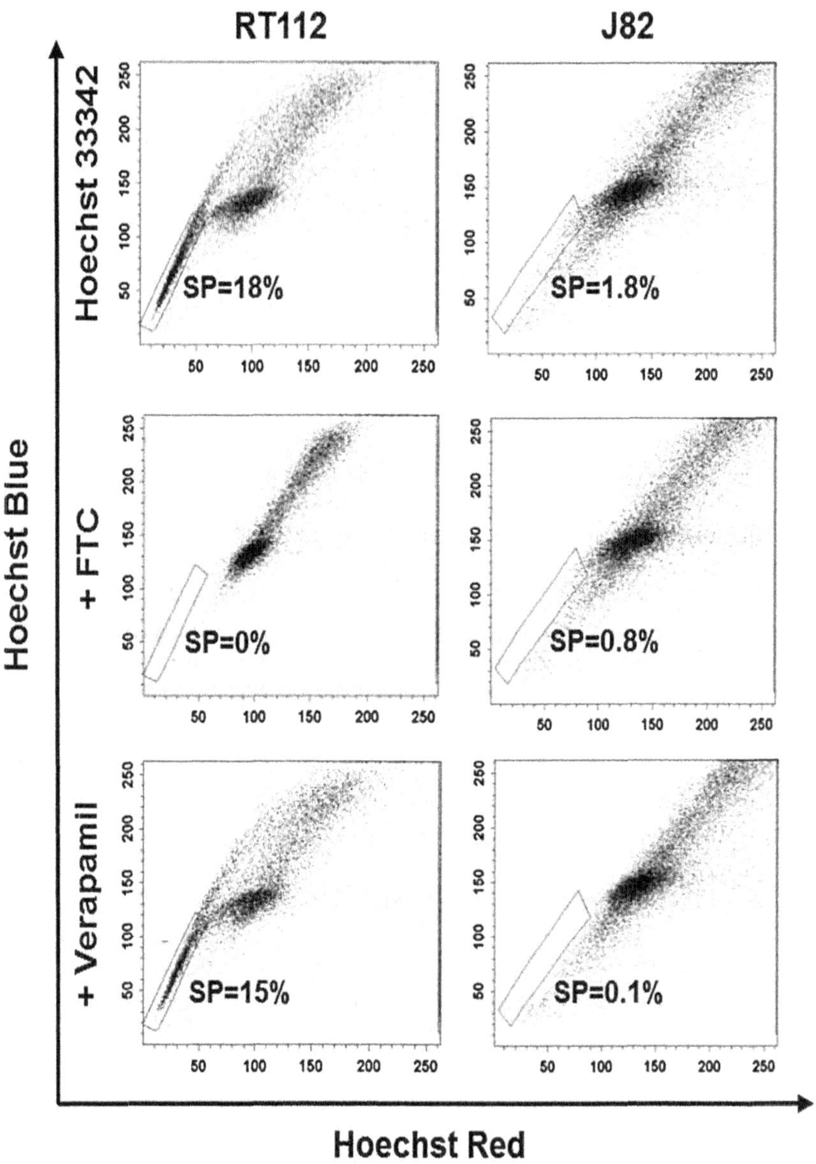

Fig. 3 SP profiles of bladder cancer cells. RT112 and J82 cells were stained with Hoechst 33342 dye alone or in the presence of ABC transporter inhibitors fumitremorgin C (FTC) and verapamil and analyzed by flow cytometry. Use of different pharmacological inhibitors of ABC-efflux pumps makes it possible to distinguish different molecular mechanisms of SP, with ABCG2 and ABCB1 being primary responsible for RT112 and J82 SP cells, respectively

often with EGF (20 ng/ml), FGF (20 ng/ml) and the specific supplement B27 (2%) [23]. Well established e.g., in brain, breast or colon cancer stem cell characterization (called accordingly neurospheres, mammospheres, or colonospheres, respectively), this sphere-forming assay has not been extensively used for urothelial stem cell characterization yet, nevertheless.

The tumorigenicity tests for the ability of sorted cell population to initiate tumor growth upon transplantation into a suitable animal host, and the quantitative threshold (i.e., the minimal amount of cells transplanted) necessary. For animal tumors and their cancer stem cells, the recipient animals have to be of the same species and the same histocompatibility genotype. The only suitable animal recipients for assessing cancer-initiating properties of human cancer stem cells are various immunodeficient mouse strains (*see* below). Also, tumorigenicity can be tested either xenotopically, most often subcutaneously, or orthotopically, i.e., by injecting cells into the bladder wall. If cell lines are used as the source of stem cells, they might be genetically manipulated to express luciferase and the tumor growth can be monitored in real time by whole-body bioluminescence imaging [21]. Finally, sorted cell populations can be transplanted either alone in a suitable liquid medium, or various supportive substances (collagen, Matrigel) or cells (fibroblasts) are cotransplanted to assess their stemness-promoting and niche-providing activity [36].

2 Materials

2.1 Hoechst 33342 Staining

1. Culture medium (*see* **Note 1**) warmed to 37 °C.
2. Hoechst 33342 powder is dissolved in distilled water at 1 mg/ml concentration and filter sterilized. Aliquots are frozen at −20 °C.
3. Verapamil is dissolved in ethanol at 5 mM. Aliquots are frozen at −20 °C.
4. Reserpine is dissolved in DMSO at 5 mM. Aliquots are frozen at −20 °C.
5. Fumitremorgin C is dissolved in DMSO at 10 mM. Aliquots are frozen at −20 °C.
6. 15 ml conical bottom polypropylene tubes.
7. Phosphate buffered saline (PBS).
8. Refrigerated centrifuge.
9. Circulating water bath at 37 °C.
10. 5 ml polypropylene round bottom tubes.
11. 40 μm cell strainers.
12. Propidium iodide dissolved at 2.5 mg/ml in distilled water, covered with aluminum foil and stored at 4 °C.
13. Flow cytometer with UV laser capable of excitation at 350 nm and detection with 450/50 and 675lp optical filters.

2.2 Clonogenic Ability Evaluated by 2D-Colony Forming Assay

1. FACS sorted cells.
2. Culture medium.
3. 6-well cell culture plate.
4. Carnoy's fixative; methanol: acetic acid, 3:1.
5. Crystal violet dissolved in distilled water at 0.4%.

2.3 Clonogenic Ability Evaluated by 3D-Colony Forming Assay in Semisolid Media

1. FACS sorted cells
2. Culture medium
3. 6-well cell culture plate, Ultra Low Attachment Surface (e.g., cat. No. 3471, Corning)
4. Methylcellulose

2.4 In Vivo Tumorigenicity Assay

1. Mice (*see* **Note 2**)
2. FACS sorted cells
3. Culture medium
4. Matrigel (e.g., cat. No. 356234, BD Biosciences)
5. Insulin syringes

3 Methods

3.1 Hoechst 33342 Staining

Hoechst 33342 staining protocol for bladder cancer cells follows [26].

1. Add ABC transporter inhibitor (reserpine 50 μM, verapamil 50 μM or fumitremorgin C 10 μM) to cell suspension (10^6 cells/ml) resuspended in pre-warmed (37 °C) culture medium in 15 ml conical bottom polypropylene tube for 15 min.
2. Add Hoechst 33342 to cell suspension to a final concentration 2.5 μg/ml.
3. Incubate sample for 90 min at 37 °C in a circulating water bath and mix every 30 min (*see* **Note 3**).
4. Following staining always keep sample at 4 °C to prevent Hoechst 33342 cell expulsion.
5. Antibody co-staining should be performed following Hoechst 33342 staining at concentrations recommended by the manufacturer or by titration at 4 °C.
6. Spin down cells in a refrigerated centrifuge for 5 min at 400 × *g* and resuspend in 1 ml iced PBS buffer.
7. Pour through cell strainer into 5 ml polypropylene round bottom tube.
8. When sample is ready for fluorescence activated cell sorting (FACS) add 2 μg/ml propidium iodide (PI) to exclude dead cells.

3.2 Clonogenic Ability Evaluated by 2D-Colony Forming Assay

1. Seed FACS sorted cells in appropriate dilutions (depending on rate of growth of cells) to form colonies in 2 weeks. Seed FACS sorted cells into six-well cell culture plates at a density of 100 cells/well.
2. Fix colonies with 1 ml Carnoy's fixative for 1 min.
3. Stain colonies with 1 ml 0.4% crystal violet (w/v) for 5 min.
4. Count colonies (omitting colonies with <64 cells as they represent early abortive colonies).
5. Colony forming efficiency (CFE, %) is calculated as [(no. colonies counted/no. cells seeded) × 100].

3.3 Clonogenic Ability Evaluated by 3D-Colony Forming Assay in Semisolid Media

1. Prepare cell suspensions of equal numbers (5×10^3–80×10^4 cells, depending on the clonogenic potential of the sample) of FACS-sorted cells to be tested (e.g., SP and non-SP cells) in 500 μl of complete media in a 15 ml tube
2. Pour 12 ml of methylcellulose solution (*see* **Note 4**) (1.5% in complete medium) into the tube.
3. Make cell suspension in the methylcellulose medium by carefully pipetting up and down (the solution will be viscous, 20–30 pipetting steps might be required). Plate 4 ml of the resulting cell suspension into a well of the Ultra-Low- Attachment 6-well plate; due to the viscosity, the actual amount of the suspension would be ~3 ml.
4. Overlay the methylcellulose layer with 0.5 ml of complete growth medium.
5. Culture the cells for 3–5 weeks, with replenishment of the upper medium layer once or twice a week to avoid drying of the cultures.
6. Count colonies under an inverted microscope

3.4 In Vivo Tumorigenicity Assay

1. Anesthetize mouse (one animal at a time) according to the local institutional animal care rules.
2. Inject 1000 FACS sorted cells mixed in 100 μl of their regular culture medium and 100 μl of Matrigel subcutaneously into the flank area.
3. Tumor growth is monitored by two dimensional measurement with electronic calipers.
4. Tumor volume is calculated using the formula $a/2 \times b/2$, where a is the smallest measurement and b the largest.
5. Terminate experiment when tumor grows to a maximum of 750 mm^3 or volume agreed in animal license.

4 Notes

1. For established urothelial carcinoma cell lines, the most frequently used culture media are the Dulbecco's Modified Eagle Medium (DMEM) and Roswell Park Memorial Institute (RPMI) 1640 Medium, both available from a number of suppliers. Specific culture media might be used for primary cancer cell cultures [37].
2. For human cancer stem cells, various immunodeficient strains (nude mouse, SCID, NOD/SCID, Rag2 −/− γc −/− or NOD/SCID γc −/−, so-called NSG mouse) have to be used, with increasing immunodeficiency directly proportional to the increasing demands on the respective animal facility. Nude mice carry a specific defect in T cell development due to a mutational disruption of the FOXN1 gene, SCID (severe combined immunodeficiency) show a practically complete absence of the adaptive immune system due to their inability to carry out the V(D)J recombination as a consequence of a mutational disruption of the gene encoding the catalytic subunit of DNA-activated protein kinase, and the same is basically true for Rag2 −/− mice. The γc −/− mice carry a gene knockout in the gene encoding a common subunit of receptors for IL-2, IL-4, IL-7, IL-9, IL-15 and IL-21 and feature another form of severe combined immunodeficiency characterized by T-, B-, an well as NK-cell deficiency [38]. NOD (nonobese diabetic) represents, on the contrary, a specific autoimmune mouse strain with polygenic etiology.
3. SP depends on Hoechst concentration, incubation time, and temperature stability. These conditions can dramatically vary with cell type. A preliminary experiment to optimize these conditions is critical for the success of this method and isolation of a pure SP.
4. As a semisolid medium, agar, agarose or methylcellulose can be used as equivalent possibilities giving the same message. From the practical point of view, the methylcellulose is probably the most easy to handle, except the solubilization, which should be made at 4 °C for 1 week upon continuous stirring.

Acknowledgments

The work has been supported by the projects of Faculty of Medicine in Pilsen SVV-2016-260283 and SVV-2017-260393, and by JGW Patterson Foundation.

References

1. Hatina J, Fernandes MI, Hoffmann M, Zeimet AG (2013) Cancer stem cells – basic biological properties and experimental approaches. In: Encyclopedia of Life Sciences. John Wiley & Sons, Chichester. doi:10.1002/9780470015902.a0021164.pub2
2. Kreso A, Dick JE (2014) Evolution of the cancer stem cell model. Cell Stem Cell 14:275–291
3. Hatina J, Schulz WA (2012) Stem cells in the biology of normal urothelium and urothelial carcinoma. Neoplasma 59:728–736
4. Ho PL, Kurtova A, Chan KS (2012) Normal and neoplastic urothelial stem cells: getting to the root of the problem. Nat Rev Urol 9:583–594
5. Kurzrock EA, Lieu DK, Degraffenried LA, Chan CW, Isseroff RR (2008) Label-retaining cells of the bladder: candidate urothelial stem cells. Am J Physiol Renal Physiol 294: F1415–F1421
6. Yamany T, Van Batavia J, Mendelsohn C (2014) Formation and regeneration of the urothelium. Curr Opin Organ Transplant 19:323–330
7. Gaisa NT, Graham TA, McDonald SA, Cañadillas-Lopez S, Poulsom R, Heidenreich A, Jakse G, Tadrous PJ, Knuechel R, Wright NA (2011) The human urothelium consists of multiple clonal units, each maintained by a stem cell. J Pathol 225:163–171
8. Shin K, Lim A, Odegaard JI, Honeycutt JD, Kawano S, Hsieh MH, Beachy PA (2014) Cellular origin of bladder neoplasia and tissue dynamics of its progression to invasive carcinoma. Nat Cell Biol 16:469–478
9. Van Batavia J, Yamany T, Molotkov A, Dan H, Mansukhani M, Batourina E, Schneider K, Oyon D, Dunlop M, Wu XR, Cordon-Cardo C, Mendelsohn C (2014) Bladder cancers arise from distinct urothelial sub-populations. Nat Cell Biol 16:982–991
10. Dancik GM, Owens CR, Iczkowski KA, Theodorescu D (2014) A cell of origin gene signature indicates human bladder cancer has distinct cellular progenitors. Stem Cells 32:974–982
11. Mysorekar IU, Isaacson-Schmid M, Walker JN, Mills JC, Hultgren SJ (2009) Bone morphogenetic protein 4 signaling regulates epithelial renewal in the urinary tract in response to uropathogenic infection. Cell Host Microbe 5:463–475
12. Shin K, Lee J, Guo N, Kim J, Lim A, Qu L, Mysorekar IU, Beachy PA (2011) Hedgehog/Wnt feedback supports regenerative proliferation of epithelial stem cells in bladder. Nature 472:110–114
13. Shin K, Lim A, Zhao C, Sahoo D, Pan Y, Spiekerkoetter E, Liao JC, Beachy PA (2014) Hedgehog signaling restrains bladder cancer progression by eliciting stromal production of urothelial differentiation factors. Cancer Cell 26:521–533
14. Chan KS, Espinosa I, Chao M, Wong D, Ailles L, Diehn M, Gill H, Presti J Jr, Chang HY, van de Rijn M, Shortliffe L, Weissman IL (2009) Identification, molecular characterization, clinical prognosis, and therapeutic targeting of human bladder tumor-initiating cells. Proc Natl Acad Sci U S A 106:14016–14021
15. He X, Marchionni L, Hansel DE, Yu W, Sood A, Yang J, Parmigiani G, Matsui W, Berman DM (2009) Differentiation of a highly tumorigenic basal cell compartment in urothelial carcinoma. Stem Cells 27:1487–1495
16. Kurtova AV, Xiao J, Mo Q, Pazhanisamy S, Krasnow R, Lerner SP, Chen F, Roh TT, Lay E, Ho PL, Chan KS (2015) Blocking PGE2-induced tumour repopulation abrogates bladder cancer chemoresistance. Nature 517:209–213
17. Cheah MT, Chen JY, Sahoo D, Contreras-Trujillo H, Volkmer AK, Scheeren FA, Volkmer JP, Weissman IL (2015) CD14-expressing cancer cells establish the inflammatory and proliferative tumor microenvironment in bladder cancer. Proc Natl Acad Sci U S A 112:4725–4730
18. Volkmer JP, Sahoo D, Chin RK, Ho PL, Tang C, Kurtova AV, Willingham SB, Pazhanisamy SK, Contreras-Trujillo H, Storm TA, Lotan Y, Beck AH, Chung BI, Alizadeh AA, Godoy G, Lerner SP, van de Rijn M, Shortliffe LD, Weissman IL, Chan KS (2012) Three differentiation states risk-stratify bladder cancer into distinct subtypes. Proc Natl Acad Sci U S A 109:2078–2083
19. Fei DL, Sanchez-Mejias A, Wang Z, Flaveny C, Long J, Singh S, Rodriguez-Blanco J, Tokhunts R, Giambelli C, Briegel KJ, Schulz WA, Gandolfi AJ, Karagas M, Zimmers TA, Jorda M, Bejarano P, Capobianco AJ, Robbins DJ (2012) Hedgehog signaling regulates bladder cancer growth and tumorigenicity. Cancer Res 72:4449–4458
20. Fei DL, Li H, Kozul CD, Black KE, Singh S, Gosse JA, DiRenzo J, Martin KA, Wang B, Hamilton JW, Karagas MR, Robbins DJ (2010) Activation of Hedgehog signaling by the environmental toxicant arsenic may

contribute to the etiology of arsenic-induced tumors. Cancer Res 70:1981–1988

21. Ferreira-Teixeira M, Parada B, Rodrigues-Santos P, Alves V, Ramalho JS, Caramelo F, Sousa V, Reis F, Gomes CM (2015) Functional and molecular characterization of cancer stem-like cells in bladder cancer: a potential signature for muscle-invasive tumors. Oncotarget 6:36185–36201
22. Aaboe M, Birkenkamp-Demtroder K, Wiuf C, Sørensen FB, Thykjaer T, Sauter G, Jensen KM, Dyrskjøt L, Ørntoft T (2006) SOX4 expression in bladder carcinoma: clinical aspects and in vitro functional characterization. Cancer Res 66:3434–3442
23. Shen H, Blijlevens M, Yang N, Frangou C, Wilson KE, Xu B, Zhang Y, Zhang L, Morrison CD, Shepherd L, Hu Q, Zhu Q, Wang J, Liu S, Zhang J (2015) Sox4 expression confers bladder cancer stem cell properties and predicts for poor patient outcome. Int J Biol Sci 11:1363–1375
24. Ikushima H, Todo T, Ino Y, Takahashi M, Saito N, Miyazawa K, Miyazono K (2011) Glioma-initiating cells retain their tumorigenicity through integration of the sox axis and Oct4 protein. J Biol Chem 286:41434–41441
25. Ling S, Chang X, Schultz L, Lee TK, Chaux A, Marchionni L, Netto GJ, Sidransky D, Berman DM (2011) An EGFR-ERK-SOX9 signaling cascade links urothelial development and regeneration to cancer. Cancer Res 71:3812–3821
26. Hepburn AC, Veeratterapillay R, Williamson SC, El-Sherif A, Sahay N, Thomas HD, Mantilla A, Pickard RS, Robson CN, Heer R (2012) Side population in human non-muscle invasive bladder cancer enriches for cancer stem cells that are maintained by MAPK signalling. PLoS One 7:e50690
27. Koch A, Hatina J, Rieder H, Seifert HH, Huckenbeck W, Jankowiak F, Florl AR, Stoehr R, Schulz WA (2012) Discovery of TP53 splice variants in two novel papillary urothelial cancer cell lines. Cell Oncol (Dordr) 35:243–257
28. Goodell MA, Brose K, Paradis G, Conner AS, Mulligan RC (1996) Isolation and functional properties of murine hematopoietic stem cells that are replicating in vivo. J Exp Med 183:1797–1806
29. Martin CM, Meeson AP, Robertson SM, Hawke TJ, Richardson JA, Bates S, Goetsch SC, Gallardo TD, Garry DJ (2004) Persistent expression of the ATP-binding cassette transporter, Abcg2, identifies cardiac SP cells in the developing and adult heart. Dev Biol 265:262–275
30. Ho MM, Ng AV, Lam S, Hung JY (2007) Side population in human lung cancer cell lines and tumors is enriched with stem-like cancer cells. Cancer Res 67:4827–4833
31. Golebiewska A, Brons NH, Bjerkvig R, Niclou SP (2011) Critical appraisal of the side population assay in stem cell and cancer stem cell research. Cell Stem Cell 8:136–147
32. Patrawala L, Calhoun T, Schneider-Broussard R, Zhou J, Claypool K, Tang DG (2005) Side population is enriched in tumorigenic, stem-like cancer cells, whereas ABCG2+ and ABCG2- cancer cells are similarly tumorigenic. Cancer Res 65:6207–6219
33. Hirschmann-Jax C, Foster AE, Wulf GG, Nuchtern JG, Jax TW, Gobel U, Goodell MA, Brenner MK (2004) A distinct "side population" of cells with high drug efflux capacity in human tumor cells. Proc Natl Acad Sci U S A 101:14228–14233
34. Locke M, Heywood M, Fawell S, Mackenzie IC (2005) Retention of intrinsic stem cell hierarchies in carcinoma-derived cell lines. Cancer Res 65:8944–8950
35. Mori S, Chang JT, Andrechek ER, Matsumura N, Baba T, Yao G, Kim JW, Gatza M, Murphy S, Nevins JR (2009) Anchorage-independent cell growth signature identifies tumors with metastatic potential. Oncogene 28:2796–2805
36. Albini A, Bruno A, Gallo C, Pajardi G, Noonan DM, Dallaglio K (2015) Cancer stem cells and the tumor microenvironment: interplay in tumor heterogeneity. Connect Tissue Res 56:414–425
37. Seifert HH, Meyer A, Cronauer MV, Hatina J, Müller M, Rieder H, Hoffmann MJ, Ackermann R, Schulz WA (2007) A new and reliable culture system for superficial low-grade urothelial carcinoma of the bladder. World J Urol 25:297–302
38. Waickman AT, Park JY, Park JH (2016) The common γ-chain cytokine receptor: tricks-and-treats for T cells. Cell Mol Life Sci 73:253–269

Chapter 11

In Vitro Differentiation and Propagation of Urothelium from Pluripotent Stem Cell Lines

Stephanie L. Osborn and Eric A. Kurzrock

Abstract

Bioengineering of bladder tissue, particularly for those patients who have advanced bladder disease, requires a source of urothelium that is healthy, capable of significant proliferation in vitro and immunologically tolerated upon transplant. As pluripotent stem cells have the potential to fulfill such criteria, they provide a critical cell source from which urothelium might be derived in vitro and used clinically. Herein, we describe the in vitro differentiation of urothelium from the H9 human embryonic stem cell (hESC) line through the definitive endoderm (DE) phase via selective culture techniques. The protocol can be used to derive urothelium from other hESCs or human-induced pluripotent stem cells.

Key words Induced pluripotent stem cells, Human embryonic stem cells, Urothelium, Bladder bioengineering, Definitive endoderm, Activin A, Uroplakins

1 Introduction

Patients with urinary bladder disease, such as bladder cancer, neuropathic bladder disorders, or trauma, often require bladder reconstruction or augmentation. The current standard for cystoplasty utilizes gastrointestinal tissue for reconstruction. Gastrointestinal tissue has inherent absorptive and secretary properties that lead to recurrent urinary infection, stone formation, and electrolyte imbalance when juxtaposed with bladder tissue. Long-term marriage of these tissues also brings about an increased incidence of adenocarcinomas [1–3].

The bladder is a luminal organ that works by deeply coordinated efforts among the muscles, nerves, vasculature, and epithelial lining to contract and expand for proper voiding. Although the concept of bioengineering bladder tissue has been at the forefront of urologic research for the last decade, the complexity of bladder function poses significant challenges to engineering functional tissue for use in reconstruction. Considerations for scaffold type and cell source are integral to ensure that the engineered tissue best

Wolfgang A. Schulz et al. (eds.), *Urothelial Carcinoma: Methods and Protocols*, Methods in Molecular Biology, vol. 1655, DOI 10.1007/978-1-4939-7234-0_11, © Springer Science+Business Media LLC 2018

mirrors the function of the native organ, as well as to provide a safer and more efficacious alternative to current clinical practices.

Cell sources for regenerating the bladder epithelium, or urothelium, are particularly important to consider. The urothelium expresses specialized proteins called uroplakins that organize into plaques at the luminal surface [4–6]. These plaques create an impenetrable barrier, which functions in concert with muscle contractions to store and void urine, all while preventing toxins and pathogens from reentering the blood stream. Thus, proper and safe function of an engineered bladder hinges on the urothelium. Autologous cells are ideal for use in bioengineering since transplant of these cells would minimize harmful immune responses and graft rejection. However, most patients needing reconstruction are those with advanced bladder disease or bladder cancer, where the use of autologous urothelium would not be prudent. Furthermore, the urothelium from many patients with benign bladder disease is weakly proliferative in vitro and may not be functional when transplanted [7]. Thus, patients with bladder disease would greatly benefit from a healthy and robust non-urologic, non-autologous source of urothelium for the creation of a neobladder [8]. Human pluripotent stem cells are able to renew and proliferate indefinitely and differentiate into any cell type and therefore have become attractive candidates for cell therapy and bioengineering applications.

The protocol herein describes the directed differentiation of urothelium from H9 hESCs through the definitive endoderm (DE) step, which is an important milestone in the development of the bladder epithelium in vivo [9]. The protocol can also be used to derive urothelium from other hESCs or human-induced pluripotent stem cells [10]. Recapitulation of the developmental process in vitro efficiently induces urothelium that may serve as a future source of urothelial cells for bioengineering of bladder tissue for patients needing cystoplasty.

2 Materials

All cell culture should be performed within a biosafety cabinet using sterile technique and cell culture-specific or sterile-filtered media, buffers, compounds, and tissue culture-treated plastic ware. All the cells are cultured in humidified incubators at 37 °C with 5% CO_2. All media should be stored at 4 °C and pre-warmed to 37 °C prior to use, unless otherwise indicated.

2.1 H9 hESC Culture

1. H9 hESC line (WA09; WiCell).
2. Irradiated mouse embryonic fibroblasts (GlobalStem, Inc.).

3. H9 medium; 80% Dulbecco's Modified Eagles Medium (DMEM)/F12 Nutrient Mix, 20% KnockOut Serum Replacement (ThermoFisher Scientific), 4 ng/mL basic fibroblast growth factor (bFGF), 1 mM GlutaMAX, 0.1 mM β-mercaptoethanol, 1% nonessential amino acids.
4. 6-well tissue culture plates.

2.2 Induction of DE

1. RPMI medium; RPMI 1640 supplemented with 1 mM GlutaMAX, penicilin/streptomycin, and FBS at varying concentrations (0%, 0.2%, or 2%, as indicated in the Methods section).
2. Activin A (human, recombinant) reconstituted as per the manufacturer's recommendation, and added to cultures, when indicated, for a final concentration of 100 ng/mL.

2.3 Induction, Propagation, and Cryopreservation of Urothelium

1. RPMI-based Uromedium (R-Uromedium); RPMI 1640 supplemented with Clonetics Singlequots™ consisting of 60 μg/mL bovine pituitary extract, 0.1 ng/mL human EGF, 5 μg/mL insulin, 0.5 μg/mL hydrocortisone, 30 μg/mL gentamycin, and 15 ng/mL amphotericin (Lonza), 30 ng/mL cholera toxin A and 2% FBS.
2. KBM-based Uromedium (K-Uromedium): same supplementation as for RPMI-based Uromedium, but use KBM (Lonza) as basal medium.
3. (*Optional*) Retinoic Acid, reconstituted as per the manufacturer's instructions (*see* **Note 1**).
4. (*Optional*) Cloning cylinders.
5. Dispase II (Life Technologies) at 0.5% (wt/vol) in PBS without Ca^{2+} or Mg^{2+}.
6. Cell lifters.
7. Cryopreservation medium: K-Uromedium with 10% FBS and 10% DMSO.
8. Cryovials.
9. Controlled-rate freezing container (i.e., Mr. Frosty™).

3 Methods

A schematic of the entire urothelial induction process is depicted in Fig. 1a, including time and culture medium.

3.1 Maintenance of the H9 Human ESC Line (See Note 2) [11]

1. Plate irradiated mouse embryonic fibroblasts (MEF), as per manufacturer's instructions, into 6-well plates.
2. On the next day, plate H9 ESCs onto MEF feeder layer in H9 medium.

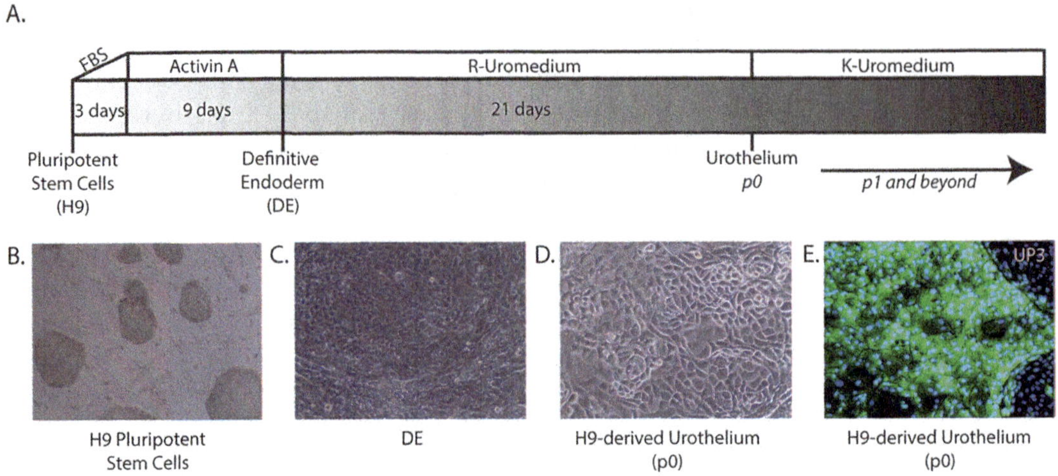

Fig. 1 The differentiation of urothelium from H9 ESCs. (**a**) Schematic of the induction protocol from ESCs to DE to urothelium, depicting culture time for each phase as well as induction media. (**b–d**) Phase contrast images of H9 ESCs, DE, and induced urothelium, respectively; 10× magnification. (**e**) Immunocytochemistry staining of an induced urothelial colony at p0 (day 21) for UP3 (*green*) and DAPI (*blue*) as the counterstain; 10× magnification

3. Incubate H9 ESCs on MEF feeders at 37 °C in 5% CO_2 and perform medium changes every day.
4. Passage H9 at a 1:4 split ratio approximately every 5–7 days using the manual passage technique, as detailed by Loring et al. [11] (*see* **Note 3**).
5. H9 ESCs will grow as tightly packed colonies on the top of the MEF feeder layer (Fig. 1b).

3.2 Induction of Pluripotent Stem Cells to Definitive Endoderm (DE) [12]

1. Prior to initiating differentiation of H9 to DE, gently wash H9 cells with PBS (with Ca^{2+} and Mg^{2+}).
2. Replace the H9 medium with RPMI medium containing 0% FBS and culture for 24 h.
3. Replace the medium with RPMI supplemented with 0.2% FBS and culture for another 24 h.
4. Replace the medium with RPMI supplemented with 2% FBS and use for all subsequent days of differentiation.
5. After 24 h in RPMI supplemented with 2% FBS, add 100 ng/mL recombinant human Activin A to the cultures. Maintain cultures in Activin A-supplemented medium for 9 days to induce differentiation to DE (*see* **Note 4** and Fig. 1c). During this culture period, replace the medium every 2 days.
6. If desired, test for the efficiency of DE induction using immunocytochemistry or intracellular flow cytometry (*see* **Note 5** and Subheading 3.5).

Table 1
Antibodies for determining efficiency of DE and urothelial induction via intracellular flow cytometry (FC) and immunocytochemistry (ICC)

Application	Antibody	Source	Dilution* (FC, ICC)
FC	Sox17 Alexa Fluor 488 conjugate	R&D Systems, mouse IgG1	1:20
FC	FoxA2	BD Biosciences, mouse IgG1	1:50
FC, ICC	UP1a	Abcam, rabbit	1:100, 1:1000
FC, ICC	UP1b	Abcam, rabbit	1:100, 1:1000
FC, ICC	UP2	Santa Cruz, goat (N-18)	1:20, 1:50
ICC	UP2	Abcam, rabbit	1:1000
FC	UP3	Santa Cruz, goat (M-20)	1:20
ICC	UP3	Abcam, rabbit	1:1000

*Dilutions for FC are based on the staining of 10^6 cells in 100 μL volume.

3.3 Differentiation and Propagation of Urothelium from DE

1. At the end of the 12 days of DE induction, replace the RPMI medium with R-Uromedium; change to R-Uromedium denotes day 0 and passage 0 (p0) of the urothelial induction phase (*see* **Note 6**).
2. (*Optional*) Add RA to the R-Uromedium at a final concentration of 10 μM (*see* **Note 1**).
3. Change the medium every 2–3 days.
4. Note the multilayered, cobblestone morphology of the induced urothelial colonies via phase contrast microscopy (Fig. 1d).
5. Urothelial fate specification can be assessed at various times during the differentiation process. Note the expression of uroplakin 3 (UP3) in colonies at day 21 by immunocytochemistry (Fig. 1e) (*see* Subheading 3.5 and Table 1).
6. At day 21 of urothelial induction, release cells from adherence using 0.5% Dispase II solution. Incubate cells at 37 °C in Dispase II for approximately 5 min. Add twofold volume of R-Uromedium to inactivate the Dispase and gently lift the cells from the plate using a cell lifter (*see* **Notes 7** and **8**).
7. Centrifuge the cell suspension for 5 min at 160 × *g*.
8. Resuspend cells in KBM-based Uromedium (K-Uromedium) and replate the cells at a split ratio of approximately 1:4. Mark the passage as p1 (*see* **Note 9**).
9. Return the cells to culture and passage the cells when they reach approximately 80% confluence (*see* **Note 10**).

3.4 Cryopreservation of Induced Urothelial Cells

1. Release cells to be cryopreserved from adherence as in Subheading 3.3.
2. After centrifugation, gently resuspend cells to a concentration of 1×10^6 cells/mL in cold cryopreservation medium.
3. Aliquot into cryovials, cap and freeze at −80 °C using a controlled-rate freezing container.
4. Store long term in a liquid nitrogen cryogenic freezer.

3.5 Quantifying the Yield of Induced DE and Urothelium in Culture

We have successfully used both quantitative immunocytochemistry and intracellular flow cytometry to quantify the amount of DE and urothelium derived from the induction protocol (*see* **Note 11**) [10]. Table 1 lists information for antibodies we have successfully used for these purposes.

4 Notes

1. While retinoic acid (RA) is a primary vitamin A derivative that is important for specification of endodermal lineages, including urothelium, we did not find exogenous RA to increase the yield of urothelium in the presence of serum (FBS). However, the addition of RA has been shown to be necessary in serum-free induction conditions [13]. Moreover, researchers may consider adding RA if the yield of urothelium is sub-par, as the concentration of RA (and other factors) in FBS varies greatly among suppliers and lots.
2. Detailed information on maintaining and passaging human ESCs can be found in *Human Stem Cell Manual: A Laboratory Guide* [11].
3. Because hESCs do not fare well upon dissociation to single cells, the manual dissection method is the preferred method for passage (versus enzymatic methods) as it allows pieces of colonies containing only a few hundred cells to be lifted from the plate. Briefly, colonies are cut and released from the plate by cross-hatching with a sterile pipet tip or needle. The colony pieces are washed from the plate, gently resuspended as a uniform solution of cell clumps (not a single cell suspension), and replated at the suggested split ratio.
4. Induction of DE is 12 days in total. The first 3 days are three 24-hour periods of increasing FBS concentrations, followed by 9 more days at the highest FBS concentration (2%). More detailed information on DE induction from hESCs can be found in the original publication by d'Amour et al. [12].
5. We routinely check the efficiency of DE induction by intracellular flow cytometry for DE markers, Sox17, and/or FoxA2 (Table 1) [10].

6. For the initial induction of DE to urothelium, we sought to minimize the stress on the DE culture. To do so, we kept RPMI as the basal medium and supplemented it with the components necessary for urothelial cell specification.
7. Our method for increasing the urothelial cell purity of the mixed culture upon passage involves transfer to a urothelial selective medium; this method routinely gave us greater than 80% purity over multiple passages. Alternatively, cobblestone, multi-layered colonies can be individually cloned, if preferred. Colonies can be morphologically identified by microscopy, marked with an objective marker and isolated with a cloning cylinder. After Dispase treatment, the individual colony within the cylinder can be gently scraped with a pipet tip, collected, centrifuged, and returned to culture as described.
8. Cells can also be released from adherence using TrypLE (Life Technologies) or Trypsin-EDTA. We prefer the use of either Dispase or TrypLE, as these solutions are less harsh on the proteins of the urothelial cell surfaces. Urothelial cells are strongly adherent cells and release best when lifted manually after a gentle and brief enzymatic treatment. In the absence of manual release, the prolonged enzymatic treatment that would be necessary to detach urothelial cells may negatively alter the expression of the ever so important uroplakin proteins on the cell surface.
9. Upon the initial passage of induced urothelium, the medium should be switched from R-Uromedium to K-Uromedium. K-Uromedium is more specifically tailored to epithelial cell culturing and is the traditional medium for growing urothelium in vitro, thus favoring and enriching for urothelial growth.
10. We have successfully cultured the induced urothelium out to passage 4 with greater than 80% purity. The urothelium continues to grow as a cobblestone monolayer, just as it did at p0 (Fig. 1d).
11. There are four subtypes of uroplakins, which assemble within intracellular vesicles and heterodimerize (UP1a/UP2, UP1b/UP3) to form the cell surface plaques that create the impenetrable urothelial lining of the bladder [5]. The expression pattern of the uroplakin subtypes also indicates the level of differentiation of the urothelial cells. Cultured urothelial cells typically take on a more undifferentiated phenotype [14], thus assessing yield is best done with UP1a or UP1b. Furthermore, uroplakins are found within intracellular vesicles, particularly prior to terminal differentiation, so it is prudent to assess the yield of urothelium by a method that accounts for both extracellular and intracellular uroplakin expression.

References

1. Kurzrock EA, Baskin LS, Kogan BA (1998) Gastrocystoplasty: long-term followup. J Urol 160(6 Pt 1):2182–2186
2. McDougal WS (1992) Metabolic complications of urinary intestinal diversion. J Urol 147(5):1199–1208
3. Nguyen HT, Kurzrock EA (2004) The effect of enterocystoplasty on skeletal development in children. In: Stone AR (ed) Urinary diversion, 2nd edn. Martin Dunitz, London
4. Khandelwal P, Abraham SN, Apodaca G (2009) Cell biology and physiology of the uroepithelium. Am J Physiol Renal Physiol 297(6):F1477–F1501. doi:10.1152/ajprenal.00327.2009
5. Wu XR, Kong XP, Pellicer A, Kreibich G, Sun TT (2009) Uroplakins in urothelial biology, function, and disease. Kidney Int 75(11):1153–1165. doi:10.1038/ki.2009.73
6. Hu P, Meyers S, Liang FX, Deng FM, Kachar B, Zeidel ML, Sun TT (2002) Role of membrane proteins in permeability barrier function: uroplakin ablation elevates urothelial permeability. Am J Physiol Renal Physiol 283(6):F1200–F1207. doi:10.1152/ajprenal.00043.2002
7. Subramaniam R, Hinley J, Stahlschmidt J, Southgate J (2011) Tissue engineering potential of urothelial cells from diseased bladders. J Urol 186(5):2014–2020. doi:10.1016/j.juro.2011.07.031
8. Horst M, Madduri S, Gobet R, Sulser T, Milleret V, Hall H, Atala A, Eberli D (2013) Engineering functional bladder tissues. J Tissue Eng Regen Med 7(7):515–522. doi:10.1002/term.547
9. Staack A, Hayward SW, Baskin LS, Cunha GR (2005) Molecular, cellular and developmental biology of urothelium as a basis of bladder regeneration. Differentiation 73(4):121–133. doi:10.1111/j.1432-0436.2005.00014.x
10. Osborn SL, Thangappan R, Luria A, Lee JH, Nolta J, Kurzrock EA (2014) Induction of human embryonic and induced pluripotent stem cells into urothelium. Stem Cells Transl Med 3(5):610–619. doi:10.5966/sctm.2013-0131
11. Loring JF, Peterson SE (eds) (2012) Human stem cell manual: a laboratory guide, 2nd edn. Elsevier, Amsterdam
12. D'Amour KA, Agulnick AD, Eliazer S, Kelly OG, Kroon E, Baetge EE (2005) Efficient differentiation of human embryonic stem cells to definitive endoderm. Nat Biotechnol 23(12):1534–1541. doi:10.1038/nbt1163
13. Kang M, Kim HH, Han YM (2014) Generation of bladder urothelium from human pluripotent stem cells under chemically defined serum- and feeder-free system. Int J Mol Sci 15(5):7139–7157. doi:10.3390/ijms15057139
14. Sun TT (2006) Altered phenotype of cultured urothelial and other stratified epithelial cells: implications for wound healing. Am J Physiol Renal Physiol 291(1):F9–21. doi:10.1152/ajprenal.00035.2006

Chapter 12

Spheroid Cultures of Primary Urothelial Cancer Cells: Cancer Tissue-Originated Spheroid (CTOS) Method

Takahiro Yoshida, Hiroaki Okuyama, Hiroko Endo, and Masahiro Inoue

Abstract

Increasingly, it has been recognized that studying cancer samples from individual patients is important for the development of effective therapeutic strategies and in endeavors to overcome therapy resistance. Primary cultures of cancer cells acutely dissected from individual patients can provide a platform that enables the study and characterization of individual tumors. To that end, we have developed a method for preparing cancer cells in the form of multi-cellular spheroids. The cells can be derived from patient tumors (primary cells), from patient-derived xenografts, or from genetically- or chemically induced animal tumors. This method of culturing spheroids composed of cells derived from cancer tissues can be applied to various types of cancer, including urothelial cancer. The method is based on the principle of retaining cell-cell contact throughout cancer cell preparation and culturing. The first step is a partial digestion of the tumor specimen into small fragments; these fragments spontaneously form spheroidal shapes within several hours. The spheroid is referred to as a cancer tissue-originated spheroid (CTOS). The advantage of the CTOS method is that it allows one to prepare pure cancer cells at high yield. CTOSs can be stably cultured in serum-free conditions. The CTOS method can be applied to drug sensitivity assays, drug screening, and analyses of intracellular signaling. Moreover, the CTOS method provides a platform for studying the nature of cancer cell clusters.

Key words Urothelial cancer, Bladder cancer, Primary cell culture, Spheroid, Organoid, CTOS

1 Introduction

Established cancer cell lines cultured in 2D conditions have served as a major platform for studying cancer cells in vitro [1, 2]. Indeed, most of our knowledge about intracellular signaling has been elucidated in vitro with cell lines. Nevertheless, compared to cells cultured in 2D conditions, multicellular spheroids, also known as 3D-cultured cancer cells, are thought to exhibit more similarity to cancer cells in vivo [1, 3]. Recent studies have reported that cancer cell clusters existed in blood and urine, and these cell clusters were found to contribute to metastasis [3–5]. Thus, more studies are emerging that focus on cell clusters, rather than on single cells.

Wolfgang A. Schulz et al. (eds.), *Urothelial Carcinoma: Methods and Protocols*, Methods in Molecular Biology, vol. 1655, DOI 10.1007/978-1-4939-7234-0_12, © Springer Science+Business Media LLC 2018

Cancer is a heterogeneous disease. Cancer characteristics vary, even between patients with the same pathological diagnosis [6, 7]. Increasingly, it has been recognized that studying cancer tissues derived from individual patients is important for developing effective therapeutic strategies and for overcoming therapy resistance [8]. Conventional cell lines cannot fulfill the requirements, due to the low success rate and the long times required to become established [8]. Thus, primary cultures, i.e., culturing cancer cells from individual patients, are necessary. Primary cultures have not been widely used, due to the technical obstacles involved, including cumbersome procedures, poor success rates, low purity, low yields, and poor reproducibility.

We recently developed a method for preparing cancer cells in the form of multi-cellular spheroids composed of cells derived from patient tumors (primary cells), from patient-derived xenografts, or from genetically- or chemically induced animal tumors [9, 10]. This method of preparing spheroids from cells that originate from cancer tissues can be applied to various types of cancer, including urothelial cancer [5, 11, 12]. The principle of this method is to retain cell-cell contact between cancer cells throughout the preparation and culturing procedures. The first step is the partial digestion of tumor specimens into small fragments, which spontaneously form a spheroidal structure within several hours. The spheroid is referred to as a cancer tissue-originated spheroid (CTOS). The advantage of the CTOS method is that it produces pure cancer cells in high yield. CTOSs can be stably cultured in serum-free conditions. In contrast to single cell cultures, CTOSs can be cultured in suspension without any extrinsic extracellular matrix. The CTOS method is applicable to drug sensitivity assays, drug screening [13], and analyses of intracellular signaling [9, 11, 13–15].

For urothelial cancer, we revealed that CTOS growth depended mostly on the heregulin-HER3-Akt pathway, but with some exceptions, which indicated that inter-patient heterogeneity existed in growth factor signaling [11]. A varied response was also observed in a sensitivity assay performed with individual patient CTOSs, where high-dose drugs used in intravesical chemotherapy were tested. That study showed that cell death was caspase-independent [12].

The multicentricity of urothelial cancer might be due to dissemination of cancer cells into the walls of the urinary tract; thus, the interaction between cancer cell clusters and urothelial cells may be an important step for implantation [16]. We previously demonstrated that, in the urine of patients with urothelial cancer, there were cell clusters that could be cultured as spheroids in vitro. Furthermore, we revealed that, once part of a floating CTOS had attached to type I collagen, the p63 protein was immediately degraded in all the cells of the urothelial cancer CTOSs. The degradation of p63, and the consequential reduction of E-cadherin, were necessary for the attachment of cell clusters to normal urothelium [5]. Thus, the CTOS method provides a platform for studying the nature of cancer cell clusters.

In this chapter, we describe the protocol for CTOS preparation from urothelial cancer tissues and the protocol for performing a drug sensitivity assay with CTOS cultures.

2 Materials

2.1 Equipment

1. Sterile forceps and scalpel.
2. Conical tube, 50 mL.
3. Water bath.
4. Glass flask (100 mL) and magnetic stir bar. Put the magnetic stir bar in the glass flask and autoclave them.
5. An Immersible Magnetic Stirring apparatus and Controller (MS-101, MC-303, Scinics, Tokyo, Japan).
6. Stainless-steel wire mesh filter, 250 μm.
7. Cell strainer, 40 μm (352340, BD Falcon, Franklin Lakes, NJ).
8. Nontreated culture dish, 60 or 10 mm.
9. Nontreated 96-well culture dish.

2.2 Materials and Reagents

1. Fresh samples from a human bladder tumor or an upper urinary tract tumor. The CTOS method is also applicable to patient-derived xenotumors, generated with a subcutaneous inoculation of a human urothelial cancer specimen into NOD-SCID mice.
2. DMEM/F-12 (11330032, Thermo Fisher Scientific, Waltham, MA, USA).
3. HBSS (14025092, Thermo Fisher Scientific, Waltham, MA, USA).
4. Penicillin-Streptomycin (15140122, Thermo Fisher Scientific, Waltham, MA, USA).
5. Liberase DH, 50 mg (5401089001, Roche Applied Science, Mannheim, Germany). For making the stock solution (5 mg/mL), dissolve the powder in 10 mL of DMEM/F12 on ice. Make aliquots of 100 μL, and store at −20 °C. Be sure to complete this procedure within 30 min.
6. 2-mercaptoethanol, 55 mM (21985023, Thermo Fisher Scientific, Waltham, MA, USA).
7. StemPro hESC SFM (A1000701, Thermo Fisher Scientific, Waltham, MA, USA). This solution consists of DMEM/F-12 with GlutaMAX, StemPro hESC Supplement (StemPro), and

25% bovine serum albumin. Make aliquots of 400 μL for StemPro, and store at −20 °C.

8. DNaseI, 100 mg (11284932001, Roche Applied Science, Mannheim, Germany). For making the stock solution (10 mg/mL), dissolve the powder in 10 mL of sterile deionized water. Make aliquots of 1 mL and store at −20 °C. Once thawed, maintain the aliquot at 4 °C to avoid repeating a freeze/thaw cycle.
9. Matrigel Matrix Growth Factor, Reduced (Matrigel) (354230, BD Falcon, Franklin Lakes, NJ). Make aliquots of 0.5 mL or 1.0 mL and store at −20 °C. Once thawed, maintain the aliquot at 4 °C to avoid repeating a freeze/thaw cycle.

3 Methods

3.1 Preparation of CTOS

1. Immediately after tumor resection or biopsy (*see* **Notes 1** and **2**), place the tissue sample in a 50 mL conical tube on ice, with 10 mL DMEM/F12 supplemented with 100 units/mL penicillin and 100 μg/mL streptomycin. Store the specimen at 4 °C until ready to proceed (*see* **Note 3**).
2. Transfer the medium and the samples to a 10 cm tissue culture dish, by inverting the tube.
3. Mince the tissue into small (1–2 mm) pieces with sterile forceps and a scalpel.
4. Resuspend the minced tissue in a 100 mL sterile glass flask with 10 mL DMEM/F12 supplemented with 100 U/mL penicillin, 100 μg/mL streptomycin, and 100 μL Liberase DH (final concentration, 50 μg/mL); add a magnetic stir bar.
5. Place the glass flask into a 37 °C water bath with constant stirring, and allow sample digestion for 1–2 h (Fig. 1) (*see* **Note 4**). Digestion times can be longer, depending on the amount of sample.
6. Prepare complete culture medium according to the manufacture's protocol, with some modifications. To make 10 mL of medium, start with 9.08 mL DMEM/F-12 with Glutamax-MAX, and add 100 U/mL penicillin, 100 μg/mL streptomycin, 200 μL StemPro, 720 μL of 25% bovine serum albumin, and 18.2 μL of 55 mM 2-mercaptoethanol. Pre-warm the complete culture medium at 37 °C (*see* **Note 5**).
7. Add 10 μL DNaseI to the glass flask (final concentration; 10 μg/mL). Digest the samples for another 15 min.
8. Filter the samples sequentially, through a 500 μm, then a 250 μm wire mesh (*see* **Note 6**). Transfer the filtrate into a 50 mL conical tube (Fig. 2).

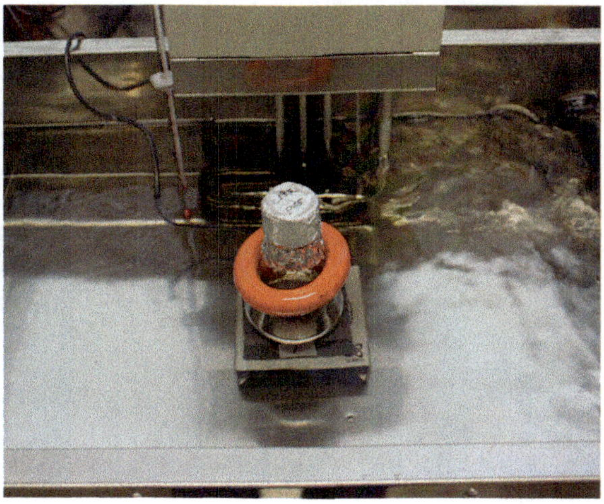

Fig. 1 A glass flask is partially immersed in a 37 °C water bath with constant stirring

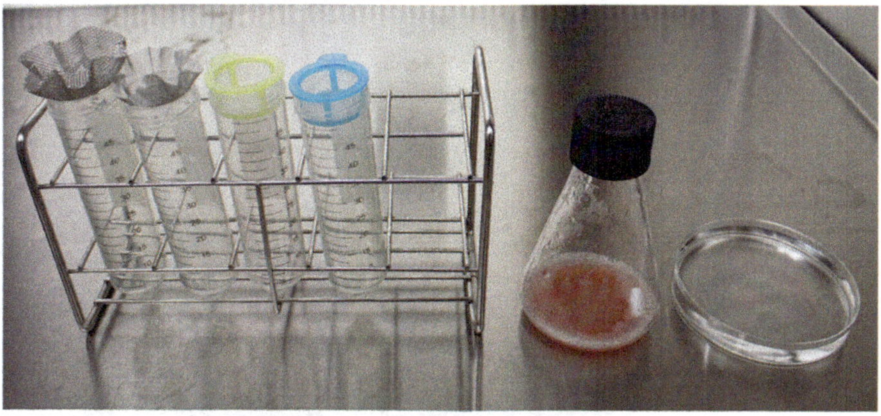

Fig. 2 Setup for the filtration procedure. On the open top of the 50 mL tube, 500 μm wire mesh, 250 μm wire mesh, 100 μm cell strainer (*yellow*), and 40 μm cell strainer (*blue*) are placed (*from left to right*). The digested sample is in the glass flask with a stir bar (*second from right*). HBSS in a 10 cm dish (*right most*)

9. Filter the flow-through fraction with a 40 μm cell strainer (*see* **Note 7**).
10. Place 30 mL of HBSS in a 10 cm tissue culture dish, and dip the bottom of the cell strainer into the solution; swirl it gently to remove the small debris, the single cells, and cell clumps with diameters <40 μm.
11. Collect the organoids that remain in the cell strainer with a 1 mL micropipette (Fig. 3).
12. Centrifuge at 100 × *g* at room temperature (RT) for 2 min. Discard the supernatant.
13. Wash the samples by pipetting with 20 mL HBSS.
14. Centrifuge at 100 × *g* at RT for 2 min.

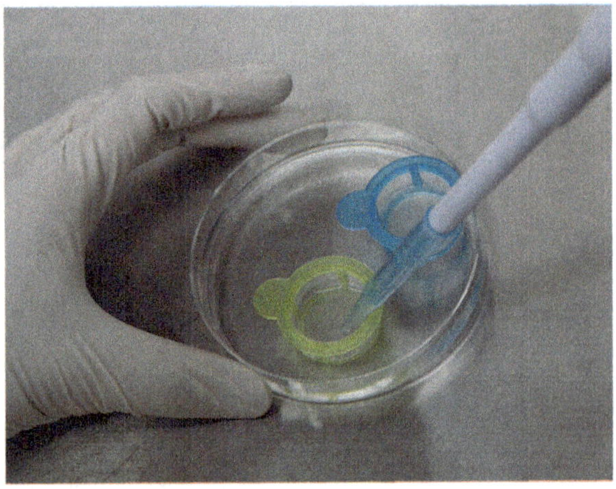

Fig. 3 Collecting the organoids for CTOS isolation. The 100 μm cell strainer (*yellow*) and 40 μm cell strainer (*blue*) are dipped in 30 mL HBSS in a 10 cm tissue culture dish. The fragments that remain in the cell strainer are collected with a 1 mL micropipette

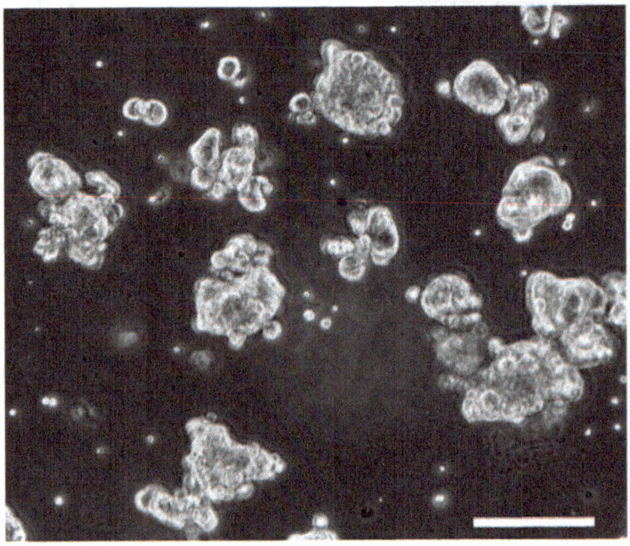

Fig. 4 CTOS culture on day 0. Phase contrast image shows organoid fractions immediately after digestion and filtration. Scale bar: 100-μm

15. Discard the supernatant.
16. Add 5 or 10 mL of the complete culture medium, depending on the amount of the sample. Pipette the pellet to disperse small clumps.
17. Transfer the organoids and medium to a 6- or 10 cm non-treated dish.
18. View under a phase-contrast microscope; organoids appear as irregular fragments (Fig. 4).

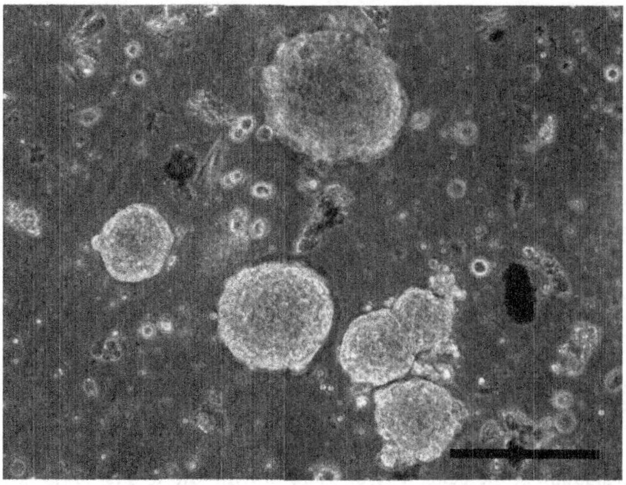

Fig. 5 CTOS formation. Phase contrast image shows organoids at 24 h after digestion. Scale bar: 100 μm

19. Incubate in a 5% CO_2 humidified chamber at 37 °C for 24 h.
20. View under a phase-contrast microscope; CTOSs appear as bright, smooth spheres (Fig. 5).

3.2 Three-Dimensional Chemosensitivity Assay with CTOS

1. Prepare CTOSs 24–48 h before performing this assay.
2. Thaw the stock Matrigel solution at 4 °C overnight, and maintain it on ice (*see* **Note 8**).
3. Prepare a drug solution at the prescribed concentration with StemPro. Warm the drug solution to 37 °C in a water bath.
4. View the CTOSs under a phase-contrast microscope. When many single cells are present, transfer the CTOSs to a 15 mL conical tube, and allow it to stand for 5 min. Discard the supernatant, resuspend the pellet in fresh complete culture medium, and transfer to a new dish.
5. Make a droplet of 10 μL Matrigel, at the center of the well of a 96-well nontreated dish.
6. Under a phase-contrast microscope, pick up a CTOS with a micropipette. The volume should be set at 0.8 μL.
7. Inject the CTOS into the Matrigel droplet.
8. Repeat **steps 5** and **6**, until you obtain the required number of wells.
9. Incubate the 96-well dish in a 5% CO_2 humidified chamber at 37 °C for 30 min to solidify the Matrigel.
10. Add 100 μL StemPro with the indicated dose of the drug.
11. Acquire a photograph of each CTOS under a phase-contrast microscope with a 10× objective lens (day 0).

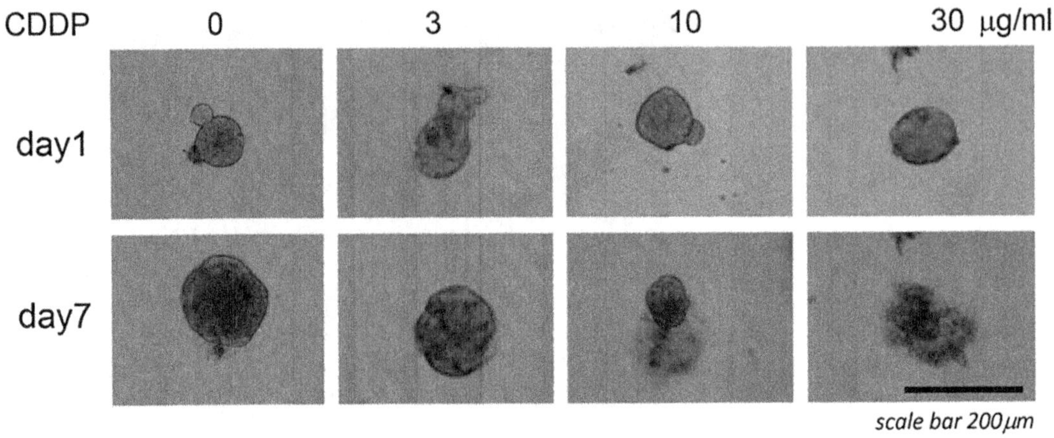

Fig. 6 Evaluation of the sensitivity of CTOS growth rate to chemotherapy drug. Images show CTOSs on day 1 and day 7 of treatment with the indicated doses of cisplatin (CDDP)

12. After 4–7 days, acquire another photograph of each CTOS under a phase-contrast microscope with a 10× objective lens.
13. Measure the CTOS areas by analyzing the photographs with image analysis software. The CTOS growth rate is calculated by dividing the area measured on days 4–7 by the area measured on day 1 (Fig. 6). Alternatively, intracellular ATP levels can be measured (*see* **Note 9**). Since ATP levels of CTOSs are proportional to the area of CTOSs, ATP levels can be adjusted by the area at day 1 [14].

4 Notes

1. CTOSs are much easier to prepare from papillary tumors than from non-papillary tumors [11, 12]. With papillary tumor tissue, a 5 mm^3 tumor sample will yield 100–300 CTOSs.
2. Sterile saline is adequate for transporting clinical samples from the operation room to the lab.
3. In DMEM/F-12 or saline, CTOS preparation can be performed within 2–3 h after the tumor is resected.
4. Enzymatic digestion can be performed in the 37 °C incubator, when the magnetic stirring system can be placed inside.
5. In general, heregulin has been the most efficient growth factor [11] examined to date, but some CTOSs respond better to other growth factors [11]. To examine the effect of a single growth factor, we do not add StemPro, which includes multiple growth factors, into the complete culture medium.
6. When the initial sample volume is very low, the entire digested sample should be cultured without filtration and wash.

7. You can use a 100 μm cell strainer (352360; BD Falcon, Franklin Lakes, NJ), depending on the desired CTOS size.
8. CTOSs generally grow in suspension. However, when CTOSs are embedded in Matrigel or type I collagen gel, growth is enhanced.
9. ATP is measured with the CellTiter-Glo® Luminescent Cell Viability Assay (G7571, Promega, Fitchburg, WI, USA).

References

1. Sharma SV, Haber DA, Settleman J (2010) Cell line-based platforms to evaluate the therapeutic efficacy of candidate anticancer agents. Nat Rev Cancer 10(4):241–253
2. Barretina J, Caponigro G, Stransky N, Venkatesan K, Margolin AA, Kim S et al (2012) The cancer cell line encyclopedia enables predictive modelling of anticancer drug sensitivity. Nature 483(7391):603–607
3. Yu M, Bardia A, Wittner BS, Stott SL, Smas ME, Ting DT et al (2013) Circulating breast tumor cells exhibit dynamic changes in epithelial and mesenchymal composition. Science 339(6119):580–584
4. Aceto N, Bardia A, Miyamoto DT, Donaldson MC, Wittner BS, Spencer JA et al (2014) Circulating tumor cell clusters are oligoclonal precursors of breast cancer metastasis. Cell 158 (5):1110–1122
5. Yoshida T, Okuyama H, Nakayama M, Endo H, Tomita Y, Nonomura N et al (2015) Dynamic change in p63 protein expression during implantation of urothelial cancer clusters. Neoplasia 17(7):574–585
6. Bedard PL, Hansen AR, Ratain MJ, Siu LL (2013) Tumour heterogeneity in the clinic. Nature 501(7467):355–364
7. Cancer Genome Atlas Research N, Weinstein JN, Collisson EA, Mills GB, Shaw KR, Ozenberger BA et al (2013) The cancer genome atlas pan-cancer analysis project. Nat Genet 45(10):1113–1120
8. Mitra A, Mishra L, Li S (2013) Technologies for deriving primary tumor cells for use in personalized cancer therapy. Trends Biotechnol 31 (6):347–354
9. Kondo J, Endo H, Okuyama H, Ishikawa O, Iishi H, Tsujii M et al (2011) Retaining cell-cell contact enables preparation and culture of spheroids composed of pure primary cancer cells from colorectal cancer. Proc Natl Acad Sci U S A 108(15):6235–6240
10. Takeda T, Okuyama H, Nishizawa Y, Tomita S, Inoue M (2012) Hypoxia inducible factor-1alpha is necessary for invasive phenotype in Vegf-deleted islet cell tumors. Sci Rep 2:494
11. Okuyama H, Yoshida T, Endo H, Nakayama M, Nonomura N, Nishimura K et al (2013) Involvement of heregulin/HER3 in the primary culture of human urothelial cancer. J Urol 190(1):302–310
12. Yoshida T, Okuyama H, Nakayama M, Endo H, Nonomura N, Nishimura K et al (2015) High-dose chemotherapeutics of intravesical chemotherapy rapidly induce mitochondrial dysfunction in bladder cancer-derived spheroids. Cancer Sci 106(1):69–77
13. Kiyohara Y, Yoshino K, Kubota S, Okuyama H, Endo H, Ueda Y et al (2016) Drug screening and grouping by sensitivity with a panel of primary cultured cancer spheroids derived from endometrial cancer. Cancer Sci 107 (4):452–460
14. Endo H, Okami J, Okuyama H, Kumagai T, Uchida J, Kondo J et al (2013) Spheroid culture of primary lung cancer cells with neuregulin 1/HER3 pathway activation. J Thorac Oncol 8(2):131–139
15. Nakajima A, Endo H, Okuyama H, Kiyohara Y, Kimura T, Kamiura S et al (2015) Radiation sensitivity assay with a panel of patient-derived spheroids of small cell carcinoma of the cervix. Int J Cancer 136(12):2949–2960
16. Knowles MA, Hurst CD (2015) Molecular biology of bladder cancer: new insights into pathogenesis and clinical diversity. Nat Rev Cancer 15(1):25–41

Chapter 13

The N-butyl-N-4-hydroxybutyl Nitrosamine Mouse Urinary Bladder Cancer Model

Paula A. Oliveira, Cármen Vasconcelos-Nóbrega, Rui M. Gil da Costa, and Regina Arantes-Rodrigues

Abstract

Urinary bladder cancer (UBC) is a common and complex malignancy, with a multifactorial etiology, like environmental factors, such as cigarette smoking, occupational exposure, and genetic factors.

UBC exhibits considerable genotypic and phenotypic heterogeneity. Among all UBC lesions, urothelial carcinoma is the most frequently observed histological type. Despite all the developments made in urologic oncology field, therapeutic options remain inadequate. There is urgency for the identification and development of new antineoplastic drugs to replace or improve current protocols and in vivo models have been proven to be essential for this step. There are different animal models of UBC: Spontaneous and experimentally induced models (genetically engineered, transplantable-xenograft and syngeneic animals- and chemically induced models). *N-butyl-N(4-hydroxybutil)nitrosamine* (BBN) is the most suitable reagent to generate chemically induced in vivo models of UBC and to study bladder carcinogenesis. BBN has proven, over the years, to be very realistic and reliable. It is bladder specific, and induces high tumor incidence.

Key words Bladder cancer, Chemical carcinogenesis, Arylamines, Animal models

1 Urinary Bladder Cancer (UBC)

Urinary bladder cancer (UBC) is a common and complex malignancy and is estimated to be the ninth most frequent cause of cancer this year worldwide, with approximately 77,000 estimated new cases and 16,390 estimated deaths, from both sexes, only in the United States [1]. It is the seventh most frequent neoplasia in men and the seventeenth in women, with a threefold higher probability of developing in men than in women, and with a ratio of 2:1 for whites and blacks, respectively [2]. UBC predominantly affects the elderly. Its incidence peaks in the 7th decade of life (from the age of 60), and about 20% of the patients are more than 80 years old [3]. Since the mid to late-1990s, incidence rates have stabilized or decreased in men from Western and Northern Europe, but kept increasing in Southern, Central, and Eastern Europe. In Southern

Wolfgang A. Schulz et al. (eds.), *Urothelial Carcinoma: Methods and Protocols*, Methods in Molecular Biology, vol. 1655, DOI 10.1007/978-1-4939-7234-0_13, © Springer Science+Business Media LLC 2018

Europe, Spain and Italy are the countries with the highest incidence rates [4]. However, the highest mortality rates are recorded in Northern Africa and the Middle East [5].

The etiology of UBC can be considered multifactorial. Environmental factors, such as cigarette smoking, and occupational exposure, do indeed contribute to a part of the UBC risk. Cigarette smoking is the primary and the most important risk factor, due to aromatic amines and hydrocarbons that can form DNA adducts [6]. No less important are the genetic factors, gene-gene or gene-environment interaction may better predict the risk of developing UBC [7]. In the Middle East and some African countries, such as Israel, Egypt, Iran, and Iraqi, chronic urothelial infections with *Schistosoma haematobium* occur, leading to a high incidence of squamous cell carcinoma of the bladder [8].

1.1 Types of UBC and Treatment

UBC exhibits considerable genotypic and phenotypic heterogeneity, with differing outcomes related to its underlying basic biology, responsiveness to therapy, and host-related factors. Consequently, the spectrum of UBC ranges from a manageable entity that may be only just a nuisance to a lethal variant with high metastatic potential [9–11]. Among all UBC lesions, urothelial carcinoma (formerly: transitional cell carcinoma) is the most frequently observed histological type [12]. Squamous cell carcinoma, adenocarcinoma, small-cell tumors, and sarcomatoid tumors are less common [13]. Nearly 70% of the patients with urothelial carcinoma have tumors confined to the mucosa or sub-mucosa, called non-muscle invasive tumors, while the remaining present with muscle invasive tumors [14].

The non-muscle invasive tumors are mostly low-grade and well-differentiated papillary lesions [15], which tend to recur locally and rarely metastasize, with a favorable prognosis [16, 17]. Low-grade papillary lesions frequently show HRAS and fibroblast growth factor receptor 3 (FGFR3) activating mutations [18, 19]. Constitutive activation of receptor tyrosine kinases (RTKs), upstream of RAS-activated pathways, in particular FGFR3, has been detected in 75% of low-grade lesions [20]. Other RTKs associated with low-grade noninvasive papillary tumors are ERBB3 and ERBB4 [21]. These lesions are generally managed with surgical resection and/or by induction and maintenance immunotherapy with intravesical Bacillus Calmette-Guérin (BCG) vaccine or intravesical chemotherapy [11]. The main goals of these therapies are to prevent recurrence and progression of UBC patients [22].

Several clinical factors, such as tumor multiplicity, diameter, concomitant carcinoma in situ (CIS), and gender, have been identified as having prognostic significance for recurrence [23]. CIS and high-grade papillary lesions are different histological entities, both associated with alterations in structural and cell adhesion molecules, such as cytokeratins and E-cadherin [24]. Molecular alterations on retinoblastoma (*RB1*) and *TP53* genes are common in these two kinds of lesions [25] and it is reported that patients with both gene defects have worse prognosis than those harboring a defect in either gene alone [26, 27]. BCG is the most adopted first-line immunotherapeutic and the most effective treatment for prophylaxis and treatment of CIS [28].

Muscle invasive tumors are the most worrying, since at the time of treatment of the primary tumor, approximately one-third of the patients have undetected nodal or distant metastases. Involving structural and functional defects also in the *TP53* and *RB1*, as well as in phosphatase and tensin homologue gene (*PTEN*) tumor-suppressors, these tumors tend to metastasize with a poor prognosis [29]. For muscle invasive UBC, multimodal treatment involving radical cystectomy with neoadjuvant chemotherapy offers the best chance for cure [11]. Selected patients with muscle invasive tumors can be offered bladder-sparing trimodality treatment consisting of transurethral resection with chemoradiation. Advanced disease is best treated with systemic cisplatin-based chemotherapy [11].

1.2 Main Challenges

The high rate of recurrence and the repeated surgical interventions make UBC treatment one of the most expensive ones among solid tumors, with a high impact in the quality of life of patients. Despite all the developments made in this area, even today therapeutic options remain inadequate. These limitations highlight the urgency for the identification and development of new antineoplastic drugs to replace or improve current protocols.

2 Animal Models

In vivo models have been a crucial tool for providing insights into the mechanisms of urothelial carcinogenesis, and are widely recognized as being essential to test the efficacy of antineoplastic drugs [30]. Under specific experimental conditions, animal models develop lesions similar to those described in human patients. Models are considered valid if they resemble the human condition in etiology, pathophysiology, symptoms, target identification, and response to therapeutic interventions [31].

2.1 Spontaneous Models of UBC

Spontaneous animal models of UBC are available and present important opportunities for research [32]. Cattle and dogs provide two spontaneous animal models of UBC. In cattle exposed to the poisonous fern *Pteridium spp.* and its toxin, ptaquiloside, the developing UBC lesions are histologically heterogeneous and differ from those found in human patients [33–35], precluding the use of this model for drug development. On the other hand, dogs spontaneously recapitulate transitional cell carcinoma development (TCC). Although TCC in dogs comprise only 2% of all canine cancers [36], this model resembles human UBC, with respect to its histopathologic appearance, biological behavior, and response to therapy and prognosis, among other advantages [37]. The use of spontaneous animal models of disease circumvents the ethic concerns related to the use of laboratory animals. For a society concerned with animal welfare it is more acceptable to treat sick animals and use the knowledge thereby obtained in favor of scientific development than to deliberately induce disease in animals for research purposes. Moreover, any comparative studies performed in pet animals clearly benefit both animals and humans [38].

2.2 Experimentally Induced UBC

Three types of experimental models are currently available for inducing urinary bladder tumors: genetically engineered, transplantable (xenograft and syngeneic animals), and chemically induced models [39].

2.2.1 Genetically Modified Models

Genetically engineered mice, generated to carry cloned oncogenes or lack tumor-suppressing genes by ever-improving techniques, provide useful systems for dissecting the roles of specific molecular events, individually or in combination, in urinary bladder tumorigenesis [32, 40]. Several genetically modified animals for UBC study are available, namely CK19-Tag, Nrf2−/−, HRas, Pten flox/flox, p53+/−, Hras 128, UPII-SV407; p53 flox/flox, and p27kip1 −/−? [41]. However, with the exception of altered p53, there are no driver mutations that are obvious candidates for transgenics. Genetically modified animals are expensive, take time to develop, and assess, and need to be normalized to a predictable pattern of tumor development, as penetrance is never 100% [42].

2.2.2 Transplantable Models

Transplantable models comprise various systems and techniques to propagate tumor cells in different hosts for controlled studies in vivo.

Xenograft models are established by transplanting human urothelial cancer cells or primary tumor fragments into immunodeficient hosts, most usually mice [43]. Syngeneic models consist of rodent UBC cells or tumor fragments transplanted into an immunocompetent host of the same species and strain, allowing researchers to monitor tumor growth and other parameters. Syngeneic models are most commonly employed when the study focuses on the immune response or gene therapy [40]. Both syngeneic and xenograft models have advantages and drawbacks to be considered. Syngeneic models take advantage of a fully functional host immune system (as opposed to the immunodeficient xenografted animals), while xenografts make use of human rather than murine cells [32]. Xenograft and syngeneic models can be further divided into orthotopic and heterotopic models. In orthotopic models, the tumor is placed in the site at which it would be expected to arise naturally in the host, simulating thus the local cancer environment and recapitulating to some extent the natural history of the disease [44, 45]. In heterotopic models, the transplants are placed in other locations, most often subcutaneously in the flank or hind leg of the animal

[40]. Heterotopic tumor models have been widely used, because subcutaneous implantation is commodious and facilitates tumor follow-up [44, 45], but their different microenvironmental conditions may limit correlations with natural disease. Besides, with both heterotopic and orthotopic models, there may be a long latency period before tumors become noticeable and the take rate is generally low when passaging tumor samples for the first time.

2.2.3 Chemically Induced (Papillary and Invasive) Models

Several animal species such as dogs, rabbits, guinea pigs, and hamsters may be used to obtain UBC tumors induced chemically. However, rats and mice are the animals most frequently employed, due to their small size, innumerable anatomical, physiological and biochemical similarities to humans, well-known genetic background and high reproductive rate. Furthermore, spontaneous bladder tumors are rare in laboratory rodents, which is another reason why they are often selected as models for the study of chemically induced UBC [46].

In early investigations of UBC, it was necessary to validate these animal models histologically [32]. Such models were used for preclinical drug development early on, and were later subjected to immunohistochemical evaluation, revealing further similarities with their human counterparts [47]. Although animal models preserve the three-dimensional tumor structure with cell-cell interactions and allow pharmacokinetic and toxicity evaluation of the compounds, these models also present significant limitations, such as the high costs involved, the long experimental protocols, difficulties in monitoring UBC development during the experimental protocol, and the fact that their molecular characteristics remain only partially understood [41].

There are several chemical carcinogens associated with bladder cancer development [48–50]. Among them are nitroso compounds, including *N-butyl-N(4-hidroxybutil)nitrosamine* (BBN) and *N-methyl-N-nitrosourea* (MNU), and nitrofuran compounds, such as *N-[4-(5-nitro-2-furyl)-2-thiazolyl]-formamide* (FANFT). When administered via the appropriate route, at the correct dosage and in the appropriate strain of animal, they all produce 100% incidence of bladder tumors.

3 Chemical Carcinogens: BBN, FANFT, MNU

The chemical carcinogens BBN, FANFT, and MNU specifically induce bladder cancer. BBN and FANFT are indirect carcinogens when administered orally, while MNU requires direct bladder instillation [51].

Being an indirect carcinogen, BBN needs to be activated, mainly in the liver, but also in the bladder. BBN is converted to *N-butyl-N-(3-carboxypropyl)nitrosamine* (BCPN) after oxidation of the alcoholic group into a carboxylic group by the enzymatic system alcohol/aldehyde dehydrogenase [52–54]. BBN is also converted to BBN-glucuronide by uridine diphosphate-glucuronosyltransferase-catalyzed conjugation but, unlike BCPN, this metabolite does not possess carcinogenic properties. BCPN reaches the urinary bladder through blood and urine and comes into contact with the urothelium, binding covalently to cellular macromolecules and initiating the carcinogenic process [54–58]. Additional metabolites, such as *N-butyl-N-(2-hydroxy-3-carboxy-propyl)nitrosamine*, *N-butyl-N-(carboxymethyl)nitrosamine*, and *N-butyl-N-(2-oxopropyl)nitrosamine*, can also be detected in urine, but in minor quantities [55, 56, 59, 60]. BBN causes DNA damage in the bladder epithelium and selectively induces urinary bladder tumors in mice and rats [57, 61], being therefore considered a genotoxic or DNA-reactive carcinogen [58, 62]. In BBN-induced bladder tumors, the clonal mutations detected were predominantly G-A or C-T transitions (15/27, 56%) and substitutions of T (10/27, 37%) [61].

FANFT is a carcinogenic agent which specifically targets the bladder in mice, rats, and dogs. It is administered on the animal's diet in doses ranging between 0.05 and 0.2%. FANFT is converted into *2-amino-4-(5-nitro-2-furyl)thiazole* (ANFT), a mutagenic and carcinogenic metabolite [48, 63–65] through a renal metabolic/excretory coupling, that enhances ANFT excretion [66].

MNU is a direct-acting carcinogen which does not need metabolic activation to exert carcinogenicity. It is instilled directly into the bladder and acts directly on the urothelium, following its spontaneous pH-dependent decomposition, and producing persistent, multiple methylation of cellular DNA. MNU is a genotoxic compound that can act both as an initiator and as a promoter [67, 68].

4 BBN Mouse Model: Practical Implementation

Due to its high potency to induce bladder cancer, BBN is the most suitable reagent to generate chemically induced in vivo models of bladder cancer and to study bladder carcinogenesis [51]. Implementing the BBN mouse bladder cancer model involves a number of technical details, which should be taken into account.

There are several ways to administer BBN to animals, but the oral route is most commonly used, in drinking water or by gavage [69–74]. The oral BBN dose usually ranges between 0.01% and 0.05% (v/v) in drinking water [75]. The administration of BBN in drinking water has major advantages over gavage, since the animals are not manipulated, are not subjected to stress or to secondary effects that can occur in gavage administration, like esophageal injury, gastric rupture when using repeated oral gavage or even aspiration pneumonia in consequence of a non-intentional tracheal intubation [76]. On the other hand, with the gavage technique, the BBN doses can be exactly calculated, whereas in the drinking water, it can only be estimated based on the daily water intake.

BBN can also be administered subcutaneously and introduced directly into the urinary bladder by intravesical instillation [46, 57, 77–80], with similar tumor incidence rates [46, 70, 81].

The carcinogen is usually administered to young adult mice, and when BBN was administered subcutaneously to infant mice, pulmonary and hepatic neoplasms were induced rather than urinary lesions [79]. Xu *et al.* [82] recently reported the use of 3–4 weeks-old male C57BL/6 mice for a BBN-induced bladder cancer study.

Intravesical instillation of BBN requires technical skill and specific training. Anesthesia is required, in order to immobilize the animal, and an experienced technician is essential, in order to perform the technique correctly, and to avoid unnecessary pain and distress for the experimental animals [81].

The route of administration must be carefully planned, since if intravesical instillation is the method of choice, female mice should be used, because the male anatomy makes this method impossible [81]. Intravesical administration has an important difference when compared with other techniques: only the urethra and bladder come into contact with the carcinogenic agent, and systemic exposure is avoided. This may be an important advantage or not, depending on the purposes of the study [77, 81, 83].

BBN is a clear yellow to reddish-yellow color liquid that is quite viscous and, for this reason, it is recommended to cut the pipette tip in order to allow a better control while pipetting, and to vigorously shake the final solution in order to obtain an homogeneous distribution. It is also a photosensitive compound and therefore opaque bottles should be used [71], or alternatively, bottles should be involved in aluminum foil or similar, to protect it from light exposure.

Since bladder cancer is much more frequent in male (rather than female) patients, some research groups prefer to employ male animals, as a way to enhance the model's realism [84]. However, and apart from the question of the route of the administration of BNN, as previously mentioned, it is important to consider that using male mice entails some animal husbandry and welfare issues [85]. Male mice are highly aggressive among themselves, and should be housed at a low density. Even so, hair clipping, skin bites, and genital lesions are commonly observed. A "normal" cage behavior may therefore be associated with high stress levels and corresponding endocrine and immune changes. Consecutive bites may also lead to prolonged and variably severe systemic inflammation. All these factors constitute new variables that may interfere with the study results and they are not always easy to control [86]. In some instances, it may be necessary to house males individually to prevent injuries, which leads to other forms of stress and may be reflected by behavioral changes (e.g., circling). Seriously wounded animals may need to be removed from the study on ethical grounds and to avoid biasing the results [87]. These problems may be minimized to some extent by keeping a low population density, providing environmental enrichment and by monitoring the animal's behavior and health status regularly [88, 89]. Using female animals is a valid strategy to circumvent these problems: bladder lesions developed by female mice have been extensively characterized and found to reproduce closely those observed in human patients [32, 41].

As mentioned in the previous paragraphs, monitoring the animals during the experimental protocol is important to assess their health status, prevent unnecessary suffering, and avoid factors that might bias the study. Monitoring the animals also provides important data concerning food and water consumption, weight gains/losses, hematological and biochemical parameters from blood and urine analysis [86]. During experimental protocols, animals undergoing bladder carcinogenesis may present with variably severe hematuria, abdominal pain (reflected by a typical "hunched" position), and severe weight loss, all of which should be considered when determining humane endpoints for each particular study. Severe hematuria may be reflected by blood drops in the animal's litter; in order to systematically detect and quantify hematuria, periodic urine analysis may be performed. Urine may be collected using light abdominal compression (a practical and efficient method for this purpose), catheterization or in metabolic cages.

Experimental mice may be sacrificed at one or more time points during the experimental protocol and, typically, at the end of the protocol. When sacrificing the animals it is important to bear in mind that the urothelium suffers very fast postmortem degradation. It is therefore essential to collect and fixate the urinary bladder as soon as possible following the animal's death [47]. The sacrifice is usually performed under deep anesthesia, using common anesthetic protocols (e.g., ketamine/xylazine), followed by exsanguination (e.g., by cardiac puncture). This also allows the collection of an additional blood sample. The bladder should be immediately fixated by instilling a standard volume (e.g., 300 μl) of 10% neutral buffered formaldehyde in the lumen and carefully tie a knot in the ventral region, using a surgical silk yarn (2/0). The identification of the ventral region of the bladder is extremely important, since this is the area where more lesions are found, in consequence of the bladder position in quadrupeds (the urine and the carcinogenic agent is kept in the ventral area for a longer time, as with the vesical trigone in humans), but this identification may also be executed using China ink. Following fixation (ideally during 12 h in formaldehyde at lower temperatures, e.g., in the refrigerator), the bladders are trimmed by performing a sagittal incision, thus obtaining two symmetrical halves. These samples are then paraffin-embedded and processed for histological examination, using a routine hematoxylin and eosin (H&E) staining. On H&E, a variety of histological lesions are usually observed [46, 47], ranging between urothelial hyperplasia and invasive urothelial carcinomas (T1 and T2). Simple and nodular hyperplasia, low- and high-grade dysplasia, squamous and adenoid metaplasias, papillomas, papillary carcinomas, in situ carcinomas (CIS), and squamous carcinomas may be present. Cystitis may be lymphocytic, with lymphoid aggregates, or mixed, often showing a neutrophilic and sometimes eosinophylic component, and is often ulcerative and accompanied by hemorrhage.

5 Conclusions

Animal models of cancer are essential to understand the pathophysiology of the disease, to discover new therapeutic targets, and to test new treatments. Although the ideal model is unreachable, combining different models with complementary characteristics is a valid strategy. Over the years, the BBN mouse model has proven to be very realistic and reliable. It is possible to choose a simple method for the administration of the chemical carcinogen; BBN only affects the urothelium and the incidence of the tumors is high and reliable, allowing for the researcher to monitor the experiment and to predict results. Also, BBN-induced lesions are similar to human bladder cancer in histology, biochemical properties, molecular and genetic characteristics, natural history, and biological behavior. For all of these reasons, we consider the BBN mouse model for bladder cancer an extremely useful tool in the experimental oncology field.

References

1. Siegel R, Naishadham D, Jemal A (2012) Cancer statistics, 2012. CA Cancer J Clin 62 (1):10–29
2. Parkin DM (2008) The global burden of urinary bladder cancer. Scand J Urol Nephrol Suppl 218:12–20
3. Bellmunt J, Mottet N, De Santis M (2016) Urothelial carcinoma management in elderly or unfit patients. EJC Suppl 14(1):1–20
4. Antoni S, Ferlay J, Soerjomataram I, Znaor A, Jemal A, Bray F (2016) Bladder cancer incidence and mortality: a global overview and recent trends. Eur Urol 71(1):96–108. doi:10.1016/j.eururo.2016.06.010
5. Mahdavifar N, Ghoncheh M, Pakzad R, Momenimovahed Z, Salehiniya H (2016) Epidemiology, incidence and mortality of bladder cancer and their relationship with the development index in the world. Asian Pac J Cancer Prev 17(1):381–386
6. Kiriluk KJ, Prasad SM, Patel AR, Steinberg GD, Smith ND (2012) Bladder cancer risk from occupational and environmental exposures. Urol Oncol 30(2):199–211
7. Chu H, Wang M, Zhang Z (2013) Bladder cancer epidemiology and genetic susceptibility. J Biomed Res 27:170–178
8. Santos J, Chaves J, Videira M, Botelho M, Costa J, Oliveira J, Santos L (2012) Schistosomiasis haematobium and bladder cancer: retrospective analysis of 145 patients admitted to the urology. Department at the Américo Boavida Hospital, Luanda. Acta Urol 1:15–20
9. Kader KA (2011) Bladder cancer. Sci World J 11:2565–2566

10. Oliveira PA, Arantes-Rodrigues R, Vasconcelos-Nóbrega C (2014) Animal models of urinary bladder cancer and their application to novel drug discovery. Expert Opin Drug Discov 9(5):485–503
11. Kamat AM, Hahn NM, Efstathiou JA, Lerner SP, Malmström PU, Choi W, Guo CC, Lotan Y, Kassouf W (2016) Bladder cancer. Lancet 388(10061):2796–2810. doi:10.1016/S0140-6736(16)30512-8
12. Chalasani V, Chin JL, Izawa JI (2009) Histologic variants of urothelial bladder cancer and non urothelial histology in bladder cancer. Can Urol Assoc J 3(6Suppl4):S193–S198
13. Shanks JH, Iczkowski KA (2009) Divergent differentiation in urothelial carcinoma and other bladder cancer subtypes with selected mimics. Histopathology 54(7):885–900
14. Anastasiadis A, de Reijke TM (2012) Best practice in the treatment of nonmuscle invasive bladder cancer. Ther Adv Urol 4(1):13–32
15. Pasin E, Josephson DY, Mitra AP, Cote RJ, Stein JP (2008) Superficial bladder cancer: an update on etiology, molecular development, classification, and natural history. Rev Urol 10 (1):31–43
16. Grignon DJ (2009) The current classification of urothelial neoplasms. Mod Pathol 22: S60–S69
17. Zuiverloon TC, van der Aa MN, van der Kwast TH, Steyerberg EW, Lingsma HF, Bangma CH, Zwarthoff EC (2010) Fibroblast growth factor receptor 3 mutation analysis on voided urine for surveillance of patients with low-grade non-muscle-invasive bladder cancer. Clin Cancer Res 16(11):3011–3018
18. Knowles MA (2007) Role of FGFR3 in urothelial cell carcinoma: biomarker and potential therapeutic target. World J Urol 25:581–593
19. Noël N, Couteau J, Maillet G, Gobet F, d'Aloisio F, Minier C, Pfister C (2013) Preliminary study of p53 and FGFR3 gene mutations in the urine for bladder tumors. Prog Urol 23 (1):29–35
20. Van Rhijn BW, Montironi R, Zwarthoff EC, Jöbsis AC, van der Kwast TH (2002) Frequent FGFR3 mutations in urothelial papilloma. J Pathol 198(2):245–251
21. Memon AA, Sorensen BS, Melgard P, Fokdal L, Thykjaer T, Nexo E (2004) Expression of HER3, HER4 and their ligand heregulin-4 is associated with better survival in bladder cancer patients. Br J Cancer 91:2034–2041
22. Jarow J, Maher VE, Tang S, Ibrahim A, Kim G, Sridhara R, Pazdur R (2015) Development of systemic and topical drugs to treat non-muscle invasive bladder cancer. Bl Cancer 1 (2):133–136
23. Palou J, Sylvester RJ, Faba OR, Parada R, Pena JA, Algaba F, Villavicencio H (2012) Female gender and carcinoma in situ in the prostatic urethra are prognostic factors for recurrence, progression, and disease-specific mortality in T1G3 bladder cancer patients treated with bacillus Calmette-Guerin. Eur Urol 62(1):118–125
24. Garcia del Muro X, Torregrosa A, Muñoz J, Castellsagué X, Condom E, Vigués F, Arance A, Fabra A, Germà JR (2000) Prognostic value of the expression of E-cadherin and beta-catenin in bladder cancer. Eur J Cancer 36 (3):357–362
25. Wu XR (2005) Urothelial tumorigenesis: a tale of divergent pathways. Nat Rev Cancer 5 (9):713–725
26. Shariat SF, Tokunaga H, Zhou J, Kim J, Ayala GE, Benedict WF, Lerner SP (2004) p53, p21, pRB, and p16 expression predict clinical outcome in cystectomy with bladder cancer. J Clin Oncol 22(6):1014–1024
27. Cordon-Cardo C, Zhang ZF, Dalbagni G, Drobnjak M, Charytonowicz E, Hu SX, Xu HJ, Reuter VE, Benedict WF (1997) Cooperative effects of p53 and pRB alterations in primary superficial bladder tumors. Cancer Res 57 (7):1217–1221
28. Braasch MR, Bohle A, O'Donnell MA (2009) Intravesical instillation treatment of non–muscle-invasive bladder cancer. Eur Urol Suppl 8:549–555
29. Rosenberg JE, Hahn WC (2009) Bladder cancer: modeling and translation. Genes Dev 23:655–659
30. Zips D, Thames HD, Baumann M (2005) New anticancer agents: in vitro and in vivo evaluation. In Vivo 19(1):1–7
31. Van Dam D, De Deyn PP (2006) Drug discovery in dementia: the role of rodent models. Nat Rev Drug Discov 5:956–970
32. Oliveira PA, Gil da Costa RM, Vasconcelos-Nóbrega C, Arantes-Rodrigues R, Pinto-Leite R (2016) Challenges with in vitro and in vivo experimental models of urinary bladder cancer for novel drug discovery. Expert Opin Drug Discov 11(6):599–607
33. Gil da Costa RM, Oliveira PA, Vilanova M, Bastos MM, Lopes CC, Lopes C (2011) Ptaquiloside-induced B-cell lymphoproliferative and early-stage urothelial lesions in mice. Toxicon 58:543–549
34. Gil da Costa RM, Bastos MMSM, Oliveira PA, Lopes C (2012) Bracken-associated human and animal health hazards: chemical, biological

and pathological evidence. J Hazard Mater 203-204:1–12
35. Gil da Costa RM, Oliveira PA, Bastos MMSM, Lopes CC, Lopes C (2014) Ptaquiloside-induced early-stage urothelial lesions: increased cell proliferation and intact β-catenin and E-cadherin expression. Environ Toxicol 29:763–769
36. Knapp DW, Ramos-Vara JA, Moore GE et al (2014) Urinary bladder cancer in dogs, a naturally occurring model for cancer biology and drug development. ILAR J 55(1):100–118
37. Knapp DW, Waters DJ (1997) Naturally occurring cancer in pet dogs: important models for developing improved cancer therapy for humans. Mol Med Today 3(1):8–11
38. Lairmore MD, Khanna C (2014) Naturally occurring diseases in animals: contributions to translational medicine. ILAR J 55(1):1–3
39. Arentsen HC, Hendricksen K, Oosterwijk E, Witjes JA (2009) Experimental rat bladder urothelial cell carcinoma models. World J Urol 27(3):313–317
40. Ding J, Xu D, Pan C, Ye M, Kang J, Bai Q, Qi J (2014) Current animal models of bladder cancer: awareness of translatability (review). Exp Ther Med 8(3):691–699
41. Arantes-Rodrigues R, Colaço A, Pinto-Leite R, Oliveira PA (2013) In vitro and in vivo experimental models as tools to investigate the efficacy of antineoplastic drugs on urinary bladder cancer. Anticancer Res 33(4):1273–1296
42. Rosenbert MP, Bortner D (1998) Why transgenic and knockout animal models should be used (for drug efficacy studies in cancer). Cancer Metastasis Rev 17:295–299
43. Russell PJ, Raghavan D, Gregory P et al (1986) Bladder cancer xenografts: a model of tumor cell heterogeneity. Cancer Res 46:2035–2040
44. Günther JH, Jurczok A, Wulf T et al (1999) Optimizing syngeneic orthotopic murine bladder cancer (MB49). Cancer Res 59:2834–2837
45. Chan ESY, Patel AR, Smith AK et al (2009) Optimizing orthotopic bladder tumor implantation in a syngeneic mouse model. J Urol 183 (6):2926–2931
46. Oliveira PA, Colaço A, De la Cruz Palomino LF, Lopes C (2006) Experimental bladder carcinogenesis–rodent models. Exp Oncol 28:2–11
47. Gil da Costa RM, Oliveira PA, Vasconcelos-Nóbrega C, Arantes-Rodrigues R, Pinto-Leite R, Colaço A, de la Cruz PLF, Lopes C (2015) Altered expression of CKs 14/20 is an early event in a rat model of multistep bladder carcinogenesis. Int J Exp Pathol 96(5):319–325. doi:10.1111/iep.12145
48. Cohen SM (1983) Promotion in urinary bladder carcinogenesis. Environ Health Perspect 50:51–59
49. Johansson SL, Cohen SM (1997) Epidemiology and etiology of bladder cancer. Semin Surg Oncol 13:291–298
50. Cohen SM (2008) Tresholds in genotoxicity and carcinogenicity: urinary bladder carcinogenesis. Genes Environ 30(4):132–138
51. Jiang T, Lui T, Li L, Yang Z, Bai Y, Liu D, Kong C (2016) Knockout of phospholipase Cε attenuates N-butyl-N-(4-hydroxybutyl) nitrosamine-induced bladder tumorigenesis. Mol Med Rep 13:2039–2045
52. Bonfanti M, Magagnotti C, Bonati M, Fanelli R, Airoldi L (1988) Pharmacokinetic profile and metabolism of N-nitrosobutyl-(4-hydroxybutyl)amine in rats. Cancer Res 48:3666–3669
53. Mirvish SS (1995) Role of N-nitroso compounds (NOC) and N-nitrosation in etiology of gastric, esophageal, nasopharyngeal and bladder cancer and contribution to cancer of known exposures to NOC. Cancer Lett 93:17–48
54. Iida K, Itoh K, Maher JM, Kumagai Y, Oyasu R, Mori Y, Shimazui T, Akaza H, Yamamoto M (2007) Nrf2 and p53 cooperatively protect against BBN-induced urinary bladder carcinogenesis. Carcinogenesis 28(11):2398–2403
55. Suzuki E, Okada M (1980) Metabolic fate of N-butyl-N-(4-hydroxybutyl)nitrosamine in the rat. Gann 71(6):856–862
56. Mochizuki M, Suzuki E, Okada M (1997) Structure and metabolic fate of N-nitrosodialkylamines in relation to their organotropic carcinogenicity with special reference to induction of urinary bladder tumors. Yakugaku Zasshi 117(10-11):884–894
57. Cohen SM (1998) Urinary bladder carcinogenesis. Toxicol Pathol 26:121–127
58. Cohen SM, Ohnishi T, Clark NM, He J, Arnold LL (2007) Investigations of rodent urinary bladder carcinogens: collection, processing, and evaluation of urine and bladders. Toxicol Pathol 35(3):337–347
59. Okada M, Suzuki E, Hashimoto Y (1976) Carcinogenicity of N-nitrosamines related to N-butyl-N-(4-Hydroxybutyl)nitrosamine and N, N-Dibutylnitrosamine in ACI/N rats. Gann 67:825–834
60. Airoldi L, Magagnotti C, Bonfanti M, Fanelli R (1987) Development of an experimental model for studying bladder carcinogen metabolism using the isolated rat urinary bladder. Cancer Res 47:3697–3700
61. Yamamoto K, Nakata D, Tada M, Tonoki H, Nishida T, Hirai A, Ba Y, Aoyama T, Hamada J, Furuuchi K, Harada H, Hirai K, Shibahara N,

Katsuoka Y, Moriuchi T (1999) A functional and quantitative mutational analysis of p53 mutations in yeast indicates strand biases and different roles of mutations in DMBA- and BBN-induced tumors in rats. Int J Cancer 83:700–705

62. Weisburger JH, Williams GM (2000) The distinction between genotoxic and epigenetic carcinogens and implication for cancer risk. Toxicol Sci 57:4–5

63. Drago JR (2004) The noble rat bladder cancer model–FANFT induced Tumours. Cancer 53:1093–1099

64. Mann AM, Asamoto M, Chlapowski FJ, Masui T, Macatee TL, Cohen SM (1992) Ras involvement in cells transformed with 2-amino-4-(5-nitro-2-furyl)thiazole (ANFT) in vitro and with N-[4-(5-nitro-2-furyl)-2-thiazoyl]formamide in vivo. Carcinogenesis 13(9):1651–1655

65. Reis LO, Pereira TC, Favaro WJ, Cagnon VH, Lopes-Cendes I, Ferreira U (2009) Experimental animal model and RNA interference: a promising association for bladder cancer research. World J Urol 27:353

66. Spry LA, Rubinstein J, Rettke C, Zenser TV, Davis BB (1988) Renal metabolic/excretory coupling. Am J Physiol 254(1):F145–F152

67. Severs NJ, Barnes SH, Wright R, Hicks RM (1982) Induction of bladder cancer in rats by fractionated intravesicular doses of N-methyl-N-nitrosourea. Br J Cancer 45:337–351

68. Steinberg GD, Brendler CB, Ichikawa T, Squire RA, Isaacs JT (1990) Characterization of an N-methyl-N-nitrosourea-induced autochthonous rat bladder cancer model. Cancer Res 50(20):6668–6674

69. Vasconcelos-Nóbrega C, Colaço A, Lopes C, Oliveira PA (2012) Review: BBN as an urothelial carcinogen. In Vivo 26(4):727–739

70. Cohen SM, Friedell GH (1982) Neoplasms of the urinary system. In: The mouse in biomedical research. Academic Press, New York, pp 439–463

71. Ito N, Shirai T, Fukushima S, Hirose M (1984) Dose-response study of urinary bladder carcinogenesis in rats by N-butyl-N-(4-hydroxybutyl)nitrosamine. J Cancer Res Clin Oncol 108:169–173

72. Ohtani M, Kakizoe T, Nishio Y, Sato S, Sugimura T, Fukushima S, Niijima T (1986) Sequential changes of mouse bladder epithelium during induction of invasive carcinomas by *N*-butyl-*N*-(4-hydroxybutyl)nitrosamine. Cancer Res 46:2011–2004

73. Wanibuchi H, Wei M, Salim EI, Kinoshita A, Morimura K, Sudo K, Fukushima S (2006) Inhibition of rat urinary bladder carcinogenesis by the antiangiogenic drug TNP-470. Asian Pac J Cancer Prev 7:101–107

74. Wang SC, Huang CC, Shen CH, Lin LC, Zhao PW, Chen SY, Deng YC, Liu YW (2016) Gene expression and DNA methylationstatus of glutathione-S-transferase Mu1 and Mu5 in urothelial carcinoma. PLoS One 11:e0159102

75. Oliveira PA, Palmeira C, Lourenço L, Lopes C (2005) Evaluation of DNA content in preneoplastic changes of mouse urinary bladder induced by N-butyl-N-(4-hydroxybutyl) nitrosamine. J Exp Clin Cancer Res 24:207–214

76. Arantes-Rodrigues R, Henriques A, Pinto-Leite R, Faustino-Rocha A, Pinho-Oliveira J, Teixeira-Guedes C, Seixas F, Gama A, Colaço B, Colaço A, Oliveira PA (2012) The effects of repeated oral gavage on the health of male CD-1 mice. Lab Anim (NY) 41(5):129–134

77. Okada M, Ishidate M (1977) Metabolic fate of N-butyl-N-(4-hydroxybutyl)-nitrosamine and its analogues: selective induction of urinary bladder tumours in the rat. Xenobiotica 7 (1):11–24

78. Hashimoto Y, Suzuki K, Okada M (1974) Induction of urinary bladder tumors by intravesicular instillation of butyl(4-hydroxybutyl) nitrosoamine and its principal urinary metabolite, butyl(3-carboxypropyl)nitrosoamine in rats. Gann 65:69–73

79. Fuji K, Odashima S, Okada M (1977) Induction of tumours by administration of N-dibutylnitrosamine and derivatives to infant mice. Br J Cancer 35:610–614

80. Tsuda H, Miyata Y, Hagiwara A, Hasegawa R, Shirai T, Ito N (1977) Damage and repair of DNA in urinary bladder epithelium of rats treated with N-butyl-N-(4-hydroxybutyl) nitrosamine. Gann 68:781–783

81. Oliveira PA, Pires MJ, Nóbrega C, Arantes-Rodrigues R, Calado AM, Carrola J, Ginja M, Colaço A (2009) Technical report: technique of bladder catheterization in female mice and rats for intravesical instillation in models of bladder cancer. Scand J Lab Anim Sci 36(1):5–9

82. Xu J, Wang Y, Hua X, Xu J, Tian Z, Jin H, Li J, Wu XR, Huang C (2016) Inhibition of PHLPP2/cyclin D1 protein translation contributes to the tumor suppressive effect of NFκB2 (p100). Oncotarget 7:34112–34130

83. Suzuki E, Anjo T, Aoki J, Okada M (1983) Species variations in the metabolism of N-butyl-N-(4-hydroxybutyl)nitrosamine and related compounds in relation to urinary bladder carcinogenesis. Gann 74:60–68

84. Shin K, Lim A, Odegaard JI, Honeycutt JD, Kawano S, Hsieh MH, Beachy PA (2014) Cellular origin of bladder neoplasia and tissue

dynamics of its progression to invasive carcinoma. Nat Cell Biol 16:469–478

85. Van Loo PLP, Kruitwagenb CLJJ, Koolhaasc JM, Van de Weerdd HA, Van Zutphena LFM, Baumansa V (2002) Influence of cage enrichment on aggressive behaviour and physiological parameters in male mice. Appl Anim Behav Sci 76:65–81
86. Danneman PJ, Suckow MA, Brayton CF (2012) The laboratory mouse, 2nd edn. Taylor and Francis, London
87. Conn PM (2013) Animal models for the study of human disease, 1st edn. Elsevier, Amsterdam
88. Wolfer DP, Litvin O, Morf S, Nitsch RM, Lipp HP, Würbel H (2004) Laboratory animal welfare: cage enrichment and mouse behaviour. Nature 432:821–822
89. Gouveia K, Hurst JL (2013) Reducing mouse anxiety during handling: effect of experience with handling tunnels. PLoS One 8:e66401

Chapter 14

Patient-Derived Bladder Cancer Xenografts

Carina Bernardo and Lúcio Lara Santos

Abstract

Patient-derived xenograft (PDX) tumors are models developed by direct transplant of human tumors into immune-compromised hosts such as nude mice. These models retain the histological and genetic characteristics of the primary tumor and are considered a valuable platform for translational cancer research. This chapter describes the methodology to establish and propagate bladder cancer PDX model.

Key words Bladder cancer, Xenograft, Animal models, Tumorgraft, In vivo, Drug testing

1 Introduction

Over the past few years, there has been increasing interest in the development and use of patient-derived xenograft (PDX) models in translational cancer research, namely, for preclinical drug evaluation, biomarker identification, and personalized medicine strategies [1]. These models are generated from human tumor samples directly implanted, with minimum manipulation, into immunodeficient rodents, typically nude mice. PDX models provide significant improvements over standard cell line xenografts, as they better represent the heterogeneity and complexity of human tumors, preserve the primary tumor architecture and gene expression patterns, and are regarded as valuable platforms to study tumor response to therapeutic agents in a more realistic background [2, 3].

PDX models were first described more than 40 years ago [4–6]. Over the years, the development of a variety of immune-deficient hosts significantly reduced the complexity of the procedure and improved the tumor engraftment rate. PDX models have been created for several types of cancers such as lung, prostate, liver, pancreatic, and colon carcinomas [7–11].

Due to the significant expansion of the field over the past years, an initiative of translational and clinical researchers, the EuroOPDX consortium, was formed in Europe to create a network for clinically relevant and annotated models of human cancer, particularly PDX

Wolfgang A. Schulz et al. (eds.), *Urothelial Carcinoma: Methods and Protocols*, Methods in Molecular Biology, vol. 1655, DOI 10.1007/978-1-4939-7234-0_14, © Springer Science+Business Media LLC 2018

models (http://www.europdx.eu/) [1]. With the optimization of the establishment process and use of PDX models in a consistent way, they are likely to gradually play a broader role in the drug development process.

A few studies have reported the establishment of bladder cancer PDX, mainly subcutaneous models, which were shown to retain the histology and genetic characteristics of the original tumors even after serial passages in mice [12–15]. Recently, bladder cancer PDX models have been used to evaluate the response of the tumors to targeted therapy based on expression analysis of target pathways and genetic mutations [16, 17].

The main limitations observed in the establishment of bladder cancer xenograft models are the modest take rate (varying between 11% and 80%) and long lag period to establish the first passage (up to 4 months) [18]. After successful establishment in the first, human to mice passage, the engraftment rate in the subsequent passages is almost 100% and the lag period becomes significantly shorter. The implantation of multiple fragments per through small dorsal incisions and the use of were associated with higher engraftment success [18]. Advanced disease stage and high-grade tumors were also associated with higher probability of successful xenograft establishment. The establishment of bladder cancer PDXs under the renal capsule, too, has recently been reported to yield a high success rate [17]. The under renal capsule space has emerged as a promising alternative to the subcutaneous compartment, especially for tumor types more difficult to grow in mice, and is generally associated with a higher success rate. However, establishing this model is technically more complex and as it requires bioimaging techniques to monitor tumor growth, this approach is less frequently employed.

Other aspects that should be considered include the replacement of stromal components and lack of immune response. Therefore, PDX models are not suitable for the evaluation of agents directed against factors in the tumor microenvironment (e.g., angiogenesis, stroma, or inflammatory cells).

In this protocol, we present methods to establish subcutaneous human bladder cancer xenografts in nude mice from patient tumor samples and for the serial transfer of xenografts grown in mice.

2 Materials

1. Human bladder cancer tissue samples or tumorgrafts (fresh or cryopreserved).
2. 5–7 weeks old male athymic (nu/nu) or NOD-SCID mice.
3. Collection medium; RPMI 1640 medium, 10% FBS, and 1% penicillin/streptomycin (cold).

4. Freezing medium; RPMI 1640 medium, 20% FBS, 10% DMSO (cold).
5. Matrigel basement membrane matrix.
6. Isoflurane.
7. 70% ethanol.
8. 50 ml tubes (sterile).
9. 1–2 ml cryovials tubes (sterile).
10. Sterile instruments (microsurgery scissors, scalpel, curved, and straight forceps, 7–9 mm surgical clips/staples or sutures).
11. Sterile gauze pads.
12. Mouse identification equipment.
13. Anesthesia chamber and equipment for euthanasia.
14. Sterile personal protective equipment.
15. Digital scale.
16. Caliper.

All animal experiments should be conducted according to the guidelines for the welfare and use of animals in research [19] and relevant national regulations. The protocol must be reviewed and approved by the animal care and use committee of the animal facility.

3 Methods

3.1 Processing the Tumor Samples

1. For each individual patient, place the freshly excised tumor tissue (one or several pieces) into a 50 ml tube containing cold sterile collection medium. The specimen should be collected by a pathologist after confirming the presence of viable tumor tissue. Immediately transport the tubes on ice to the animal facility (*see* **Note 1**).

The following steps and all the in vivo procedures should be undertaken in a class 2 biological safety cabinet using the sterile personal protective equipment. The working area must be previously disinfected with 20% bleach solution or another adequate disinfectant followed by 70% ethanol.

2. Transfer the tumor tissue to a Petri dish containing cold sterile 10% RPMI 1640 medium so that enough medium is present to cover the tumor.
3. Remove all adjacent normal tissue from the tumor, using curved/straight forceps and scissors. Cut in half and remove any necrotic tissue if present. The necrotic human tissue is generally white and softer compared to the surrounding tumor or present as liquefied tissue at the center of a large tumor.

4. Gently wash the tumor in the medium-containing dish and transfer to a new Petri dish containing collection medium.
5. Cut the tumor into small fragments (3 × 3 × 3 mm) as uniform as possible.
6. Place the tumor fragments into a cold sterile 2 ml tube with 1 ml Matrigel and incubate for about 10 min before implantation. The use of Matrigel is optional. Alternatively, place the tumor fragments into a cold sterile 2 ml tube with 1 ml collection medium. Maintain the tubes on ice until implantation.

3.2 Transplant

1. Place the animals in the anesthesia induction chamber following the manufacturer's recommendations settings where they are exposed to vaporized isoflurane. Once sedated, transfer the animal to the surgical platform with the dorsal side facing upward and place it in a nose cone with isoflurane to maintain anesthesia. Pinch the footpad to confirm that the mouse is in the proper plane of anesthesia to start the procedure and monitor throughout the procedure.
2. Using a gauze saturated with 70% ethanol, sanitize the area where the tumor will be implanted, usually the flanks.
3. Make a small skin incision (1–1.5 cm) on one of the flanks using the surgical scissors.
4. Insert the tip of straight forceps into the incision and open to create a pocket in the subcutaneous space.
5. Place a tumor fragment into the pocket created using forceps.
6. Close the incision with wound clips or suture. Make sure the tumor fragment does not come into contact with the clips. Wipe the incision site with sterile gauze.
7. Repeat **steps 8–12** on the contralateral flank.
8. Identify each mouse and place the animal in a clean cage. Observe to ensure recovery from the anesthetic.
9. Repeat **steps 7–14**. Depending on the tumor availability, use up to 6–8 mice per tumor specimen to increase the probability of successful take in the first passage.

3.3 Mouse Monitoring

1. Carefully monitor the mice during the immediate postoperative period and daily for 3–5 days thereafter. Monitor body weight, temperature and for signs of suffering. Remove clips within 7–9 days.
2. Check for tumor growth weekly and begin making tumor measurements when a consistent mass is noticeable. Use a caliper to measure the longest and shortest diameter two times per week.
3. Calculate the tumor volume using the following formula [20].

$$\text{Tumor volume} = \frac{[\text{length} \times \text{width}^2]}{2}$$

3.4 In Vivo Passaging and Treatment Cohort

When the tumorgraft reaches approximately 1.5 cm^3 in volume, it must be excised for analysis or transplantation into additional mice generating subsequent passages that can be used to expand the tumor material or to create a treatment cohort (*see* **Note 2**).

1. Euthanize the mouse by CO_2 asphyxiation.
2. Sanitize the mouse skin over the tumor with 70% ethanol.
3. Make an incision to expose the tumor using forceps and surgical scissors. Carefully remove all skin and attached tissues from the surface of the tumor and remove the tumor.
4. Proceed as described in Subheadings 3.1 and 3.2 (*see* **Notes 3** and **5**).
5. When using the tumors in treatment cohorts, wait until tumors reach a volume of ~200 mm^3 before allocating mice to treatment groups and initiating treatment. The average tumor size should be similar across all treatment groups at the time of randomization. The number of tumors per arm can vary depending on the characteristics of the study, typically 5–10 tumors per study group are used to evaluate response.
6. Measure the tumors using calipers and weigh mice two to three times per week. Calculate the tumor volume using the formula presented above (*see* **Note 4**).
7. Sacrifice the mice at the end of the experiment, when tumor volumes reach the maximum acceptable tumor load or if the mice present any other humane endpoint [19].
8. Collect the tumor and any other organs needed for analysis (*see* **Note 5**).

4 Notes

1. To maintain viability, tumor samples must be kept on ice and transplanted as soon as possible, ideally in less than 2 h. Prolonged time between tumor excision and transplant can contribute for low take rate [21].
2. Characterization of the xenografts in terms of histology, molecular and genetic profile and comparison with the primary human tumor is important to confirm tumor integrity. This analysis should be performed at each passage and in the cohort of the tumors used for drug testing. Morphology of the primary tumors and tumors grown in mice can be compared by H&E staining including the histological subtype, differentiation grade, and cellular components of the tumors. Gene expression

and mutation analysis can be evaluated using several methodologies including microarray, exome sequencing, and immunohistochemistry. Genotype, karyotype, and copy number variation analysis by comparative genome hybridization are also commonly used to evaluate the genetic integrity of the xenografts.

3. In the second passage, the cohort is expanded to obtain sufficient material to establish the treatment cohort. During the establishment and expansion phase, the implant of two tumors per mouse, one in each flank, is advised to minimize the number of animals required and cost [22]. The same approach can be used in the treatment cohort, considering each tumor graft as an independent tumor unit. However, the application of this method to generate the treatment cohort will depend on the ability to generate tumors growing at the same rate in previous passages.
4. To minimize measure variations, the same well-trained investigator should be involved for the duration of one study. Efficacy of the treatments can be evaluated using several methods. Common measures of efficacy include the ratio of the mean tumor volume in control VS-treated mice at a specified time (T/C ratio), the relative tumor growth inhibition (TGI) index, defined as (1-(mean volume of treated tumors)/(mean volume of control tumors))*100, and the tumor growth delay (TGD) defined as the difference in days for treated VS control tumors to reach as specified volume or to double their volume.
5. For histological and immunohistochemistry analysis, the tumor samples can be fixed in 10% paraformaldehyde and processed into paraffin blocks. For genomic and protein analysis, collect tumor fragments in cryovials, place in liquid nitrogen or dry ice until frozen and store at −80 °C.

   For cryopreservation of tumor samples, cut the specimen into 4 × 4 × 4 mm fragments and place them in cryovials containing cold Freezing medium, up to 5 fragments per vial. Freeze the samples by slowly decreasing the temperature in a slow freezing container and store at −80 °C for one night before transferring to liquid nitrogen for long-term storage.

References

1. Hidalgo M, Amant F, Biankin AV et al (2014) Patient-derived Xenograft models: an emerging platform for translational cancer research. Cancer Discov 4:998–1013. doi:10.1158/2159-8290.CD-14-0001
2. Tentler JJ, Tan AC, Weekes CD et al (2012) Patient-derived tumour xenografts as models for oncology drug development. Nat Rev Clin Oncol 9:338–350. doi:10.1038/nrclinonc.2012.61
3. Voskoglou-nomikos T, Pater JL, Seymour L (2003) Clinical predictive value of the in vitro cell line, human Xenograft, and mouse allograft preclinical cancer models. Clin Cancer Res 9:4227–4239
4. Cobb LM (1973) The behaviour of carcinoma of the large bowel in man following transplantation into immune deprived mice. Br J Cancer 28:400–411

5. Houghton JA, Houghton PJ, Green AA (1982) Chemotherapy of childhood rhabdomyosarcomas growing as xenografts in immune-deprived mice. Cancer Res 42:535–539
6. Fiebig HH, Schuchhardt C, Henss H et al (1984) Comparison of tumor response in nude mice and in the patients. Behring Inst Mitt:343–352
7. Hidalgo M, Bruckheimer E, Rajeshkumar NV et al (2011) A pilot clinical study of treatment guided by personalized tumorgrafts in patients with advanced cancer. Mol Cancer Ther 10:1311–1316. doi:10.1158/1535-7163.MCT-11-0233
8. Fichtner I, Slisow W, Gill J et al (2004) Anticancer drug response and expression of molecular markers in early-passage xenotransplanted colon carcinomas. Eur J Cancer 40:298–307. doi:10.1016/j.ejca.2003.10.011
9. Merk J, Rolff J, Becker M et al (2009) Patient-derived xenografts of non-small-cell lung cancer: a pre-clinical model to evaluate adjuvant chemotherapy? Eur J Cardiothorac Surg 36:454–459. doi:10.1016/j.ejcts.2009.03.054
10. Whittle JR, Lewis MT, Lindeman GJ, Visvader JE (2015) Patient-derived xenograft models of breast cancer and their predictive power. Breast Cancer Res 17:17. doi:10.1186/s13058-015-0523-1
11. Mattie M, Christensen A, Chang MS et al (2013) Molecular characterization of patient-derived human pancreatic tumor Xenograft models for preclinical and translational development of cancer therapeutics 1,2. Neoplasia 15:1138–1150. doi:10.1593/neo.13922
12. Park B, Jeong BC, Choi Y-LL et al (2013) Development and characterization of a bladder cancer xenograft model using patient-derived tumor tissue. Cancer Sci 104:1–8. doi:10.1111/cas.12123
13. Bernardo C, Costa C, Amaro T et al (2014) Patient-derived sialyl-Tn-positive invasive bladder cancer xenografts in nude mice: an exploratory model study. Anticancer Res 34:735–744
14. McCue PA, Gomella LG, Veltri RW et al (1996) Development of secondary structure, growth characteristics and cytogenetic analysis of human transitional cell carcinoma xenografts in scid/scid mice. J Urol 155:1128–1132
15. Abe T, Tada M, Shinohara N et al (2006) Establishment and characterization of human urothelial cancer xenografts in severe combined immunodeficient mice. Int J Urol 13:47–57. doi:10.1111/j.1442-2042.2006.01220.x
16. Pan C, Zhang H, Tepper CG et al (2015) Development and characterization of bladder cancer patient-derived Xenografts for molecularly guided targeted therapy. PLoS One 10:e0134346. doi:10.1371/journal.pone.0134346
17. Jäger W, Xue H, Hayashi T et al (2015) Patient-derived bladder cancer xenografts in the preclinical development of novel targeted therapies. Oncotarget 6:21522–21532. doi:10.18632/oncotarget.3974
18. Bernardo C, Costa C, Sousa N et al (2015) Patient-derived bladder cancer xenografts: a systematic review. Transl Res 166:324–331. doi:10.1016/j.trsl.2015.02.001
19. Workman P, Aboagye EO, Balkwill F et al (2010) Guidelines for the welfare and use of animals in cancer research. Br J Cancer 102:1555–1577. doi:10.1038/sj.bjc.6605642
20. Rubio-Viqueira B, Jimeno A, Cusatis G et al (2006) An platform for translational drug development in pancreatic cancer. Clin Cancer Res 12:4652–4661. doi:10.1158/1078-0432.CCR-06-0113
21. Choi YY, Lee JE, Kim H et al (2016) Establishment and characterisation of patient-derived xenografts as paraclinical models for gastric cancer. Sci Rep 6:22172. doi:10.1038/srep22172
22. Calles A, Rubio-Viqueira B, Hidalgo M (2013) Primary human non-small cell lung unit and pancreatic tumorgraft models-utility and applications in drug discovery and tumor biology. Curr Protoc Pharmacol:1–21. doi:10.1002/0471141755.ph1426s61

Chapter 15

Orthotopic Mouse Models of Urothelial Cancer

Wolfgang Jäger, Igor Moskalev, Peter Raven, Akihiro Goriki, Samir Bidnur, and Peter C. Black

Abstract

Orthotopic mouse models of urothelial cancer are essential for testing novel therapies and molecular manipulations of cell lines in vivo. These models are either established by orthotopic inoculation of human (xenograft models) or murine tumor cells (syngeneic models) in immunocompromised or immune competent mice. Current techniques rely on inoculation by intravesical instillation or direct injection into the bladder wall. Alternative models include the induction of murine bladder tumors by chemical carcinogens (BBN) or genetic engineering (GEM).

Key words Chemical carcinogens, Intramural injection, Intravesical instillation, Orthotopic models, Transgenic models, Tumor cell inoculation, Xenografts

1 Introduction

In vivo models of human cancer are essential for analysis of tumor biology by molecular manipulation, identification of relevant diagnostic and predictive biomarkers, and preclinical testing of novel antineoplastic therapeutic agents. Although multiple models of human tumors have been developed in different animal species, mice constitute the gold standard due to their ease of housing, suitable size for surgical procedures, and cost effectiveness [1]. The favored location for growth of murine tumor models is the organ of origin of that tumor. These orthotopic tumor models optimally mimic the physiological, organ-specific microenvironment and allow consistent local tumor growth, vascular and lymphatic invasion, tumor cell seeding, and metastasis to organ-specific sites [2].

For bladder cancer research orthotopic murine tumor models can be established either in immunocompromised or immune competent hosts. Immunocompromised mice (especially athymic nude and NOD-SCID mice) are used for the inoculation of human tumor cell lines by either intravesical instillation or intramural injection. These orthotopic xenografts are a valuable tool for

Wolfgang A. Schulz et al. (eds.), *Urothelial Carcinoma: Methods and Protocols*, Methods in Molecular Biology, vol. 1655, DOI 10.1007/978-1-4939-7234-0_15, © Springer Science+Business Media LLC 2018

preclinical testing of novel therapeutic agents [2, 3]. The main limitation of these models is the absence of stroma from the original bladder tumor, which has been shown to highly influence tumor biology and growth [4]. Xenograft models retaining stromal cells and particular architectural features of human tumors can be achieved by transplantation of representative tissue fragments from human tumors into favorable organ sites of immunocompromised mice (patient-derived primary xenografts; PDX) [5]. PDX models have been established for bladder cancer [6, 7]. They best represent the heterogeneous genetic landscape of human bladder cancers and are the closest model to the human disease.

The major shortcoming of all xenograft tumor models, whether derived from cell lines or patient tumors, is the absence of a competent immune system in the host. Therefore, the effect of the immune system in cancer progression or regression cannot be assessed, and immunotherapies cannot be adequately tested. Bladder tumor models in immunocompetent mice can be induced either by inoculation of murine tumor cell lines into the bladder of immunocompetent mice [8], exposure of mice to carcinogen chemicals [9], or genetic engineering [9, 10]. The major drawback of these models pertains to the differences in the biology between murine and human tumors, as well as the environment of murine and human hosts.

1.1 Intravesical Orthotopic Bladder Xenograft Model

Intravesical instillation of tumor cells into the lumen of the bladder establishes tumors that grow primarily on the surface of the urothelium and secondarily invade into the bladder wall [11]. This "superficial" model is suitable for preclinical testing of intravesical therapies. Intravesical therapies avoid many potential toxicities of systemic treatment, but it is critical to test the propensity of candidate agents to penetrate the intact urothelium. The typical cell lines used in this model, however, tend to be highly invasive and even metastatic, so that the biology of xenografts generated in the intravesical model is not necessarily representative of non-muscle invasive bladder cancer.

Many variations of the basic method for intravesical instillation of bladder cancer cells have been described. This is because it has proven to be extraordinarily challenging using these methods to achieve reliable tumor take with any cell lines other than KU7, which we have recently demonstrated to be HeLa [12]. Furthermore, intravesical cell inoculation is time consuming and can lead to uncontrolled tumor growth in other segments of the urinary tract (urethra, ureter, renal pelvis) [13]. Finally, tumor location within the bladder is unpredictable, such that growth around the ureteral orifices can cause severe upper tract obstruction before mice reach therapeutic endpoints.

The same methods can also be used for the instillation of murine bladder cancer cells into the murine bladder to generate a model of non-muscle invasive bladder cancer in an immune competent host [8].

1.2 Intramural Orthotopic Xenograft Model: Open Technique

Direct injection of human tumor cells into the bladder wall of immunocompromised mice leads to the formation of invasive bladder tumor xenografts that are suitable for systemic treatments [14]. The utilized cell lines have usually been transduced with a lentiviral construct carrying the luciferase gene, which allows measurement of tumor burden longitudinally during the study by monitoring luminescence, although monitoring by ultrasound or other imaging modality is an alternative. Most cell lines grow reliably as xenografts in this model.

Intramural tumor inoculation can be conducted either after laparotomy and surgical exposure of the bladder [15], or percutaneously by ultrasound guidance [16]. The same procedures can be performed using murine bladder tumor cells into the bladder wall of immunocompetent mice.

Direct injection of tumor cells into the bladder wall after laparotomy and mobilization of the bladder is a well-established and reproducible method of orthotopic xenograft inoculation [14, 15]. Limitations include the invasiveness of the procedure which can inflict significant morbidity on the host mouse [15], and the technical challenge of ensuring adequate injection into the bladder wall. This method is associated with a significant learning curve.

1.3 Intramural Orthotopic Xenograft Model: Percutaneous Ultrasound-Guided Technique

The percutaneous, ultrasound-guided approach for the injection of bladder cancer cells into the bladder wall addresses existing limitations of the open technique (*see* Subheading 1.2). The major advantages of this model lie in the rapidity and ease of tumor inoculation, low morbidity inflicted on the mice, accurate localization of xenograft tumors, as well as reproducibility of the model [16]. Consequently, this technique has superseded the open procedure in research facilities with the capacity to use this model.

1.4 Ultrasound-Guided Intratumoral Injection of Therapeutic Agents

This section describes an experimental treatment modality in which therapeutic agents are locally delivered into bladder tumors by injection. Potential treatment strategies using this methodology include oncolytic viruses, gene therapies, immune-modulating agents, and nanoparticles [16–18]. As an example of the relevance of intratumoral injection in the treatment of human cancers, the intratumoral injection of DNA plasmid has recently been tested in the therapy of unresectable pancreatic cancers [19]. The advantage of an ultrasound-guided minimally invasive approach consists in the excellent visualization of the targeted bladder tumor and low morbidity inflicting on the host mouse. Accordingly, multiple cycles of treatment are feasible.

1.5 Chemical Carcinogen-Induced Model of Urothelial Cancer

Murine models of urothelial cancer induced by chemical carcinogens provide the opportunity to mimic bladder cancer in an immune-competent host, at the cost of having tissue of murine, and not human, origin. Strong evidence supports a similar series of oncogenic events in carcinogen-induced models of murine carcinoma and human urothelial carcinoma [9, 20–23]. These models represent an ideal in vivo platform to assess novel therapies that depend on an active and unaltered immune system. The most common carcinogen used in these studies is N-butyl-N-(4-hydroxybutyl)-nitrosamine (BBN). BBN appears to be highly specific to the bladder, reliably inducing bladder cancer while sparing other organ systems, as opposed to other carcinogens like 2-aminoacetylfluorene (AAF) which are potent inducers of carcinogenesis in multiple tissue types [22]. As a natural carcinogen, BBN also induces a degree of tumor heterogeneity that may mimic natural carcinogenesis in humans. This distinguishes BBN-induced tumors from the genetically engineered models described below.

BBN is provided in the drinking water of mice at 0.05% v/v ad libitum for a period of 8–12 weeks, after which it is discontinued and mice are observed for clinical signs of tumor growth (hematuria, ultrasound findings, lower abdominal mass) which can take up to 6 months to develop. High-grade tumors develop through stages from carcinoma in situ, through superficially invasive tumors to muscle invasive and metastatic tumors. While the dose of BBN cannot be reliably measured, approaches including gastric gavage have been described but tend to be associated with unnecessary mouse distress and trauma.

The natural history of BBN-induced tumors also makes these suitable for studies of chemoprevention [23]. Most recently, they have been used to study the cellular origin of bladder cancer [24]. Similar carcinogen-induced bladder cancer in rats is a frequently used alternative model [25].

1.6 Genetically Engineered Model of Urothelial Cancer

Activation of oncogenes such as H-Ras or loss of function in tumor suppressor genes such as RB1 and TP53 in the urothelium is considered critical for the development of urothelial tumors [26, 27]. These alterations can be exploited to generate genetically engineered models (GEM) of bladder cancer. GEMs are now used widely for many applications in cancer biology, including analyses of tumor phenotypes, modeling disease subtypes, mechanistic investigations of candidate genes and signaling pathways, and preclinical evaluation of potential therapeutic agents [28–30]. GEM models complement non-autochthonous mouse models, as tumors arise de novo in the native tissue microenvironment, and they also complement carcinogen-based models, as they are based on defined genetic alterations.

1.6.1 Transgenic Models

The earliest GEM models of bladder cancer were transgenic mice in which simian virus 40 (SV40) large T antigen was expressed in the urothelium under the control of the tissue-specific uroplakin-2 (*Upk2*) promoter[32]. SV40 induces loss of both TP53 and RB1. These transgenic mice develop CIS and invasive bladder cancer, with some progressing to metastasis [30, 31], and their molecular profiles are similar to human bladder cancer [32].

Activation of the oncogenes H-Ras [33] or EGFR [34] leads to hyperplasia and papillary, noninvasive tumors. In this respect, GEMs recapitulate the dual pathway of bladder cancer development that distinguishes papillary tumors from CIS and invasive, non-papillary tumors [35]. Some of the combined alterations (e.g., H-Ras activation and loss of TP53) also show noninvasive bladder cancer [35–38]. As discussed above in the context of intravesical and intramural xenograft inoculation, different types and stages of disease are suitable for different types of experiments, depending on the proposed clinical context in patients.

1.6.2 Conditional Transgenic Models

The majority of recent GEM models of cancer involve tissue-specific conditional or inducible gene targeting by using Cre-lox recombination. Conditional activation of β-catenin (*Ctnnb1*) in the bladder using a Cre driver based on the expression of the *Upk2* promoter results in hyperplasia [39], and together with activation of H-Ras or K-Ras or loss of function of PTEN, results in papillary noninvasive carcinoma [39, 40]. However, with an alternative, non-bladder-specific Cre driver, activation of β-catenin alone results in papillary noninvasive cancer [41]. Moreover, suppression of Notch pathway by the inactivation of nicastrin (*Ncstn*) results in hyperplasia and CIS, whereas inactivation of nicastrin using a ubiquitously expressed promoter results in muscle invasive bladder cancer [42]. Certainly, these differences may be due to the actions of Notch outside of the urothelium.

Another method using tissue-specific Cre alleles to target gene recombination is the delivery of Cre-recombinase-expressing adenovirus (adeno-Cre) directly into the bladder lumen. This method has been used to inactivate TP53 and PTEN in the urothelium, resulting in invasive bladder cancer with metastasis [43]. This approach has also been used to inactivate RB1 and p130, resulting in papillary noninvasive cancer [44].

The main limitation of GEMs is the lack of tumor heterogeneity compared to human bladder tumors. This means that any given GEM likely only represents a subset of tumors, or even a subset of clones within a given tumor. Furthermore, since both the tumor cells and the host are murine, the model may not adequately represent the human disease [45].

2 Materials

2.1 Intravesical Orthotopic Bladder Xenograft Model

1. Angiocatheter 24G (BD Bioscience; 381112).
2. 2% Chlorhexidine gluconate (Aplicare; 82–319).

3. Dulbecco's modified Eagle's medium (DMEM) (Thermo Scientific;SH3008101).
4. Fetal bovine serum (FBS) (Thermo Scientific; SH3007103).
5. Isoflurane (Baxter Corporation; 402–069-02).
6. IVIS Spectrum In Vivo Imaging System (PerkinElmer; 124262).
7. Prolene 6–0 (Ethicon; EH7226H).
8. Sterile filtered phosphate buffered saline (PBS) (Sigma; P4417).
9. 1 ml Syringe (BD Bioscience; 309659).
10. 0.25% Trypsin (Thermo Scientific; SH3004202).
11. Vascu-statt midi (straight) (Scanlan; #1001–500).
12. Xenolight D-Luciferin –K+ Salt bioluminescent substrate (PerkinElmer; 122799).

2.2 Intramural Orthotopic Xenograft Model: Open Technique

1. Angiocatheter 24G n(BD Bioscience; 381112).
2. 2% Chlorhexidine gluconate (Aplicare; 82–319).
3. Dulbecco's modified Eagle's medium (DMEM) (Thermo Scientific; SH3008101).
4. Fetal bovine serum (FBS) (Thermo Scientific; SH3007103).
5. Hypodermic needle (30G; ¾ in.) (Kendall; 830340).
6. Isoflurane (Baxter Corporation; 402–069-02).
7. Sterile cotton tip applicators (Medline; MDS202000).
8. Sterile filtered phosphate buffered saline (PBS) (Sigma; P4417).
9. Surgical instruments (scissors, forceps, needle driver).
10. Syringe (1 ml) (BD Bioscience; 309659).
11. 0.25% Trypsin (Thermo Scientific; SH3004202).
12. Vicryl 4–0 (Ethicon; V326H).

2.3 Intramural Orthotopic Xenograft Model: Percutaneous Ultrasound Guided Technique

1. Angiocatheter (24G) (BD Bioscience; 381112).
2. 2% Chlorhexidine gluconate (Aplicare; 82–319).
3. Dulbecco's modified Eagle's medium (DMEM) (Thermo Scientific; SH3008101).
4. Fetal bovine serum (FBS) (Thermo Scientific; SH3007103).
5. Hypodermic needle (30G; ¾ in.) (Kendall; 830340).
6. Isoflurane (Baxter Corporation; 402–069-02).
7. Matrigel®* (BD Bioscience; 356234).
8. Vevo 770® small animal imaging platform (Visual Sonics).
9. RMV 706 ultrasound scanhead (Visual Sonics).

10. Syringe (1 ml) (BD Bioscience; 309659).
11. 0.25 Trypsin (Thermo Scientific; SH3004202).
12. Ultrasound gel.

2.4 Ultrasound Guided Intratumoral Injection of Therapeutic Agents

See Subheading 2.3, additionally any dissolvable therapeutic agent dissolved in an appropriate volume.

2.5 Chemical Carcinogen Induced Model of Urothelial Cancer

1. BBN (N-butyl-N-(4-hydroxybutyl)nitrosamine) (TCI America; B0938).
2. Isoflurane (Baxter Corporation; 402–069-02).
3. RMV 706 ultrasound scanhead (Visual Sonics).
4. Vevo 770® small animal imaging platform (Visual Sonics).

3 Methods

3.1 Intravesical Orthotopic Bladder Xenograft Model

3.1.1 Preparation of Cell Lines

1. Confirm the identity of the respective human bladder cancer cell lines by DNA fingerprinting [12] prior to any further actions.
2. For growth analysis of xenograft tumors by bioluminescence perform a transfection of cell lines with a lentiviral construct carrying the firefly luciferase gene, such as UM-UC-3luc [11].
3. Thaw and expand the existing cell lines in Dulbecco's modified Eagle's medium (DMEM) with 10% fetal bovine serum (FBS) at 37 °C in a humidified, 5% CO_2 atmosphere. Make sure to perform at least three passages but avoid culture times exceeding 3 months.

3.1.2 Preparation of Cell Suspension

1. Trypsinize luciferase transduced cells at a confluence of 70%, suspend them in normal growth media.
2. Calculate the absolute cell number.
3. Spin the cell suspension for 5 min at 180 × *g*. Remove the supernatant and resuspend in PBS at a concentration of 5×10^5 cells per 50 μl (*see* **Note 1**).
4. Immediately place cells on ice until use.

3.1.3 Preparation of Animals

1. Always keep and house mice according to the guidelines of the respective national animal care committee. Make sure that all interventions are described in detail and approved prior to any further actions.
2. Weigh the mouse prior to surgery.

3. Anesthetize with an inhalational agent (isoflurane) applied through a nose cone. Anesthesia is induced with 2.0–3.0% isoflurane and maintained with 1.5–2.0% isoflurane. Preoperative analgesia is provided with buprenorphine (0.10 mg/kg) and meloxicam (2 ml/kg) injected under the skin of the scruff of the neck after induction of anesthesia. Adequate depth of anesthesia is confirmed by lack of toe pinch reflex. The ears are notched or marked with ink for identification. Eye lubricant is applied to each eye.

3.1.4 Tumor Cell Instillation

1. Mount the animal in supine position on a heated table with the limbs fixed to the table with adhesive tape (Fig. 1).
2. Disinfect the lower abdomen and urethral meatus with 2% chlorhexidine gluconate and wipe the skin with a sterile cotton tip.
3. Place a superficial 6–0 monofilament purse-string suture around the urethral meatus with three stitches using a cutting needle in order to temporarily obstruct the urethra in **step 10** (Fig. 1). Alternatively, an atraumatic bulldog clamp can be used after instillation of tumor cells.
4. Palpate the lower abdomen above the bladder gently to empty the bladder of urine.
5. Grasp the urethral meatus with atraumatic forceps and carefully extend it.
6. Pass a 24G angiocatheter transurethrally into the bladder. Allow the bladder to empty if urine drains through the catheter.

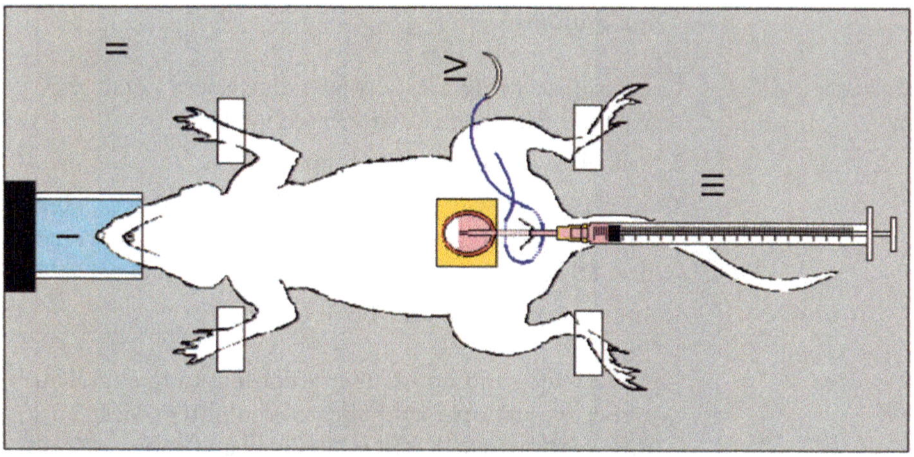

Fig. 1 Orthotopic superficial bladder xenograft model: illustration of the experimental setup. The anesthetized mouse (nose cone; I) is mounted on the heated operation table (II). A 1 ml syringe with attached 24G angiocatheter is inserted through urethra (III). A purse-string suture using Prolene 6–0 with an oval needle is placed around the urethral meatus with three stitches (IV)

7. Attach a 1 ml syringe preloaded with 0.25% trypsin and inject 20 μl into the bladder lumen.
8. Leave the angiocatheter and syringe in place and let the trypsin dwell for 15 min. Then detach the syringe and express the bladder as described in four. The trypsin should exit the angiocatheter.
9. Attach a 1 ml syringe preloaded with UM-UC3-luc cell suspension and inject 50 μl cell suspension into the bladder. Some protocols add a step to irrigate the bladder with PBS or FBS-containing medium to clear the bladder of trypsin prior to cell instillation, but we have found this to be unnecessary.
10. Tighten the suture as the angiocatheter is removed and tie it off to temporarily obstruct the urethra.
11. Let the cells dwell for 1.5 h with the mice under maintenance anesthesia (*see* **Note 2**).
12. Release the suture and express the cell suspension from the bladder.

3.1.5 Post-interventional Supportive Care

1. Dismount the mouse from the operating table.
2. Keep the animal in a warm and comfortable environment under continuous surveillance.
3. After the animal has regained consciousness and resumed normal ambulation, place it back in its home cage.

3.1.6 Tumor Imaging

(*See* **Notes 3** and **4**)

1. If using this protocol in mice with fur, shave the abdominal area of the mouse 1 day prior to imaging to maximize light transmission through the skin.
2. Anesthetize mice with isoflurane and inject 150 mg/kg of luciferin intra-peritoneally using a 30G½ needle.
3. Place mice in a supine position in a bioluminescent imager (IVIS Spectrum or like system) while under maintenance anesthesia.
4. Capture an image of the abdominal area at 10 min following luciferin injection. Quantify the tumor burden by defining the abdominal area as a region of interest and recording the photons/s.
5. Allow the mice to recover in a heated chamber and return to cage when normal behavior resumes.

3.1.7 Intravesical Administration of Therapeutic Agents

1. Follow the procedure as described in "Tumor cell instillation" up to **step 6**.
2. Attach a 1 ml syringe preloaded with the compound of interest to the angiocatheter and inject a volume of not more than 100 μl into the bladder.

3. Tighten the suture as the angiocatheter is removed and tie it off to temporarily obstruct the urethra. Alternatively, an atraumatic bulldog clamp can be used.
4. Let the compound dwell for an appropriate time not to exceed 2.5 h with the mice under maintenance anesthesia.
5. Release the suture and express the agent from the bladder.
6. Allow the mice to recover in a heated chamber and return to cage when normal behavior resumes.

3.2 Intramural Orthotopic Xenograft Model: Open Technique

3.2.1 Preparation of Cell Lines

Prepare cell lines as described in Subheading 3.1.1.

3.2.2 Preparation of Cell Suspension

Prepare cell suspension as described in Subheading 3.1.2.

3.2.3 Preparation of Animals

Prepare animals as described in Subheading 3.1.3.

3.2.4 Experimental Setup

1. Mount the animal on a heated operating table with continuous monitoring of vital signs.
2. Use sterile surgical instruments (autoclaving before inoculation and sterilization with bead sterilizer between animals).
3. Scrub the abdominal wall of mouse three times with chlorhexidine followed by one wipe with alcohol.

3.2.5 Surgical Procedure

1. Make a 1 cm horizontal incision on the lower abdomen just above the pubic bone (Pfannenstiel incision). The bladder is readily found in the pelvis.
2. Bring the bladder up into the incision using sterile cotton-tip applicators.
3. Compress the bladder with the cotton tip in order to empty its contents.
4. Inject the bladder cancer cells directly into the front wall and dome of the bladder. Use a 30G needle attached to a 1 ml syringe. The total volume injected is 100 μl. Prior experience has shown that this volume gives the most reliable and easily recognizable (by visual inspection) bleb in the bladder wall, indicating a successful intramural (and not intravesical) injection.
5. Allow the bladder to fall back into the pelvis.

6. Infiltrate a 0.075% (75 μg/ml) bupivicaine solution with a 30G needle locally around the incision in the subcutaneous layer and abdominal wall musculature in a quantity of 10 μl per gram mouse body weight (7.5 mg/kg; maximum recommended dose is 8 mg/kg). The maximum injected volume should be 250 μl.
7. Close the abdominal wall in two layers. Both the muscle layer and the skin are closed with a running buried Vicryl 4–0 suture (no exposed knot/suture upon which mouse can gnaw). Take care not to injure bowel during the closure.
8. Inject warm phosphate buffered saline (1 ml) subcutaneously at the end of the procedure. Keep the mouse warm on a heating pad and observe until it awakens and moves about the cage. This usually happens within several minutes.
9. Provide postoperative analgesia with buprenorphine (0.10 mg/kg) and meloxicam (2 ml/kg) injected under the skin of the scruff of the neck. This is done once (meloxicam) or twice (buprenorphine) daily for 3 days starting with the preoperative dose.

3.2.6 Tumor Imaging by Bioluminescence

Image tumors as described in Subheading 3.1.6.

3.2.7 Bladder Examination by Ultrasound

1. Induce anesthesia with 2.0–3.0% isoflurane in an induction chamber. When the mouse is immobile, transfer to imaging platform and maintain anesthesia through nose cone on imaging platform with 1.5–2.0% isoflurane.
2. Apply eye lubricant to each eye.
3. Monitor heart rate of mouse through electrodes on imaging platform.
4. Insert thermometer into the rectum of mouse for temperature measurement only if imaging is to last more than 5 min (generally not needed if imaging is <5 min). The imaging platform is heated.
5. Apply depilatory cream to the skin overlying the region of interest and scrub the skin with a plastic spoon 90 s later. Wipe off residual depilatory cream with alcohol swab after fur removal.
6. Apply sterile ultrasound gel from tube to the skin overlying the region of interest.
7. Gently lower the mounted scanhead onto the abdominal wall and adjust to allow visualization of the bladder. The scanhead is mounted on an adjustable arm. A motor for 3-D imaging can be interposed on this arm to allow for automatic 3-D imaging. Imaging is performed according to usual practices as outlined in the users' manual.
8. After imaging, transfer the mouse to a recovery cage lined with paper towel and placed on a heating pad. After 5–10 min, the

awake and ambulatory mouse can be transferred back to its home cage with cage mates.

9. Repeat imaging usually once weekly for the duration of the study. This frequency can be increased to once every 4 days in rapidly growing tumors, and the duration can be extended as long as 12 weeks in slowly growing xenografts.

3.3 Intramural Orthotopic Xenograft Model: Percutaneous Ultrasound Guided Technique

3.3.1 Preparation of Cell Lines

Prepare cells as described in Subheading 3.1.1.

3.3.2 Preparation of Cell Suspension

1. Thaw Matrigel®. Keep on ice in order to avoid increased viscosity observed at higher temperature.
2. Trypsinize luciferase transduced cells at a confluence of 70%, suspend them in normal growth media.
3. Calculate the absolute cell number.
4. Spin the cell suspension for 5 min at 180 × *g*. Remove the supernatant.
5. Add the appropriate volume of Matrigel® in order to reach the required cell concentration. The maximal injectable volume of tumor cell suspension is 40 μl (*see* justification under "Notes"). Similar cell numbers are used here as described above for the open method of tumor inoculation.
6. Mix well by pipetting up and down (P1000), avoid creating air bubbles in the suspension.

3.3.3 Preparation of Animals

Prepare animals as described in Subheading 3.1.3.

3.3.4 Experimental Setup

1. Mount the animal on the heated imaging table (Fig. 2 I) of the Vevo 770® small animal imaging platform with continuous monitoring of vital signs. Fix the lower limbs with a rubber band (Fig. 2 III).
2. Remove the fur of the lower abdomen by usage of an electric razor and application of depilatory cream (not necessary for nude mice).
3. Disinfect the abdomen with 2% chlorhexidine gluconate and wipe the skin with a sterile cotton tip.
4. Immobilize the bladder with the bladder stabilization strap (Fig. 3 I, II).
5. Apply sterile ultrasound gel to the lower abdomen.

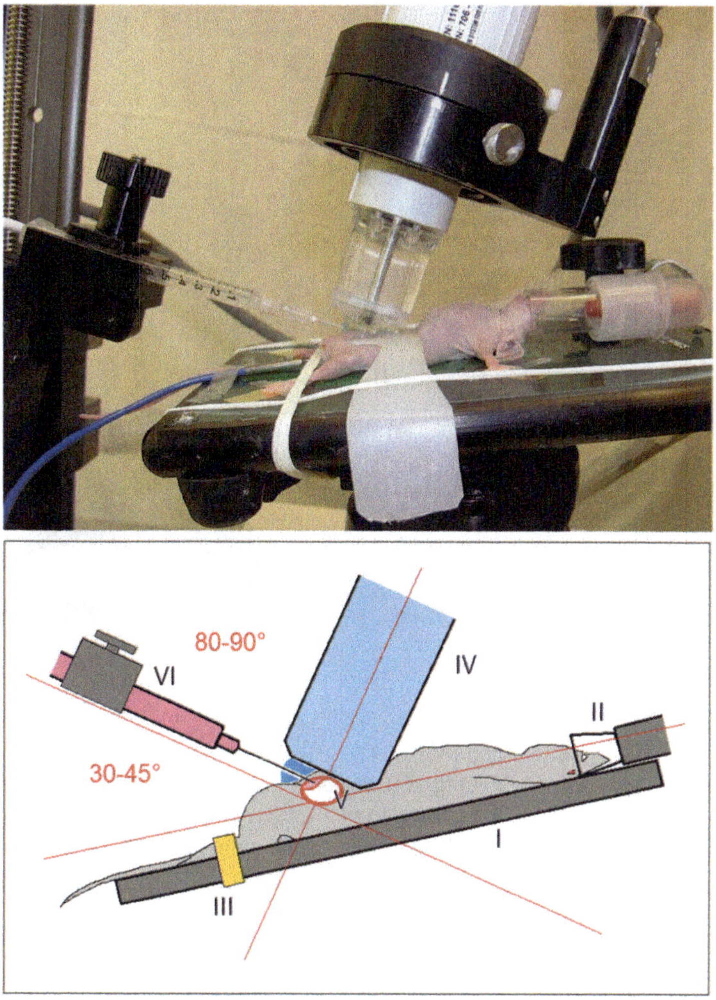

Fig. 2 Ultrasound-guided minimally invasive inoculation of bladder cancer cells: image and schematic illustration of the experimental setup. The mouse is mounted on the heated operation table (I) and held under anesthesia (II) with 3% isoflurane/oxygen mixture. The lower limbs are fixed with a rubber band (III). After approaching the ultrasound scanhead (IV) to the skin (longitudinal alignment with a cranial angle of 45–70°) the bladder (V) is visualized on the ultrasound screen. A syringe with a 30G needle (VI) is guided to the skin in an angle of 30–45° (80–90° relative to the longitudinal axis of the ultrasound scanhead)

6. Slowly approach the RMV 706 ultrasound scanhead (Fig. 2 IV) to the skin (longitudinal with a cranial angle of 45–70°) and visualize the bladder on the ultrasound screen (Fig. 4 I).
7. If the bladder is flaccid fill it with 50 μl sterile, warm phosphate buffered saline (PBS) through a transurethral 24G angiocatheter (*see* Subheading 2.2 for technique).

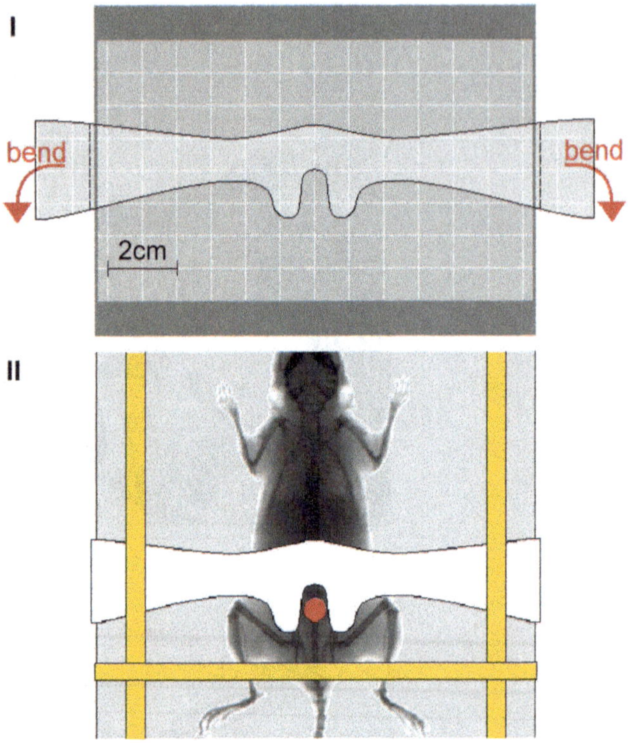

Fig. 3 Ultrasound-guided minimally invasive inoculation of bladder cancer cells: immobilization of the bladder. Dimensions and illustration to construct the bladder stabilization strap (I). The strap is attached to the lower abdomen and immobilizes the bladder (II). Thus, an evasion of the bladder during intramural injection is avoided

3.3.5 Separation of Bladder Wall Layers

1. Attach to the syringe clamp a 1.0 ml syringe filled with PBS and connected to a 30 gauge, ¾ in. needle.
2. Direct the bevel of the needle upward and bring the needle to the skin surface just above the pubic bone at a 30–45° angle to the abdominal wall, or 80–90° relative to the longitudinal axis of the ultrasound scanhead (Fig. 2).
3. Detect the needle on the ultrasound screen.
4. Slowly perforate the skin and the abdominal wall (Fig. 4 II).
5. Turn the bevel of the needle 180° (now directed posteriorly in the mouse).
6. Insert the tip of the needle into the bladder wall without penetrating the mucosa (Fig. 4 III).
7. Slowly inject 50 μl of PBS between the muscular layer and the mucosa to create an artificial space (Fig. 4 IV; *see* **Note 5**).
8. Withdraw the needle.

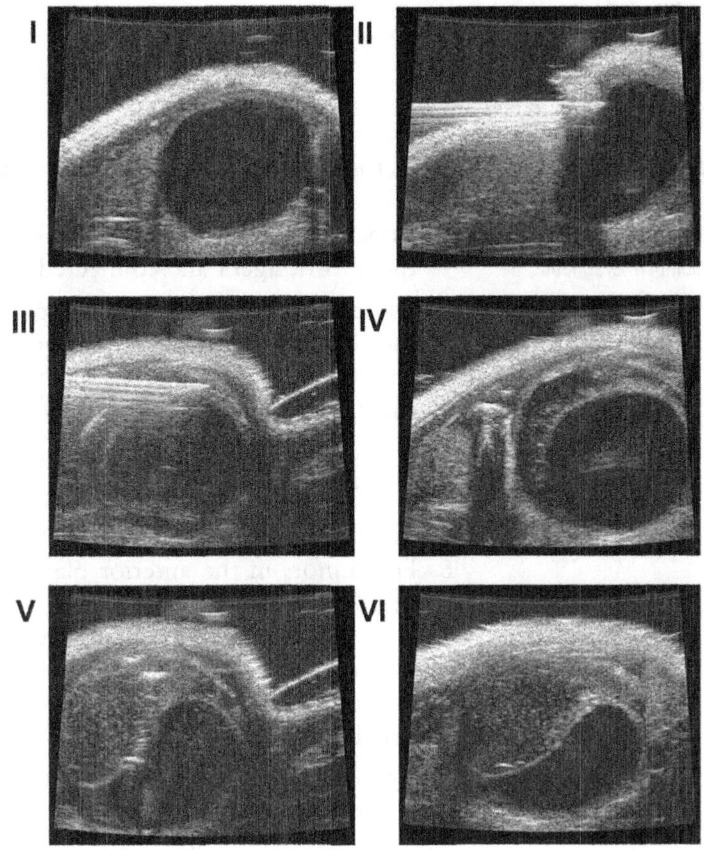

Fig. 4 Ultrasound-guided minimally invasive inoculation of bladder cancer cells: Intramural injection. Visualization of the bladder on the ultrasound screen (I). Perforation of the skin and abdominal wall muscles (II). Needle insertion into the bladder wall without penetration of the mucosa (III). PBS (50 μl) between the muscular layer and the mucosa after slow injection (IV). Tumor cells suspended in Matrigel in the intramural artificially created space (V, VI)

3.3.6 Intramural Inoculation of Bladder Cancer Cells

1. Attach to the syringe clamp a second 1.0 ml syringe filled with cancer cells suspended in Matrigel® and connected to a 30 gauge, ¾ in. needle.
2. Guide the tip of the needle to the space created with the PBS injection described above.
3. Inject 40 μl of the cell suspension into this space (Fig. 4 V, VI; *see* **Note 6**).
4. Withdraw the needle.

3.3.7 Post-interventional Supportive Care

Handle mice as described in Subheading 3.1.6.

3.3.8 Tumor Imaging

Image tumors as described in Subheaing 3.1.6.

3.4 Ultrasound Guided Intratumoral Injection of Therapeutic Agents

3.4.1 Experimental Setup

Set up the experiment as described in Subheading 3.3.4.

3.4.2 Intratumoral Injection of Therapeutic Agents

1. Attach to the syringe clamp a 1.0 ml syringe filled with the therapeutic agent and connected to a 30 G, ¾ in. needle.
2. Direct the bevel of the needle upward and bring the needle to the skin just above the pubic bone at a 30–45° angle to the abdominal wall, or 80–90° relative to the longitudinal axis of the ultrasound scanhead.
3. Detect the bladder tumor and the needle longitudinally on the ultrasound screen.
4. Slowly perforate the skin and the abdominal wall.
5. For tumors in the anterior bladder wall insert the tip of the needle into the adjacent bladder wall. Perforate the serosa and guide the tip of the needle to the center of the tumor (Fig. 5). For tumors in the posterior bladder wall perforate all the layers of the opposing anterior bladder wall and guide the tip of the needle to the center of the tumor.
6. Slowly inject an appropriate volume of therapeutic agent (maximum 25 μl) in the center of the tumor.
7. Withdraw the needle.

3.4.3 Post-interventional Supportive Care

Handle mice as described in Subheading 3.1.5.

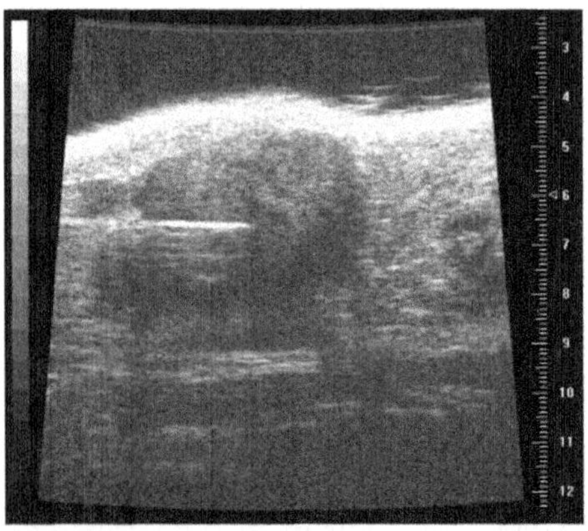

Fig. 5 Ultrasound-guided intratumoral injection of treatment agents. A xenograft tumor is visualized by ultrasound and the treatment agent is injected through a 30G needle into the center of the tumor

3.5 Chemical Carcinogen Induced Model of Urothelial Cancer

3.5.1 Handling of BBN

1. BBN is a carcinogen. It must be stored securely in the animal facilities of an accredited laboratory, and cytotoxic precautions must be observed at all times.
2. As BBN is photosensitive it has to be stored in opaque vessels.
3. All handling of BBN should be done in the fume hood with chemical-resistant gloves (nitrile) and facemask.
4. All containers and contents of animal cages coming into contact with BBN should be appropriately labeled and disposed of as hazardous.

3.5.2 Preparation of BBN

1. Reconstitute the thick yellow stock solution of BBN (2 g/2 ml) in 4 l of drinking water to reach a solution of 0.05%.
2. Store the diluted solution in an opaque vessel and label as hazardous chemical.

3.5.3 Administration of BBN

1. All mouse cages intended to come into contact with BBN-water must be clearly labeled.
2. Provide mice with BBN-water (solution of 0.05%) ad libitum for 8–12 weeks. Assuming a daily fluid intake of 5 ml per mouse (≙35 ml/mouse/week), a cage of five mice (≙175 ml/cage/week) should be given 100 ml of 0.05% BBN drinking water twice weekly.
3. Following 8–12 weeks of BBN-water only, regular water is provided.

3.5.4 Clinical Mouse Evaluation

Observe mice for clinical signs of tumor growth (loss of weight, hematuria, formation of lower abdominal masses; *see* **Note 7**) on a regular basis (every 4 weeks for first 20 weeks, then weekly). Development of intravesical tumors can take up to 6 months (*see* **Note 8**).

3.5.5 Bladder Examination by Ultrasound

Examine bladder as described in Subheading 3.2.6.

4 Notes

1. Different bladder cancer cell lines have different growth kinetics. The study extends for 6 weeks with slow growing cells, but only 4 weeks for more rapidly growing cells. More tumorigenic cells, such as UM-UC3 or T24, are injected at lower numbers (100,000 or 250,000) compared to less tumorigenic cells, such as

UM-UC13 (500,000 or 1,000,000 cells). In general, it is important to conduct a pilot experiment to establish the optimal cell number for both tumor take and growth kinetics.

2. It is important that mice remain under maintenance anesthesia throughout the specified dwell time. If mice reach a shallower anesthetic plane there is a high risk of spontaneous voiding and the loss of the test therapeutic. Dwell times in excess of 2.5 h may cause severe stress on the mice and potentially result in morbidity. Prolonged dwell times and high instilled volumes appear also to cause reflux into the intrarenal collecting system, which at the time of tumor cell instillation can lead to upper tract tumor engraftment.
3. The presence of instilled cancer cells should be apparent on bioluminescent imaging the day following instillation. Engraftment suitable for initiation of treatment for most studies should be achieved by 4 days post procedure. In order to reduce variability all tumors should be measured and mice allocated by tumor size prior to treatment.
4. Tumor burden can also be measured by ultrasound or other imaging modalities (e.g., MRI or CT [11]). In the intravesical model tumor growth can initially be spread across the urothelial surface, making definition of a circumscribed tumor volume difficult. Discrepancies may arise between tumor burden determined by luminescence and tumor volume determined by imaging, which may be attributable to tumor hypoxia and necrosis [15].
5. The key step of this procedure is the creation of an artificial submucosal space in the bladder wall with saline. Once this space is created appropriately and without perforation of the mucosa, it remains stable for several minutes. The guidance of the second needle into this space to inoculate the tumor cells is relatively uncomplicated. If the tip of the needle perforates the mucosa into the lumen of the bladder, the creation of a submucosal space is still feasible. The needle has to be withdrawn slowly through the bladder wall and the saline injected just at the moment when the mucosal layer flips over the tip of the needle. After this maneuver the submucosal space is less stable (saline will escape to the bladder lumen within 30–60 s) and the injection of the tumor cells has to be performed quickly.
6. Another theoretical concern with this model is the spillage of tumor cells into the peritoneal cavity through the needle tract. This complication can be avoided by restricting the volume of tumor cell suspension to 40 μl (in addition to 50 μl PBS injection to establish submucosal space). Spillage of tumor cells into the bladder lumen is observed when the needle perforates through the bladder mucosa. Although the loss of

tumor cells might lead to a decreased tumor volume during follow-up, intravesical tumor growth has not been observed.

7. BBN administration may be withheld if there is evidence of intolerance or rapid development of intravesical changes.
8. Once intravesical changes are observed, and confirmed histologically, mice can be allocated to treatment groups for treatment studies.

References

1. Ding J, Xu D, Pan C, Ye M, Kang J, Bai Q, Qi J (2014) Current animal models of bladder cancer: awareness of translatability (Review). Exp Ther Med 8:691–699
2. Kubota T (1994) Metastatic models of human cancer xenografted in the nude mouse: the importance of orthotopic transplantation. J Cell Biochem 56:4–8
3. Chan E, Patel A, Heston W, Larchian W (2009) Mouse orthotopic models for bladder cancer research. BJU Int 104:1286–1291
4. Bhowmick NA, Neilson EG, Moses HL (2004) Stromal fibroblasts in cancer initiation and progression. Nature 432(7015):332–337
5. Cutz JC, Guan J, Bayani J, Yoshimoto M, Xue H, Sutcliffe M, English J, Flint J, LeRiche J, Yee J, Squire JA, Gout PW, Lam S, Wang YZ (2006) Establishment in severe combined immunodeficiency mice of subrenal capsule xenografts and transplantable tumor lines from a variety of primary human lung cancers: potential models for studying tumor progression-related changes. Clinical Cancer Res 12(13):4043–4054
6. Jäger W, Xue H, Hayashi T, Janssen C, Awrey S, Wyatt AW, Anderson S, Moskalev I, Haegert A, Alshalalfa M, Erho N, Davicioni E, Fazli L, Li E, Collins C, Wang Y, Black PC (2015) Patient-derived bladder cancer xenografts in the preclinical development of novel targeted therapies. Oncotarget 6(25):21522–21532
7. Pan CX, Zhang H, Tepper CG, Lin TY, Davis RR, Keck J, Ghosh PM, Gill P, Airhart S, Bult C, Gandara DR, Liu E, de Vere White RW (2015) Development and characterization of bladder cancer patient-derived Xenografts for molecularly guided targeted therapy. PLoS One 10(8):e0134346
8. Summerhayes IC, Franks LM (1979) Effects of donor age on neoplastic transformation of adult mouse bladder epithelium in vitro. J Natl Cancer Inst 62:1017–1023
9. Arantes-Rodrigues R, Pinto-Leite R, da Costa RG, Colaço A, Lopes C, Oliveira P (2013) Cytogenetic characterization of an N-butyl-N-(4-hydroxybutyl) nitrosamine-induced mouse papillary urothelial carcinoma. Tumour Biol 34:2691–2696
10. Zhang ZT, Pak J, Shapiro E, Sun TT, Wu XR (1999) Urothelium-specific expression of an oncogene in transgenic mice induced the formation of carcinoma in situ and invasive transitional cell carcinoma. Cancer Res 59:3512–3517
11. Hadaschik BA, Black PC, Sea JC, Metwalli AR, Fazli L, Dinney CP, Gleave ME, So AI (2007) A validated mouse model for orthotopic bladder cancer using transurethral tumour inoculation and bioluminescence imaging. BJU Int 100:1377–1384
12. Jäger W, Horiguchi Y, Shah J, Hayashi T, Awrey S, Gust KM, Hadaschik BA, Matsui Y, Anderson S, Bell RH, Ettinger S, So AI, Gleave ME, Lee IL, Dinney CP, Tachibana M, McConkey DJ, Black PC (2013) Hiding in plain view: genetic profiling reveals decades old cross contamination of bladder cancer cell line KU7 with HeLa. J Urol 190 (4):1404–1409
13. Horiguchi Y, Larchian WA, Kaplinsky R, Fair WR, Heston WD (2000) Intravesical liposome-mediated interleukin-2 gene therapy in orthotopic murine bladder cancer model. Gene Ther 7:844–851
14. Dinney CP, Fishbeck R, Singh RK, Eve B, Pathak S, Brown N, Xie B, Fan D, Bucana CD, Fidler IJ, Killion JJ (1995) Isolation and characterization of metastatic variants from human transitional cell carcinoma passaged by orthotopic implantation in athymic nude mice. J Urol 154:532–1538
15. Black PC, Shetty A, Brown GA, Esparza-Coss E, Metwalli AR, Agarwal PK, McConkey DJ, Hazle JD, Dinney CP (2010) Validating bladder cancer xenograft bioluminescence with magnetic resonance imaging: the significance of hypoxia and necrosis. BJU Int 106:1799–1804

16. Jager W, Moskalev I, Janssen C, Hayashi T, Awrey S, Gust KM, So AI, Zhang K, Fazli L, Li E, Thuroff JW, Lange D, Black PC (2013) Ultrasound-guided intramural inoculation of orthotopic bladder cancer xenografts: a novel high-precision approach. PLoS One 8(3): e59536
17. Hadaschik BA, Zhang K, So AI, Fazli L, Jia W, Bell JC, Gleave ME, Rennie PS (2008) Oncolytic vesicular stomatitis viruses are potent agents for intravesical treatment of high-risk bladder cancer. Cancer Res 68(12):4506–4510
18. Adam L, Black PC, Kassouf W, Eve B, McConkey D, Munsell MF, Benedict WF, Dinney CP (2007) Adenoviral mediated interferon-alpha 2b gene therapy suppresses the pro-angiogenic effect of vascular endothelial growth factor in superficial bladder cancer. J Urol 177:1900–1906
19. Cho EJ, Yang J, Mohamedali KA, Lim EK, Kim EJ, Farhangfar CJ, Suh JS, Haam S, Rosenblum MG, Huh YM (2011) Sensitive angiogenesis imaging of orthotopic bladder tumors in mice using a selective magnetic resonance imaging contrast agent containing VEGF121/rGel. Investig Radiol 46:441–449
20. Ding J, Xu D, Pan C, Ye M, Kang J, Bai Q, Qi J (2014) Current animal models of bladder cancer: awareness of translatability (Review). Exp Ther Med 8:691–699
21. Vasconcelos-Nobrega C, Colaco A, Lopes C, Oliveira PA (2012) Review: BBN as an urothelial carcinogen. In Vivo 26:727–739
22. He Z, Kosinska W, Zhao ZL, Wu XR, Guttenplan JB (2012) Tissue-specific mutagenesis by N-butyl-N-(4-hydroxybutyl)nitrosamine as the basis for urothelial carcinogenesis. Mutat Res 742:92–95
23. Lubet RA, Huebner K, Fong LY, Altieri DC, Steele VE, Kopelovich L, Kavanaugh C, Juliana MM, Soong SJ, Grubbs CJ (2005) 4-Hydroxybutyl(butyl)nitrosamine-induced urinary bladder cancers in mice: characterization of FHIT and survivin expression and chemopreventive effects of indomethacin. Carcinogenesis 26(3):571–578
24. Shin K, Lim A, Odegaard JI, Honeycutt JD, Kawano S, Hsieh MH, Beachy PA (2014) Cellular origin of bladder neoplasia and tissue dynamics of its progression to invasive carcinoma. Nat Cell Biol 16(5):469–478
25. Hicks RM, Wakefield JS (1972) Rapid induction of bladder cancer in rats with N-methyl-N-nitrosourea. Chem Biol Interact 5(2):139–152
26. Ayala de la Peña F, Kanasaki K, Kanasaki M, Tangirala N, Maeda G, Kalluri R (2011) Loss of p53 and acquisition of angiogenic microRNA profile are insufficient to facilitate progression of bladder urothelial carcinoma in situ to invasive carcinoma. J Biol Chem 286:20778–20787
27. Wu XR (2009) Biology of urothelial tumorigenesis: insights from genetically engineered mice. Cancer Metastasis Rev 28:281–290
28. Sharpless NE, Depinho RA (2006) The mighty mouse: genetically engineered mouse models in cancer drug development. Nat Rev Drug Discov 5:741–754
29. Politi K, Pao W (2011) How genetically engineered mouse tumor models provide insights into human cancers. J Clin Oncol 29:2273–2281
30. Zhang ZT, Pak J, Shapiro E, Sun TT, Wu XR (1999) Urothelium-specific expression of an oncogene in transgenic mice induced the formation of carcinoma in situ and invasive transitional cell carcinoma. Cancer Res 59:3512–3517
31. Ayala de la peña F, Kanasaki K, Kanasaki M, Tangirala N, Maeda G, Kalluri R (2012) Loss of p53 and acquisition of angiogenic microRNA profile are insufficient to facilitate progression of bladder urothelial carcinoma in situ to invasive carcinoma. Biol Chem 286 (23):20778–20787
32. Stone R 2nd, Sabichi AL, Gill J, Lee IL, Adegboyega P, Dai MS, Loganantharaj R, Trutschl M, Cvek U, Clifford JL (2010) Identification of genes correlated with early-stage bladder cancer progression. Cancer Prev Res 3:776–786
33. Zhang ZT, Pak J, Huang HY, Shapiro E, Sun TT, Pellicer A, Wu XR (2001) Role of ha-ras activation in superficial papillary pathway of urothelial tumor formation. Oncogene 20 (16):1973–1980
34. Cheng J, Huang H, Zhang ZT, Shapiro E, Pellicer A, Sun TT, Wu XR (2002) Overexpression of epidermal growth factor receptor in urothelium elicits urothelial hyperplasia and promotes bladder tumor growth. Cancer Res 62:4157–4163
35. Spiess PE, Czerniak B (2006) Dual-track pathway of bladder carcinogenesis: practical implications. Arch Pathol Lab Med 130 (6):844–852
36. Gao J, Huang HY, Pak J, Cheng J, Zhang ZT, Shapiro E, Pellicer A, Sun TT, Wu XR (2004) p53 deficiency provokes urothelial proliferation and synergizes with activated ha-ras in promoting urothelial tumorigenesis. Oncogene 23:687–696
37. Mo L, Zheng X, Huang HY, Shapiro E, Lepor H, Cordon-Cardo C, Sun TT, Wu XR (2007)

Hyperactivation of ha-ras oncogene, but not Ink4a/Arf deficiency, triggers bladder tumorigenesis. J Clin Invest 117:314–325

38. Zhang ZT, Pak J, Huang HY, Shapiro E, Sun TT, Pellicer A, Wu XR (2001) Role of ha-ras activation in superficial papillary pathway of urothelial tumor formation. Oncogene 20:1973–1980
39. Ahmad I, Patel R, Liu Y, Singh LB, Taketo MM, Wu XR, Leung HY, Sansom OJ (2011) Ras mutation cooperates with β-catenin activation to drive bladder tumourigenesis. Cell Death Dis 2:e124
40. Ahmad I, Morton JP, Singh LB, Radulescu SM, Ridgway RA, Patel S, Woodgett J, Winton DJ, Taketo MM, Wu XR, Leung HY, Sansom OJ (2011) β -catenin activation Synergises with PTEN loss to cause bladder cancer formation. Oncogene 30:178–189
41. Lin C, Yin Y, Stemler K, Humphrey P, Kibel AS, Mysorekar IU, Ma L (2013) Constitutive β-catenin activation induces male-specific tumorigenesis in the bladder urothelium. Cancer Res 73:5914–5925
42. Rampias T, Vgenopoulou P, Avgeris M, Polyzos A, Stravodimos K, Valavanis C, Scorilas A, Klinakis A (2014) A new tumor suppressor role for the Notch pathway in bladder cancer. Nat Med 20:1199–1205
43. Puzio-Kuter AM, Castillo-Martin M, Kinkade CW, Wang X, Shen TH, Matos T, Shen MM, Cordon-Cardo C, Abate-Shen C (2009) Inactivation of p53 and Pten promotes invasive bladder cancer. Genes Dev 23:675–680
44. Santos, M. et al. (2015) NIH Public Access 74:6565–6577.
45. Ahmad I, Sansom OJ, Leung HY (2012) Exploring molecular genetics of bladder cancer: lessons learned from mouse models. Dis Model Mech 5:323–332

Part IV

Biomarkers

Chapter 16

Quantification of MicroRNAs in Urine-Derived Specimens

Susanne Fuessel, Andrea Lohse-Fischer, Dana Vu Van, Karsten Salomo, Kati Erdmann, and Manfred P. Wirth

Abstract

MicroRNAs are small noncoding RNAs which regulate the expression of genes involved in a multitude of cellular processes. Dysregulation of microRNAs and—in consequence—of the affected pathways is frequently observed in numerous pathologies including cancers. Therefore, tumor-related alterations in microRNA expression and function can reflect molecular processes of tumor onset and progression qualifying microRNAs as potential diagnostic and prognostic biomarkers.

In particular, microRNAs with differential expression in bladder cancer (BCa) might represent promising tools for noninvasive tumor detection in urine. This would be helpful not only for diagnostic and monitoring purposes but also for therapeutic decisions. Detection and quantification of BCa-associated microRNAs in urine can be performed using the cellular sediment, which also contains BCa cells, or in exosomes originating from those cells. Methods for isolation of exosomes from urine, extraction of total RNA from cells and exosomes as well as techniques for RNA quantification, reverse transcription, and qPCR-based quantification of microRNA expression levels are described herein.

Key words Bladder cancer, Exosomes, MicroRNA, Microvesicles, Quality control, Quantitative PCR, Reverse transcription, RNA isolation, Urothelial carcinoma

1 Introduction

MicroRNAs are of high functional importance in a multitude of physiological and pathological processes such as cellular proliferation and differentiation, control of developmental timing, stem cell maintenance and many more [1, 2]. This class of small noncoding RNAs, comprising over 2500 known members in humans (mirbase.org, release 21), is described to posttranscriptionally regulate the expression of numerous genes [3, 4]. The expression and function of microRNAs can be altered in numerous pathological conditions and might, therefore, serve as mirror of these deregulated processes. Particularly tumor-associated alterations in microRNA expression patterns were analyzed intensively in the last years to evaluate their value as potential tumor markers and to investigate their functional role in development and progression of tumors.

Wolfgang A. Schulz et al. (eds.), *Urothelial Carcinoma: Methods and Protocols*, Methods in Molecular Biology, vol. 1655, DOI 10.1007/978-1-4939-7234-0_16,

Several microRNAs were also identified as promising diagnostic or prognostic biomarkers for human bladder cancer (BCa) [2, 4–6]. Exemplarily, the microRNAs miR-21, miR-96, miR-125b, miR-145, miR-183, and miR-210 showed altered expression in BCa tissues compared to nonmalignant bladder tissues [7–12]. For selected microRNAs an association with tumor stage and grade or with prognosis was observed [8, 12–18].

Currently, the sensitive determination of altered microRNA expression in urine-derived specimens is one of the main issues of translational BCa research since there is an urgent need for reliable BCa biomarkers. Such markers should allow the noninvasive detection of primary and recurrent BCa as well as the discrimination between tumors of different grade and stage to assess the presence and aggressiveness of tumors with the final aim to reduce frequent invasive diagnostics [2, 6, 19]. A number of studies describe the quantification of promising BCa-associated microRNA candidates in urine comprising miR-21, miR-96, miR-125b, miR-126, miR-146a, miR-183, and miR-210 [16, 20–29]. In most of these studies, microRNA expression was assessed in the cellular sediment of urine specimens or in whole urine from patients with BCa [21–24, 26–28, 30]. Additionally, exosomes might also serve as diagnostic tool for BCa detection due to their function as cargo carriers of cellular components including microRNAs [2, 19]. These exosomes, which are released from BCa cells into the urine, can be utilized as starting material for the quantification of BCa-associated microRNAs [20].

Herein, we describe approaches for the preparation of cellular sediments and exosomes from urine specimens as well as the isolation of total RNA from these compartments by different methods. Furthermore, several techniques for quantification of the isolated total RNA, for microRNA-specific reverse transcription (RT) and quantification of microRNA expression levels by quantitative polymerase chain reaction (qPCR) are presented. Fig. 1 gives an overview of the different steps and methods within this workflow.

2 Materials

2.1 Collection and Preservation of Urine Specimens

1. Ice-cold phosphate-buffered saline (PBS).
2. *Qiazol lysis reagent* (Qiagen) (*see* **Note 1**).
3. Urine collection devices (*see* **Note 2**).
4. Conical centrifuge tubes (15 and 50 ml).
5. Cryogenic tubes (2 ml).
6. Refrigerated centrifuge with holders for 15 and 50 ml tubes.

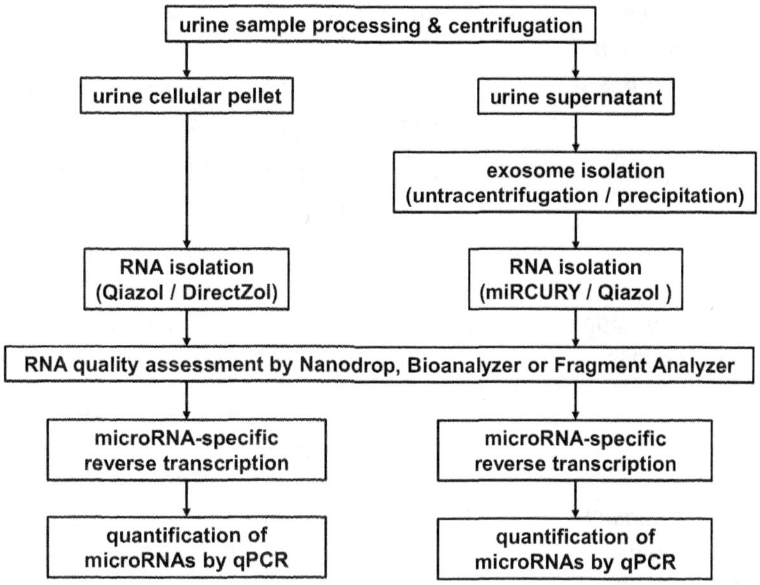

Fig. 1 Scheme of the described methods for urine sample processing, isolation and quality assessment of RNA, reverse transcription, and PCR-based quantification of microRNAs

2.2 RNA Isolation from Cellular Pellets by Conventional and Kit-Based Methods

1. *Direct-zol RNA MiniPrep Kit* (Zymo Research).
2. Disinfectant and *RNaseZap*.
3. Chloroform.
4. Isopropyl alcohol.
5. Ethanol (75% or 95–100%).
6. Nuclease-free water.
7. Nuclease-free tubes (1.5 ml).
8. Thermoblock.
9. Microcentrifuge.

2.3 Isolation of Exosomes from Urine by Ultracentrifugation

1. PBS.
2. Polycarbonate centrifuge tubes suitable for ultracentrifugation (e.g., 10 ml).
3. RNase-free tubes (1.5 ml).
4. Vortex shaker.
5. Weighing scale.
6. Microcentrifuge.
7. Ultracentrifuge.

2.4 Isolation of Exosomes from Urine by Kit-Based Methods

1. *miRCURY Exosome Isolation Kit—Cells, urine, and CSF* (Exiqon).
2. *miRCURY RNA Isolation Kit—Cell & Plant* (Exiqon).
3. RNase-free tubes (1.5 ml).
4. Conical centrifuge tubes (15 ml).
5. Vortex shaker.
6. Swing bucket centrifuge.

2.5 RNA Isolation from Exosomes

1. *miRCURY RNA Isolation Kit—Cell & Plant* (Exiqon).
2. Ethanol (95–100%).
3. β-Mercaptoethanol (recommended).
4. Microcentrifuge.

2.6 Assessment of RNA Quantity and Quality by NanoDrop 2000c System

1. Lint-free lab wipes.
2. Disinfectant and *RNaseZap*.
3. Nuclease-free water.
4. *NanoDrop 2000c* system (Thermo Fisher Scientific).

2.7 Assessment of RNA Quantity and Quality by Agilent 2100 Bioanalyzer

1. *Agilent RNA 6000 Pico Kit* and/or *Agilent RNA 6000 Nano Kit* (Agilent Technologies).
2. Disinfectant and *RNaseZap*.
3. Nuclease-free safe-lock tubes (0.5 ml).
4. Vortex shaker.
5. IKA vortex shaker.
6. Microcentrifuge.
7. Thermal cycler for heat-denaturation.
8. Priming station.
9. *Agilent 2100 Bioanalyzer* (Agilent Technologies).

2.8 Assessment of RNA Quantity and Quality by AATI Fragment Analyzer

1. *Standard Sensitivity RNA Analysis Kit* (DNF-471) or *High Sensitivity RNA Analysis Kit* (DNF-472) (Advanced Analytical Technologies).
2. Disinfectant and *RNaseZap*.
3. Deionized, sub-micron filtered water.
4. Nuclease-free water.
5. Conical centrifuge tubes (50 ml).
6. Nuclease-free PCR tubes (0.2 ml).
7. Nuclease-free 96-well PCR sample plates.
8. 96-DeepWell (1 ml) plates (natural polypropylene, Fisherbrand).

9. Reagent reservoir (50 ml).
10. Vortex shaker.
11. Electronic pipette (optional).
12. Microcentrifuge.
13. Centrifuge with plate holders.
14. Thermal cycler for heat-denaturation.
15. *AATI Fragment Analyzer* (Advanced Analytical Technologies).

2.9 Reverse Transcription of MicroRNAs

1. *TaqMan MicroRNA Reverse Transcription Kit* (Thermo Fisher Scientific) containing *MultiScribe Reverse Transcriptase*, *10× Reverse Transcription Buffer*, *RNase Inhibitor*, and dNTP mix.
2. *TaqMan microRNA assays* containing microRNA-specific RT primers (Thermo Fisher Scientific) (*see* **Note 3**).
3. Nuclease-free water.
4. PCR tubes (0.2 or 0.5 ml).
5. Microcentrifuge.
6. Thermal cycler.

2.10 Quantitative PCR

1. *TaqMan Universal PCR Master Mix* (Thermo Fisher Scientific) (*see* **Note 4**).
2. *TaqMan microRNA assays* containing PCR primers and FAM-labeled *TaqMan MGB probes* (Thermo Fisher Scientific) (*see* **Note 3**).
3. Nuclease-free water.
4. Polypropylene tubes (0.5 or 1.5 ml).
5. 96-well PCR plates (e.g., *96-Well Thin-Wall Multititer Plate* from Biozym) with adhesive optical film (e.g., *BZO Seal Film* from Biozym).
6. Microcentrifuge.
7. Centrifuge with plate holders.
8. Real-time PCR instrument (*see* **Note 5**).

3 Methods

3.1 Processing of Urine Specimens

1. Collect 20–80 ml of random non-first-morning urine from patients or suitable control subjects before any therapeutic intervention and process the urine immediately. Otherwise, the urine specimens can be stored at 4–8 °C for up to 4 h without impairment of final readouts (*see* **Note 2**).
2. If a later comparison of the analyzed microRNA patterns with clinical urinary parameters is planned, urine dipstick and

sediment analysis as well as urine cytology should be performed applying standard procedures (*see* **Note 6**).

3. Distribute the remaining urine specimen to one or (if applicable) more 50 ml tubes and centrifuge it at 1,500 × *g* for 10 min at 4 °C to remove dead cells and debris which could interfere with the later isolation of exosomes. Decant the supernatant and keep it frozen at −80 °C in 8 ml aliquots (*see* **Note 7**).
4. Resuspend the pellet(s) with 1 ml ice-cold PBS and combine them in one 50 ml tube (if applicable). Fill it up with ice-cold PBS to 50 ml and centrifuge the sample again (860 × *g* for 5 min at 4 °C). A second wash step is done in the same way with a final volume of 10 ml ice-cold PBS.
5. Remove the supernatant carefully using a micropipette and resuspend the pellet in 700 μl *Qiazol lysis reagent* (*see* **Note 8**). Transfer the lysate to a 2 ml cryogenic tube and store it until RNA extraction at −80 °C.

3.2 Isolation of Total RNA from Cellular Pellets

3.2.1 Conventional RNA Isolation

1. Prepare the work area for RNA handling, i.e., use separate pipets, tips, and vessels. Disinfect and clean the bench and to be used tools with *RNaseZap* before start of the work.
2. Heat the thermoblock to 60 °C.
3. Thaw frozen cellular pellets lysed in *Qiazol* at room temperature. Mix the samples thoroughly (e.g., using a vortex shaker) and let them equilibrate at room temperature for 5 min before the start of RNA isolation (*see* **Note 9**).
4. Add 200 μl chloroform per 1,000 μl *Qiazol*, i.e., 140 μl chloroform per 700 μl *Qiazol*. Vortex the samples vigorously for 15 s and incubate them 5 min at room temperature.
5. Centrifuge the tubes at 12,000 × *g* for 5 min at room temperature to allow the phase separation.
6. Transfer the upper aqueous phase into nuclease-free 1.5 ml tubes. Discard the tubes with the remaining interphase and lower phenolic phase according to rules for waste disposal of organic solvents.
7. RNA precipitation occurs by adding of 500 μl isopropyl alcohol per 1,000 μl *Qiazol*, i.e., 350 μl isopropyl alcohol per 700 μl *Qiazol*. Mix the samples thoroughly and incubate them for 10 min at −20 °C (*see* **Note 10**). Centrifuge the tubes at 12,000 × *g* for 10 min at 4 °C.
8. Discard the isopropyl alcohol and add 1,000 μl 75% ethanol per 1,000 μl *Qiazol*, i.e., 700 μl ethanol per 700 μl *Qiazol* to the RNA pellet. Vortex or flick the tubes to detach the pellet from the tube wall and continue with another centrifugation at 12,000 × *g* for 10 min at 4 °C.

9. Repeat this washing step and remove the ethanol afterwards carefully with a micropipette to facilitate the subsequent drying of the pellet in the opened tube under an exhaust hood for 30–60 min.
10. Finally, dissolve the dried RNA pellet in 40–50 μl nuclease-free water by incubation at 60 °C for 10 min (*see* **Note 11**).
11. Transfer the RNA immediately to cooled conditions (e.g., on ice), if applicable aliquot small volumes for assessment of RNA quantity and quality and freeze the remaining volume at −80 °C until further processing such as reverse transcription.

3.2.2 RNA Isolation Using the Direct-zol RNA MiniPrep Kit

Alternatively to the conventional RNA isolation you can use the *Direct-zol RNA MiniPrep kit* which provides an easier and faster, spin column-based method without phase separation and precipitation steps (*see* **Note 12**, Figs. 2 and 3).

1. Prepare the work area for RNA handling as described above.
2. Add the needed volumes of 95–100% ethanol to the *Direct-zol RNA PreWash concentrate* and to the *RNA Wash Buffer concentrate* as described in the kit manual. Reconstitute the lyophilized DNase I in nuclease-free water as indicated and store it as frozen aliquots. All other reagents provided with the kit are ready to use.
3. Thaw frozen cellular pellets lysed in *Qiazol* at room temperature. Mix the samples thoroughly (e.g., using a vortex shaker) and let them equilibrate at room temperature for 5 min (*see* **Note 9**).
4. Add an equal volume of 95–100% ethanol to the lysates, i.e., 700 μl per 700 μl *Qiazol* and mix thoroughly.
5. Transfer 700 μl of this mixture onto a *Zymo-Spin IIC Column* which is placed in a collection tube and centrifuge it at 10,000–16,000 × *g* for 30 s. Discard the flow-through, load the remaining lysate in aliquots of up to 700 μl onto the column and repeat the centrifugation.
6. Transfer the column into a new collection tube and discard the flow-through.
7. It is recommended to include a DNA digestion step. For this, add 400 μl *RNA Wash Buffer* to the column and centrifuge as described above. Discard the flow-through. Mix 75 μl *DNA Digestion Buffer* with 5 μl *DNase I* by gentle inversion and add this mix directly to the column. After incubation at room temperature for 15 min continue with the next step. Alternatively, the DNA digestion step can be omitted by immediately proceeding with the next step (*see* **Note 13**).

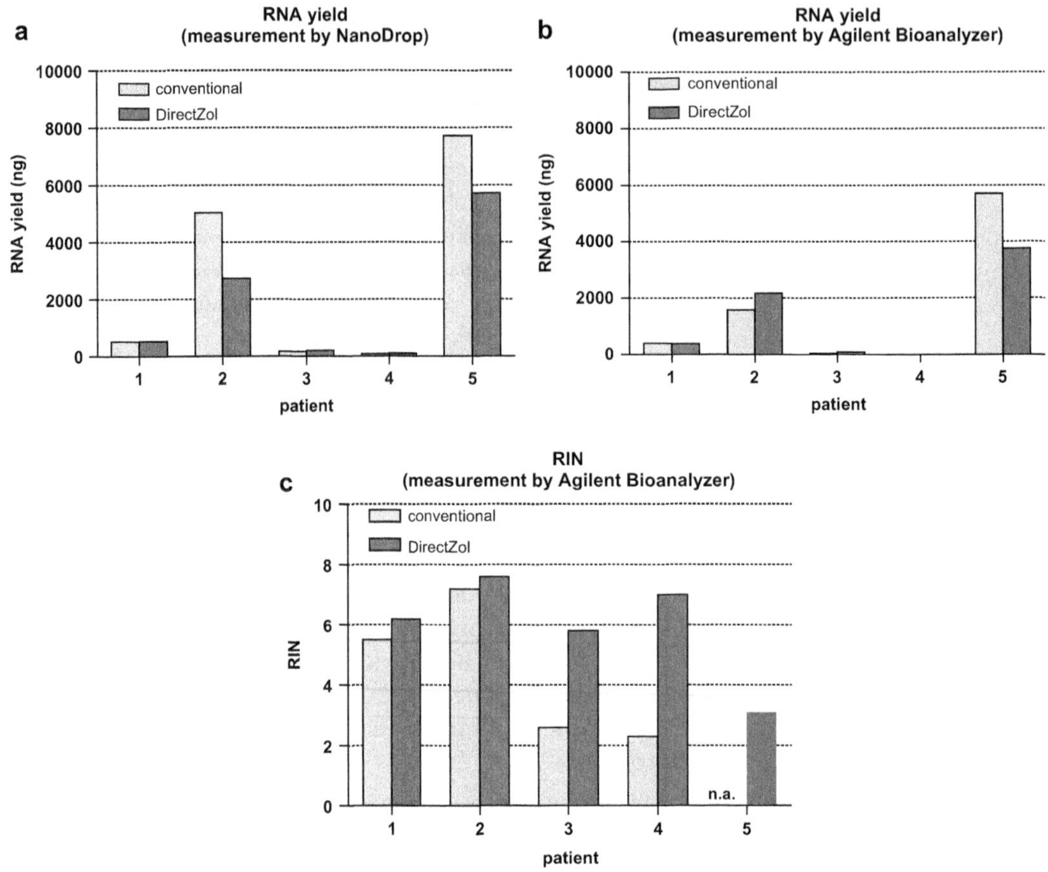

Fig. 2 Comparison of RNA yield and quality between isolation of RNA from urinary sediments by the conventional *Qiazol* method and the kit-based *Direct-zol* method. RNA was isolated from urinary sediments by the conventional *Qiazol* method and the kit-based *Direct-zol* method. Concentration and quality of the isolated RNA was assessed by spectrophotometric analyses using the *NanoDrop 2000c* instrument (**a**) and the *Agilent Bioanalyzer* (**b**). RNA yield in the elution volume of 40 μl was comparable for both isolation methods in both measurement techniques. It differed between the urine samples and was in general very low. RIN values appeared to be higher when using the *Direct-zol* kit (**c**). *n.a.:* not available, *RIN:* RNA integrity number

8. Add 400 μl *Direct-zol RNA PreWash* to the column and centrifuge. Discard the flow-through and repeat this prewash step.
9. After adding 700 μl *RNA Wash Buffer* to the column and centrifugation for 2 min transfer the column into a nuclease-free 1.5 ml tube.
10. Elute the RNA with 25–50 μl nuclease-free water which should be added directly onto the column matrix. Remove the column after centrifugation at 10,000–16,000 × *g* for 30 s and proceed with the RNA as described above.

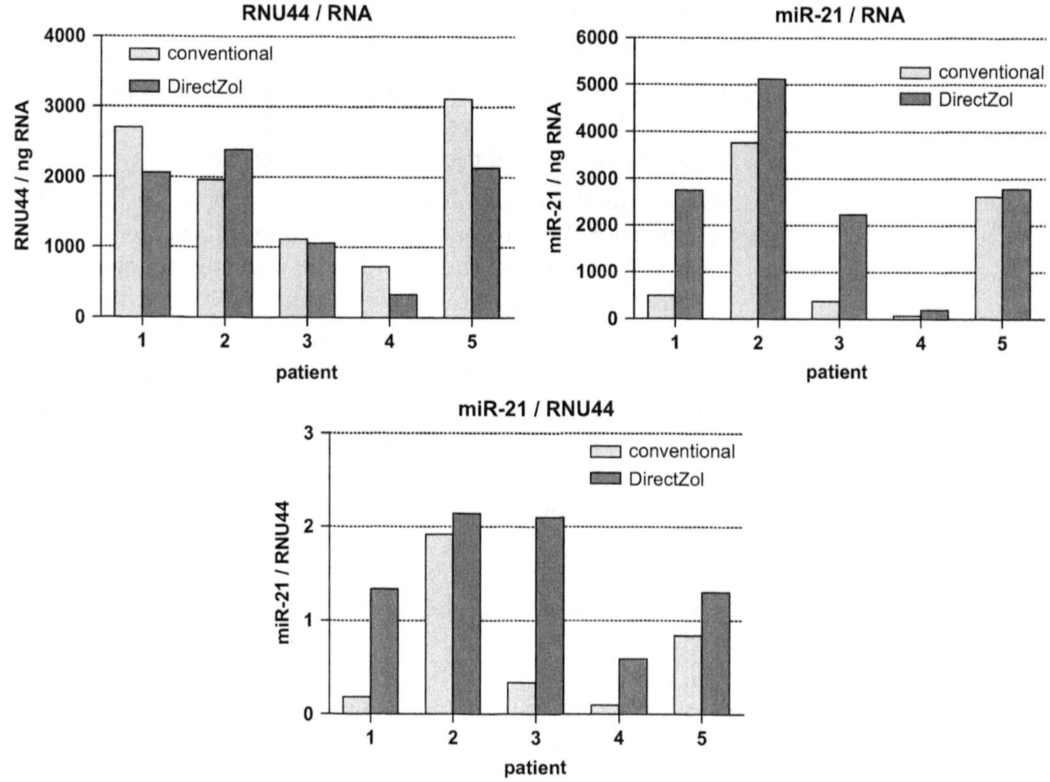

Fig. 3 Comparison of microRNA quantification in urinary sediments after RNA isolation by the conventional *Qiazol* method and the kit-based *Direct-zol* method. Total RNA was isolated form urinary sediments by the conventional *Qiazol* method and the kit-based *Direct-zol* method. After specific reverse transcription the expression levels of the microRNA miR-21 and the reference RNA RNU44 were determined by qPCR. Levels of RNU44 were comparable for both RNA isolation methods. This was also true for other reference RNAs such as RNU48 or RNU6B (data not shown). However, levels of miR-21 differed between both techniques showing higher amounts in RNA isolated by the kit-based *Direct-zol* method. Similar results were obtained for the microRNA miR-210 (data not shown). In summary, *Direct-zol* represents an easier, faster, and more standardizable technique for RNA isolation compared to the conventional *Qiazol* technique

3.3 Isolation of Exosomes from Urine

3.3.1 Isolation of Exosomes from Urine by Ultracentrifugation

1. Thaw the frozen 8 ml aliquots of the pre-centrifuged urine supernatant at room temperature and mix the samples by gentle inversion.
2. Transfer the supernatants to polycarbonate centrifuge tubes and tare the tubes very carefully (*see* **Note 14**).
3. Centrifuge the samples in an ultracentrifuge at 10,000 × *g* for 30 min at 4 °C.
4. Transfer the supernatants carefully to new polycarbonate centrifuge tubes using a 10 ml pipette without touching the pellet. If necessary, use a 100–200 μl micropipette for complete transfer of the remaining supernatant. Again, tare the tubes very carefully.

5. Perform the next ultracentrifugation step with the supernatants at 200,000 × *g* for 60 min at 4 °C.
6. Remove the supernatants carefully using a 10 ml pipette without touching the pellet. Use a 100–200 μl micropipette for complete removal of the remaining supernatant.
7. Resuspend the pellets containing the exosomes in 50 μl PBS and transfer them to nuclease-free 1.5 ml tubes. Do not apply aggressive reagents such as *Qiazol* directly to the pellets because the polycarbonate centrifuge tubes are chemically unstable if exposed to phenol and other reagents.
8. Depending on the applied method for RNA isolation from the exosomes, add 350 μl *Lysis Solution* from the *miRCURY RNA Isolation Kit—Cell & Plant* or 1,000 μl *Qiazol*, mix the lysates by pipetting or vortexing, store them at −80 °C until further processing or proceed with RNA isolation (Subheadings 3.4.1 or 3.4.2).

3.3.2 Isolation of Exosomes from Urine Using the miRCURY Exosome Isolation Kit

Alternatively, exosomes can be isolated from biofluids such as urine by precipitation, e.g., with the *miRCURY Exosome Isolation Kit* (Exiqon). This procedure is based on capturing of water molecules which otherwise form the hydrate envelope of particles. This reduction of the hydration allows the precipitation of the subcellular particles by low speed centrifugation (*see* **Note 15**, Fig. 4)

1. Thaw the frozen 8 ml aliquots of the pre-centrifuged urine supernatant (*see* Subheading 3.1) on ice or at 4 °C. Mix the samples by gentle inversion. Centrifuge them at 3,200 × *g* for 5 min at 4 °C. Transfer 7 ml of the supernatant into a new 15 ml tube (*see* **Note 16**, Fig. 5a).
2. Add 0.3 or 0.4 ml of the *Precipitation Buffer B* contained in the *miRCURY Exosome Isolation Kit (for Cells, urine, and CSF)* per 1 ml urine supernatant, i.e., 2.1 or 2.8 ml per 7 ml urine supernatant (*see* **Note 17**, Fig. 5b).
3. Incubate the mixture for 1 h or overnight at 4 °C (*see* **Note 18**).
4. Afterwards, centrifuge the precipitates at 3,200 × *g* for 30 min at 20 °C.
5. Remove the supernatants completely and centrifuge the pellets again under the same conditions as before. Remove residual supernatants carefully using a micropipette.
6. Resuspend the pellets by addition of 350 μl *Lysis Solution* from the *miRCURY RNA Isolation Kit—Cell & Plant* and by vortexing for 15 s. Transfer the lysates to nuclease-free 1.5 ml tubes. Continue with RNA isolation with this kit immediately or store the samples at −80 °C until further processing (*see* Subheading 3.4.1) (*see* **Note 19**).

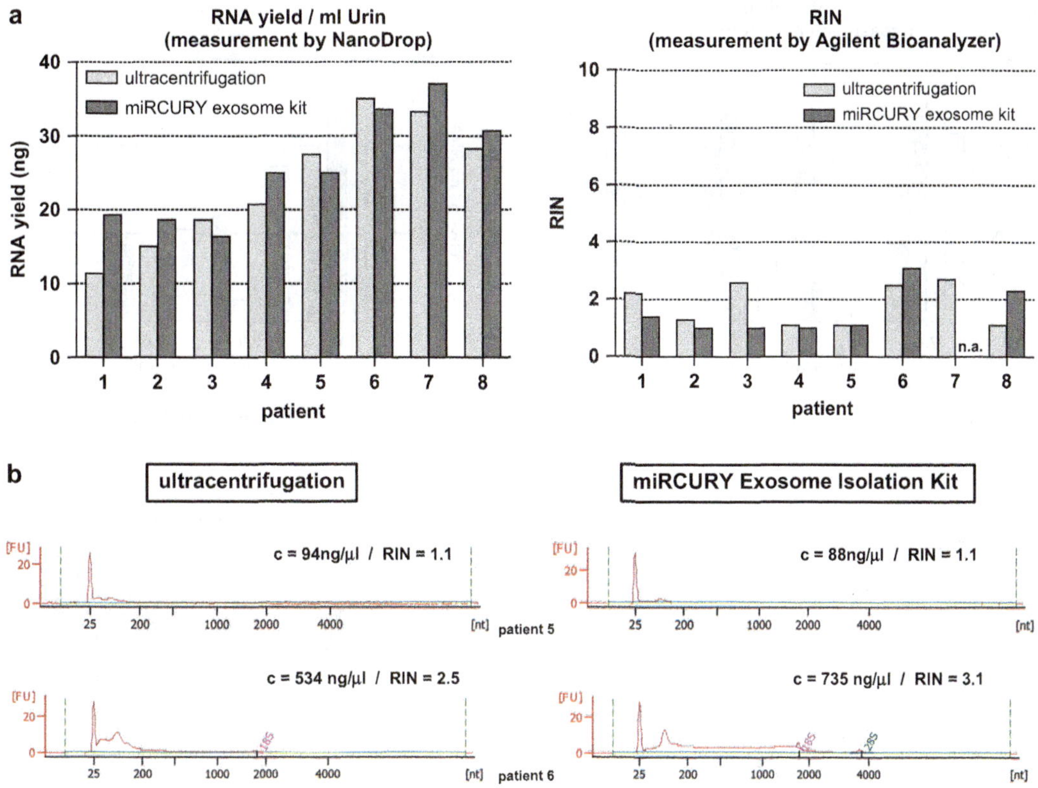

Fig. 4 Comparison of yield and quality of RNA isolated from exosomes after isolation by ultracentrifugation and the miRCURY Exosome Isolation Kit. Exosomes were isolated from 7 ml urine of 8 patients by ultracentrifugation and the *miRCURY Exosome Isolation Kit*. Subsequently, RNA was isolated using the *miRCURY RNA Isolation Kit*. RNA yield and quality was assessed by the *NanoDrop 2000c* spectrophotometer (concentration) and the *Agilent Bioanalyzer* (**a**). The electropherograms were used for determination of RNA concentration and RIN values (**b**). Both methods for isolation of exosomes from urine gave similar results. Therefore, the easier kit-based method can be used instead of the time-consuming and labor-intensive ultracentrifugation. *n.a.:* not available, *RIN:* RNA integrity number

7. Alternatively, resuspend the pellet containing exosomes in 1,000 µl *Qiazol*, store it at −80 °C or continue with RNA isolation by the conventional method (*see* Subheading 3.4.2).

3.4 RNA Isolation from Exosomes

3.4.1 RNA Isolation from Exosomes Using the miRCURY RNA Isolation Kit—Cell and Plant

1. Prepare the work area for RNA handling as described above.
2. Add the needed volume of 95–100% ethanol to the concentrated *Wash Solution* as described in the kit manual. Equilibrate all reagents at room temperature.
3. Use the lysates of exosomes prepared in 350 µl *Lysis Solution* as described in Subheadings 3.3.1 or 3.3.2 for RNA isolation (*see* **Note 19**).
4. Add 200 µl 95–100% ethanol to the lysates and mix them thoroughly by vortexing for 10 s.

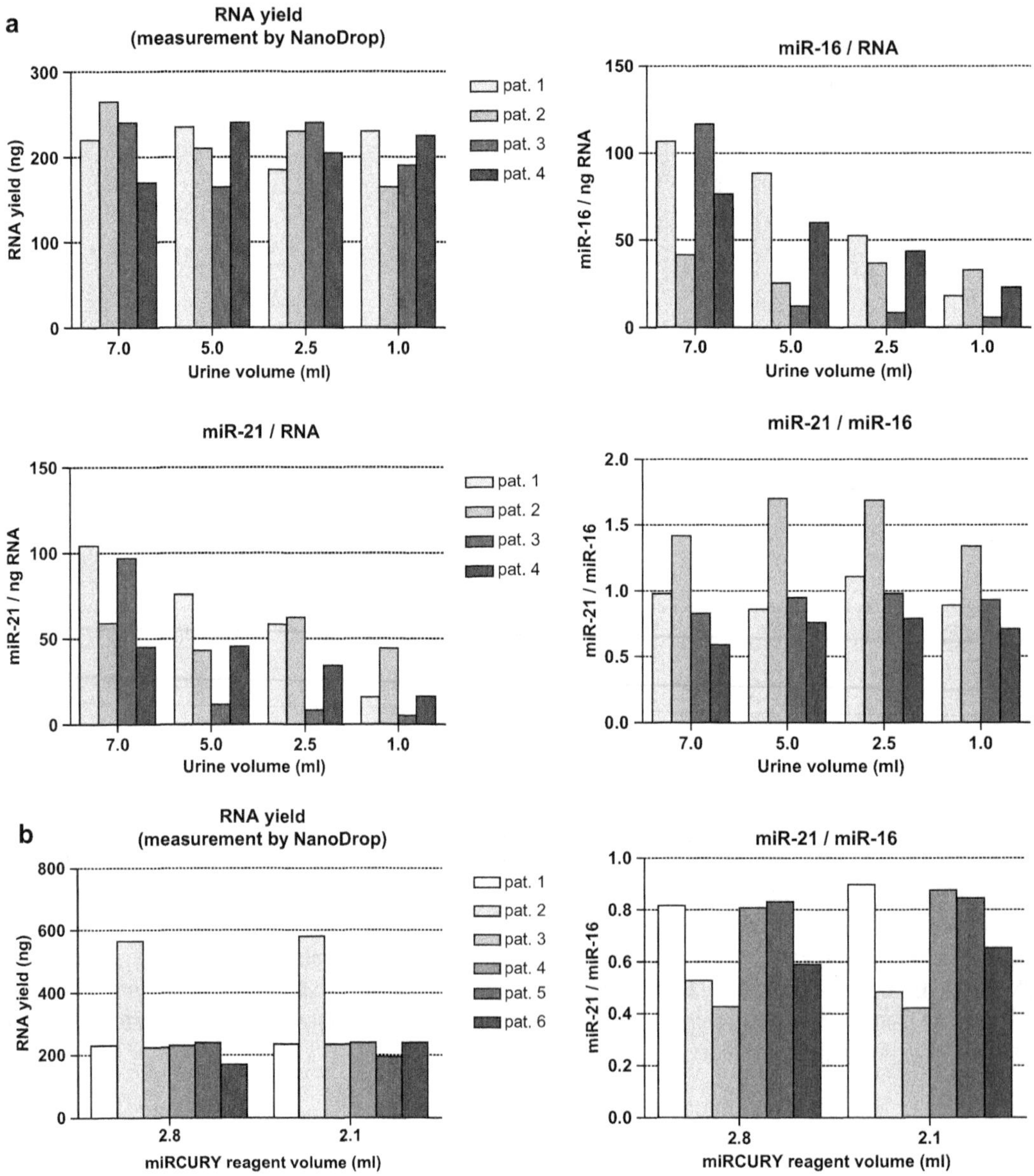

Fig. 5 RNA yield and microRNA quantification after optimization of experimental conditions for exosomes isolation by the *miRCURY Exosome Isolation Kit*. (**a**) The urine volume used for exosomes isolation was reduced maintaining a constant ratio of urine to the *Precipitation Buffer* of the *miRCURY Exosome Isolation Kit* (1.0 ml : 0.4 ml). Subsequently, RNA was isolated using the *miRCURY RNA Isolation Kit*. The RNA yield (determined by the *NanoDrop* spectrophotometer) and ratios of miR-21/miR-16 (measured by qPCR) appeared to be stable over the tested range of urine volumes. Nevertheless, at least 5–7 ml urine should be used if possible. (**b**) The volume of the *Precipitation Buffer* of the *miRCURY Exosome Isolation Kit* was reduced from 0.4 to 0.3 ml per ml urine corresponding to 2.8 ml and 2.1 ml, respectively, when using 7 ml urine. The RNA yield and ratios of miR-21/miR-16 appeared similar for both experimental conditions. Therefore, the amount of the *Precipitation Buffer* can be diminished without loss

5. Apply the lysates mixed with ethanol onto the columns prior assembled with collection tubes and centrifuge at >3,500 × *g* for 1 min at room temperature (*see* **Note 20**).
6. Discard the flow-through, add 400 μl *Wash Solution* and centrifuge at 14,000 × *g* for 1 min at room temperature.
7. Discard the flow-through and repeat the washing step twice in the same manner. Finally, centrifuge the columns at 14,000 × *g* for 2 min at room temperature in order to dry the resin thoroughly.
8. Discard the collection tubes and transfer the columns to 1.7 ml elution tubes from the kit. After addition of 50 μl *Elution Buffer* onto the columns centrifuge for 2 min at 200 × *g* followed by 1 min at 14,000 × *g* at room temperature (*see* **Note 21**).
9. Transfer RNA immediately to cooled conditions, if applicable aliquot small volumes for assessment of RNA quantity and quality and freeze the remaining volume at −80 °C for further processing.

3.4.2 RNA Isolation from Exosomes Using the Conventional Qiazol Method

1. RNA isolation from exosomes by the conventional *Qiazol* method is performed in the same way as described in Subheading 3.2.1. Since the exosomes are lysed in 1,000 μl *Qiazol*, the volumes of chloroform, isopropyl alcohol, and ethanol have to be adjusted as described in Subheading 3.2.1.
2. Finally, dissolve the dried RNA pellet in 50 μl nuclease-free water by incubation at 60 °C for 10 min (*see* **Note 11**).
3. Transfer RNA immediately to cooled conditions (e.g., on ice), if applicable aliquot small volumes for RNA quantity and quality assessment and freeze the remaining volume at −80 °C for further processing such as reverse transcription.

3.5 Assessment of RNA Quantity and Quality

3.5.1 RNA Assessment by Analyses by NanoDrop Spectrophotometer

1. First clean the sample retention system in the *NanoDrop 2000c* instrument by pipetting 2–3 μl of deionized water onto the lower optical surface. Close the lever arm enabling the upper pedestal to come in contact with the water. After lifting the lever arm wipe off both optical surfaces with a clean, dry, lint-free lab wipe.
2. Start the *NanoDrop 2000c* software and select the application "*Nucleic Acid*".
3. For blanking, apply 1 μl of the appropriate buffer or water onto the lower optical surface. Lower the lever arm and start "Blank" in the software. Afterwards, clean both optical surfaces as described above.
4. Choose the appropriate type of nucleic acid (RNA) and of the desired concentration unit for the sample that is to be measured.

5. Pipet 1 μl of the RNA sample onto the lower optical pedestal, close the lever arm and start "Measure" in the software. The software automatically calculates the RNA concentration and the ratio $A_{260nm/280nm}$ for evaluation of RNA quality. Review the spectrum to evaluate the accuracy of the measurement and to assess the sample quality (*see* **Note 22**).
6. Clean the sample retention system between all samples measured and after the last sample as described above.

3.5.2 RNA Assessment by Agilent 2100 Bioanalyzer

1. To assess the quantity and quality of the RNA isolated from cellular pellets or from exosomes, the microfluidic "lab-on-a-chip" systems from Agilent Technologies can be utilized. Depending on the yield of RNA you can choose between the *Agilent RNA 6000 Pico Kit* (for 50–5,000 pg/μl total RNA) and the *Agilent RNA 6000 Nano Kit* (for 5–500 ng/μl total RNA). You should keep in mind that the *Agilent RNA 6000 Pico Kit* is not recommended for quantitative analyses and that the quantitative range of the *Agilent RNA 6000 Nano Kit* is only between 25 and 500 ng/μl total RNA (*see* **Note 23**).
2. Prepare the work area for RNA handling as described above. Let the kit equilibrate at room temperature for 30 min. Start the *Agilent 2000 Bioanalyzer* software and select the appropriate conditions.
3. Decontaminate the electrodes of the *Agilent 2000 Bioanalyzer* using *RNaseZAP* filled into the *Electrode Cleaner* for 1 min followed by incubation with water filled in another *Electrode Cleaner* for 1 min. Check the priming station and use a new syringe for each kit.
4. Transfer the RNA ladder into a 0.5 ml PCR tube. When using the *Agilent RNA 6000 Pico Kit* add 90 μl RNase-free water to 10 μl of the RNA ladder and mix gently. The next step is a heat denaturation for 2 min at 70 °C followed by immediate cooling on ice. Due to the instability of the RNA ladder it is recommended to prepare aliquots with the required amount for the typical daily use (e.g., 1 or 2 μl) stored at −70 °C in 0.5 ml nuclease-free tubes (*see* **Note 24**).
5. To prepare the gel, pipette 550 μl of the RNA gel matrix into a spin filter, centrifuge it at 1,500 × *g* for 10 min at room temperature. This filtered gel should be stored at 4 °C and used within 4 weeks. Transfer 65 μl of the filtered gel into a nuclease-free 0.5 ml tube and add 1 μl of the dye, mix it thoroughly by vortexing and centrifuge the tube at 13,000 × *g* for 10 min at room temperature. The prepared gel–dye mix should be kept in the dark and has to be used within 1 day.

6. Next, put a RNA chip on the chip priming station, apply 9 μl gel–dye mix in the appropriate well and close the priming station. The plunger should be pressed until it is held by the clip. After exactly 30 s the clip can be released and after further 5 s the plunger can be pulled back to the 1 ml position. After opening the chip priming station 9 μl of the gel–dye mix are pipetted into the marked wells.
7. Only applicable for the *Agilent RNA 6000 Pico Kit*: Pipette 9 μl of the RNA conditioning solution into the appropriate well.
8. Pipette 5 μl of the RNA marker, 1 μl of the prepared ladder and 1 μl of the RNA samples in the appropriate wells, which are marked in the kit manual.
9. Subsequently, vortex the chip for 1 min at 2,400 rpm using a special IKA vortex shaker and start the chip run in the *Agilent 2100 Bioanalyzer* instrument within 5 min.
10. Evaluate the electropherograms for the RNA concentration, the RNA integrity number (RIN; between 1 and 10) and the peak ratio of the 28S to 18S rRNAs (*see* **Note 25**, Figs. 4 and 6a).

3.5.3 RNA Assessment by AATI Fragment Analyzer

1. The quantity and quality of the isolated RNA can alternatively be assessed using the *AATI Fragment Analyzer* instrument (Advanced Analytical Technologies), which is based on the separation of nucleic acids by automated capillary electrophoresis. Capillary arrays combined with automated sample handling and data analysis allow multiple applications.
2. Depending on the yield of RNA you can choose between the *High Sensitivity RNA Analysis Kit* (for 50–5,000 pg/μl total RNA) and the *Standard Sensitivity RNA Analysis Kit* (for 5–500 ng/μl total RNA) (*see* **Note 26**).
3. Prepare the work area for RNA handling as described above. Bring the *RNA Separation Gel* and the *Intercalating Dye* to room temperature. Mix appropriate volumes of both components, which are necessary for 1 day, in a 50 ml centrifuge tube and place it onto the instrument (*see* **Note 27**).
4. Mix 20 ml of the *5× 930 dsDNA Inlet Buffer*, equilibrated at room temperature beforehand, with 80 ml of deionized, sub-micron filtered water. Prepare a mix of 10 ml of the 5× *Capillary Conditioning Solution* and of 40 ml deionized, sub-micron filtered water and place it onto the instrument (*see* **Note 27**).
5. Check fluid levels of the waste bottle and waste tray in the instrument and empty it if necessary. Apply a fresh 96-DeepWell plate filled with 1 ml/well of *1× 930 dsDNA Inlet Buffer*. Prepare a sample plate with 200 μl/well of the 0.25×

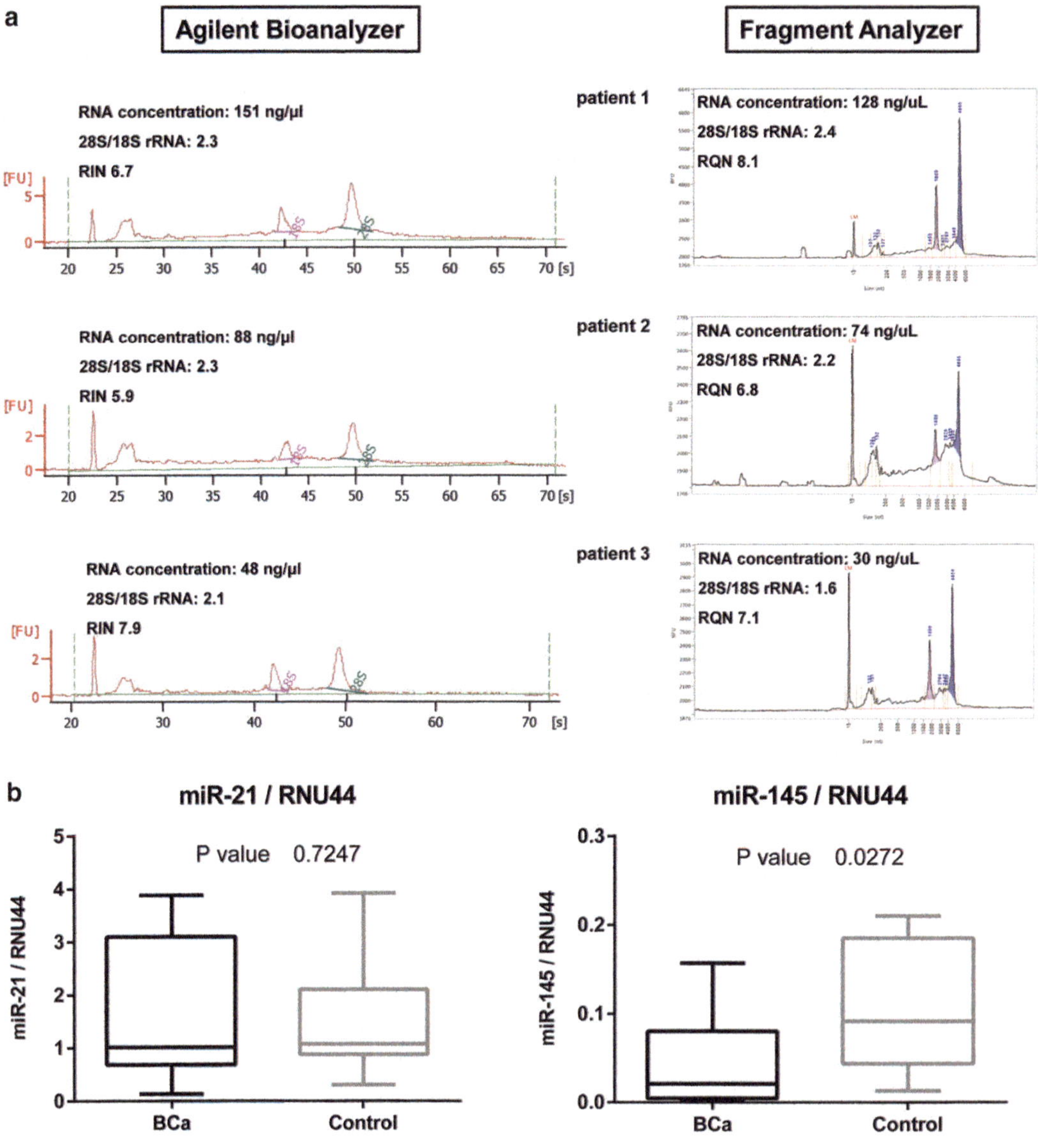

Fig. 6 Quantification of microRNAs in cellular pellets from urine of bladder cancer patients and controls. (**a**) Urine specimens were obtained from 10 patients with bladder cancer prior to TUR-BT and from 10 patients with urolithiasis as controls. RNA was isolated from urinary sediments using the Direct-zol kit. RNA concentration and quality (28S/18S rRNA ratio, RIN and RQN) was assessed by Agilent Bioanalyzer and Fragment Analyzer. Results for the presented samples are similar for both methods. (**b**) RNA (5 µl) was used for specific reverse transcription and subsequent qPCR-based quantification of the microRNAs miR-21 and miR-145 with RNU44 as reference. Significance of differences in the relative microRNA-expression levels in this test cohort was assessed by the Mann-Whitney U tes. *RIN:* RNA integrity number, *RQN:* RNA quality number, *TUR-BT:* transurethral resection of the bladder tumor

TE rinse buffer. Place solutions and plates in the appropriate trays and drawers as described in the manual of the instrument.

6. Transfer the *Standard Sensitivity RNA Diluent Marker (15 nt)* from −20 °C to ice before use. Thaw the *Standard Sensitivity*

RNA ladder, which should be aliquoted and stored at ≤−70 °C, on ice. After spinning down briefly heat-denature the ladder in a nuclease-free PCR tube for 2 min at 70 °C and cool it immediately on ice to 4 °C.

7. Perform a heat-denaturation of all RNA samples for 2 min at 70 °C followed by immediate cooling on ice in the same way.
8. Pipette 22 μl of the *Standard Sensitivity RNA Diluent Marker (15 nt) solution* into each well destined for RNA samples or the RNA ladder. Unused wells within the row have to be filled with 24 μl/well of the *BF-25 Blank Solution* (*see* **Note 28**).
9. Add 2 μl of the denatured RNA samples or of the RNA ladder into the appropriate wells and mix the content thoroughly by pipetting up and down (*see* **Note 29**).
10. Spin the filled plate briefly to remove any air bubbles which could lead to injection errors.
11. Due to the potential instability of the RNA the plate should be measured as soon as possible, otherwise it should be sealed and stored at 4 °C and used within 20 h. Place the unsealed plate into one of the sample plate trays of the *Fragment Analyzer* instrument and start the measurement in the software as described in the manual.
12. After completion of the measurements evaluate the capillary electropherograms with regard to the RNA concentration, the RNA quality number (RQN; between 1 and 10) and the peak ratio of the 28S to 18S rRNAs (*see* **Note 30**).

3.6 Reverse Transcription of MicroRNAs

1. The *TaqMan microRNA Assays* (Thermo Fisher Scientific), which are designed to quantify mature microRNAs based on looped-primer RT-PCR, comprise one tube containing a miRNA-specific stem-loop RT primer used for reverse transcription of the microRNA. The second tube containing a mix of the miRNA-specific forward PCR primer, the specific reverse PCR primer and the miRNA-specific FAM-labeled *TaqMan MGB probe* will be utilized for the subsequent quantification of the specific microRNA by qPCR (Subheading 3.7).
2. You can apply 1–10 ng total RNA for reverse transcription in a reaction volume of 15 μl using the *TaqMan MicroRNA Reverse Transcription Kit*. Thaw RNA and the kit components on ice. Prepare a RT master mix for one or up to five different microRNAs calculating the number of RNA samples and a sufficient surplus to account for variations in pipetting.
3. In case of multiplex RT the concentration of the miRNA-specific RT primers can be reduced without impairment of the subsequent quantification by qPCR. Calculate the following components per RT reaction (final volume 15 μl) in

Table 1
Composition of reaction mixtures for reverse transcription of 1–5 microRNAs

Component	Volume (μl) for reverse transcription as				
	Singleplex	Duplex	Triplex	Quadruplex	Pentaplex
dNTPs (100 mM each)	0.15	0.15	0.15	0.15	0.15
MultiScribe Reverse Transcriptase (50 U/μl)	1.00	1.00	1.00	1.00	1.00
Reverse Transcription Buffer (10×)	1.50	1.50	1.50	1.50	1.50
RNase Inhibitor (20 U/μl)	0.19	0.19	0.19	0.19	0.19
nuclease-free water	4.16	1.16	0.00	0.00	0.00
miRNA RT primer(s) (5×)	3.00	each 3.00	each 2.39	each 1.79	each 1.43
Total volume	10.00	10.00	10.00	10.00	10.00

Table 2
Temperature profile for reverse transcription of microRNAs

Step	Temperature	Time
1	16 °C	30 min
2	42 °C	30 min
3	85 °C	5 min
4	4 °C	hold

dependence on the intended number of microRNAs to be analyzed in parallel (*see* **Note 31**; Table 1).

4. Dilute the total RNA to a final concentration of 0.2–2 ng/μl and give 5 μl (up to 10 ng total RNA) in a polypropylene tube on ice. Add 10 μl of the RT master mix per tube and mix gently. Spin the mix briefly down and incubate it on ice until loading the thermal cycler.
5. Apply the temperature program listed in Table 2.
6. Store the cDNA product from this microRNA-specific RT reaction at 4 °C or −20 °C and use it undiluted for quantification of the mature microRNAs by qPCR as described in Subheading 3.7.

3.7 Quantitative PCR

1. First prepare the master mix for PCR reactions with a final volume of 10 or 20 μl (depending on the qPCR instrument). Keep the *TaqMan MicroRNA Assays* (Thermo Fisher Scientific) protected from light and frozen until use.

Table 3
Composition of the PCR master mix for different reaction volumes

Component	Volume (µl) per 10 µl reaction	Volume (µl) per 20 µl reaction
TaqMan MicroRNA Assay (20×)	0.50	1.00
TaqMan Universal PCR Master Mix (2×)	5.00	10.00
Nuclease-free water	3.50	7.00
Total volume per reaction	**9.00**	**18.00**

2. You can use the *TaqMan Universal PCR Master Mix, No AmpErase UNG* (Thermo Fisher Scientific) as recommended for *TaqMan MicroRNA Assays* or alternative PCR master mixes (*see* **Note 4**)
3. Prepare a PCR master mix consisting of the components listed in Table 3 for the intended number of PCR reactions (including a positive and a negative control) and a surplus for 1–5 additional reactions (depending on the total number of PCR reactions). Calculate necessary volumes of the PCR ingredients (Table 3). Keep in mind that a separate PCR run has to be performed for each microRNA even if the prior RT was done as multiplex.
4. Distribute the appropriate volumes of the PCR master mix to the reaction vessels (e.g., wells of the PCR plate) and add 1 µl per 10 µl reaction or 2 µl per 20 µl reaction, respectively, of the undiluted microRNA-specific cDNAs from the different samples to the wells. Apply this approach to all microRNAs to be analyzed and the appropriate reference RNAs (*see* **Note 32**).
5. After preparation of the experimental protocol in the qPCR software insert the PCR plate into the instrument and start the PCR run. Select the appropriate fluorescence channel and acquisition mode for detection of the FAM-labeled TaqMan MGB probe (depending on the qPCR instrument). Apply the temperature program listed in Table 4.
6. After completion of the run analyze the microRNA expression by calculation of the C_T or C_P values and continue with the evaluation of the expression levels (*see* **Note 33**, Fig. 6b).

4 Notes

1. You can use any analog ready-to-use reagent consisting of phenol, guanidine isothiocyanate and proprietary components depending on the provider. Best-known reagents applicable for

Table 4
Temperature profile for qPCR measurements

Step	Temperature	Time
initial denaturation	95 °C	10 min
45 amplification cycles of denaturation annealing/extension	95 °C 60 °C	15 s 60 s
Cooling	40 °C	1 min

the acid guanidinium thiocyanate-phenol-chloroform extraction of total RNA are *TRIzol* (Thermo Fisher Scientific), *TRI Reagent* (Sigma-Aldrich), *QIAzol Lysis Reagent* (Qiagen), *Tri-Fast* (VWR), *TriPure Isolation Reagent* (Roche) or *TriSure* (Bioline).

2. Use of sterile urine beakers is recommend, but not necessary. Nevertheless, processing of the urine specimens should start as soon as possible after collection. Otherwise, urine can be stored at 4 °C for few hours and/or RNA-stabilizing reagents could be added directly into the urine collection vessel. It should be validated in the specific setting whether longer storage of the urine specimens at 4 °C or the addition of potential stabilizers has an influence on the results of microRNA expression analyses.

3. Herein, the application of *TaqMan microRNA assays* based on microRNA-specific stem-loop reverse transcription (RT) primers and amplification primers is described. Alternatively, other qPCR assays may be applied for quantification of microRNA expression. Thermo Fisher Scientific offers a new assay generation, the so-called *TaqMan Advanced miRNA Assays*, which use a Poly(A) tailing reaction and adapter ligation reaction followed by an universal RT step for all assays instead of miRNA-specific RT primers. Furthermore, other qPCR-based assay systems can be used for microRNA quantification such as the SYBR Green-based *miScript PCR System* from Qiagen or the *miRCURY LNA Universal RT microRNA PCR system* from Exiqon. Pools and panels for RT and qPCR-based quantification of multiple microRNAs are also available from different providers.

4. The use of other master mixes, e.g., the *TaqMan Gene Expression Master Mix* (Thermo Fisher Scientific) or the *GoTaq Probe qPCR Master Mix* (Promega), is also possible. They should be validated regarding their performance and costs in the specific setting.

5. Different real-time PCR instruments, such as the *Applied Biosystems 7900HT Fast Real-Time PCR System* (Thermo Fisher Scientific) or the *LightCycler 480 Instrument* (Roche), can be utilized for microRNA expression analyses. Their performance in these analyses should be validated in advance.
6. For urine cytology prepare a cellular pellet from up to 10 ml urine and prefix it with 10 ml Esposti's fixative overnight. Centrifuge the prefixed cells on glass slides at 1,000 × *g* for 4 min at 20 °C and remove the supernatant carefully. After fixation, e.g., with *Cytofix N* (Niepötter Labortechnik, Bürstadt, Germany), slides are stained according to the Papanicolaou protocol. The preparations should be examined by an experienced pathologist or urologist. Other procedures, such as urine dipstick and sediment analysis, are done according to standard protocols for clinical chemistry.
7. Other volumes of urine supernatant can be aliquoted, but 8 ml are sufficient for the preparation of exosomes and the subsequent microRNA expression analyses (*see* also **Note 16**).
8. If the cellular pellet is very large and difficult to resuspend, apply 1,400 μl *Qiazol.*
9. Incubation of the thawed lysates for 5 min is necessary to permit the complete dissociation of nucleoprotein complexes.
10. Alternatively the RNA can be precipitated over 10 min at room temperature or at 4 °C. The precipitated RNA should appear at the bottom of the tube as gel-like or white pellet.
11. You can use water treated with diethylpyrocarbonate (DEPC) for resuspension of the RNA. Furthermore, some providers recommend a further clean-up of the RNA by column-based kits.
12. Isolation of RNA by the *Direct-zol RNA MiniPrep kit* is easier, faster, and less dependent on the experience and skills of the person preparing the RNA. Additionally, the use of chloroform is dispensable. According to the provider, the *Direct-zol* method allows the unbiased recovery of small RNAs including microRNAs whereas RNA isolation by conventional phase separation has been shown to selectively enrich some species of microRNAs leading to bias in downstream analysis. In our analyses, both methods delivered comparable results with regard to the yield and quality of RNA (Fig. 2). Nevertheless, enrichment of some microRNAs (e.g., miR-21) may differ between both techniques as shown in Fig. 3.
13. DNA digestion is recommended to remove contaminations with genomic DNA which might impair sensitive downstream applications. Whether DNase treatment is necessary should be evaluated in the specific setting.

14. The centrifuge tubes have to be filled at least half-full (best at 2/3), but not filled up completely due to the risk of overflow. In case of an urine sample volume below 50% of the tube volume add PBS.
15. Differential centrifugation is considered to be the "gold standard" for isolation of exosomes. However, it is a very time-consuming method and possibly not available. Precipitation of exosomes represents an attractive and easy-to-perform alternative. Own electron-microscopic analyses revealed that the microvesicles isolated by both techniques were similar in output and particle size (data not shown). The observed particle diameter between 50 and 140 nm (median values of 50–70 nm depending on the urine specimen) corresponded to the range typical for exosomes. Furthermore, exosomal protein markers, such as CD9, ALIX, and flotilin-1, were detected in both types of microvesicle preparations indicating that mainly exosomes were isolated (data not shown). Yield and quality of the RNA extracted from exosomes isolated by both methods were also comparable (Fig. 4) implying their equivalence.
16. Precipitation of exosomes is relatively expensive, independent of the provider of the precipitation reagents. Therefore, the optimization of the needed volumes of the urine sample and of the precipitation buffer seems to be meaningful to save costs and to retain sufficient yield. During the optimization of the current protocol processing of different urine volumes was compared. The stepwise reduction of urine volumes from 28 to 7 ml revealed sufficient output regarding RNA yield and microRNA quantification (data not shown). However, further diminishment of the urine volume to 1 ml resulted in a clear decrease of microRNA amplificates even if the normalized relative microRNA levels were still comparable (Fig. 5a).
17. To save money in this very expensive process, the *Precipitation Buffer* of the *miRCURY Exosome Isolation Kit* can be reduced from the recommended 0.4 to 0.3 ml per ml urine without any impairment of the output (Fig. 5b). In contrast, the addition of 0.2 ml *Precipitation Buffer* per ml urine was not sufficient (data not shown).
18. Both variants are possible according to the manufacturer's recommendations. It can be adapted depending on the optimal time setting.
19. According to the provider, β-mercaptoethanol can be used optionally in lysis. It is highly recommended for tissues known to have a high RNAse content and for sensitive downstream applications. For this purpose, 10 μl β-mercaptoethanol have to be added per 1 ml of *Lysis Solution*. In the protocol described herein *Lysis Solution* was used without β-mercaptoethanol.

20. Since minimal amounts of genomic DNA are isolated together with total RNA by the *miRCURY RNA Isolation Kit* an optional on-column DNA digestion step is recommend if necessary. For details see the manufacturer's protocol.
21. If not the entire volume of 50 μl has been eluted from the column, spin the column for another minute at 14,000 × *g*. For maximum RNA recovery the elution step can be repeated. In this case, it is recommended to elute the remaining RNA into a separate tube to avoid dilution of the previously eluted RNA sample.
22. Pure RNA should result in an $A_{260nm/280nm}$ ratio of ~2.0. Different purity ratios may indicate the presence of protein, phenol or other contaminants strongly absorbing at or near 280 nm.
23. RNA quantification using the *Agilent Bioanalyzer* is superior to conventional spectrophotometric analyses since more information on RNA integrity and size distribution is available from the electropherograms. The calculated RNA integrity number (RIN) ranging from 1 to 10 is an estimate for RNA degradation. The presence of small RNAs in the RNA preparation can be assessed as well as the ratio of the 28S/18S rRNA. You can analyze 11 or 12 RNA samples per chip in parallel depending on the selected assay.
24. The frozen aliquots do not require repeated heat denaturation after initial heat denaturation. Thaw the RNA ladder aliquots on ice before use and avoid extensive warming.
25. RNA extracts from urine-derived cellular pellets and exosomes mainly contain small RNA species due to strong degradation processes. Nevertheless, microRNAs are relatively stable and still quantifiable despite impaired overall quality of the total RNA (Figs. 4 and 6a). However, the *Agilent 2100 expert* software possibly is not able to calculate a RIN value in case of large amounts of small RNAs and the absence of 28S and 18S rRNAs resulting in an error indication.
26. Please keep in mind that the quantitative range of the *Standard Sensitivity RNA Analysis Kit* only lies between 25 and 500 ng/μl total RNA. Furthermore, the quantification accuracy of the *Standard Sensitivity RNA Analysis Kit* varies by ±20% and up to 30% for the *High Sensitivity RNA Analysis Kit*. Nevertheless, the *Agilent Bioanalyzer* displays similar disadvantages and RNA quantification should only be performed with the *Agilent RNA 6000 Nano Kit*. Furthermore, measurement by the *Fragment Analyzer* is automated and faster at similar costs per analysis. Depending on the capillary cartridge (with 12, 48 or 96 capillaries) larger numbers of RNAs samples can be analyzed in parallel.

27. Always update solution levels in the *Fragment Analyzer* software.
28. The expected RNA concentration should range between 5 and 500 ng/μl to be quantified correctly. If RNA concentration is higher than this range it should be diluted accordingly with RNase-free water. In case of lower expected RNA concentrations you can add 4 μl RNA to 20 μl of the *Standard Sensitivity RNA Diluent Marker solution*. Do the same with the RNA ladder (prior diluted 1:2) for all samples applied in the same row.
29. Thorough mixing is very important for accurate quantification. For this purpose, seal the plate with an adhesive film and vortex the plate for 2 min at 3,000 rpm. The plate has to be centrifuged briefly afterwards. Alternatively, a separate pipette tip or an electronic pipettor set to a volume >20 μl can be used for mixing the mixtures in the wells. Supply at least one well with the RNA ladder per run.
30. The results are normalized automatically to the lower marker and calibrated to the RNA ladder. If RNA samples have been pre-diluted, the settings for the dilution factor have to be changed accordingly.
31. Multiplexing can be performed for up to 96 RT primers. Suitable protocols are available from Thermo Fisher Scientific. Examples of pipetting schemes for multiplexed RT reactions with one to five RT primers are given in Table 1. Nevertheless, the feasibility should be tested in advance for the specific combinations of RT primers and be compared between the monoplex and multiplex RT reactions.
32. Appropriate reference RNAs have to be selected carefully. The small nuclear and nucleolar RNAs RNU6B, RNA44, and RNA48 are frequently used for the normalization of microRNA expression levels. For analyses of exosome-derived microRNAs these reference RNA might not work. Therefore, suitable microRNAs without differential expression should be identified and used for normalization. According to the literature [31], we used miR-16 for this purpose in the described experiments. Spiking of the synthetic reference microRNA cel-miR-39 from *Caenorhabditis elegans* into the urine lysate and its quantification after the whole processing workflow can represent a suitable alternative.
33. Apply the normalized $\Delta\Delta C_T$ or fold-change for analysis. Alternatively, standard curves can be produced to calculate the molecule numbers of microRNA transcripts. After normalization to those of the reference RNAs, the same results are obtained as for the fold-change calculations (Fig. 6b).

References

1. Carrington JC, Ambros V (2003) Role of microRNAs in plant and animal development. Science 301(5631):336–338. doi:10.1126/science.1085242
2. Mlcochova H, Hezova R, Stanik M, Slaby O (2014) Urine microRNAs as potential noninvasive biomarkers in urologic cancers. Urol Oncol 32(1):41 e41–41 e49. doi:10.1016/j.urolonc.2013.04.011
3. Fendler A, Stephan C, Yousef GM, Jung K (2011) MicroRNAs as regulators of signal transduction in urological tumors. Clin Chem 57(7):954–968. doi:10.1373/clinchem.2010.157727
4. Schubert M, Junker K, Heinzelmann J (2016) Prognostic and predictive miRNA biomarkers in bladder, kidney and prostate cancer: where do we stand in biomarker development? J Cancer Res Clin Oncol 142(8):1673–1695. doi:10.1007/s00432-015-2089-9
5. Catto JW, Alcaraz A, Bjartell AS, De Vere WR, Evans CP, Fussel S, Hamdy FC, Kallioniemi O, Mengual L, Schlomm T, Visakorpi T (2011) MicroRNA in prostate, bladder, and kidney cancer: a systematic review. Eur Urol 59 (5):671–681. doi:10.1016/j.eururo.2011.01.044
6. Ouyang H, Zhou Y, Zhang L, Shen G (2015) Diagnostic value of microRNAs for urologic cancers: a systematic review and meta-analysis. Medicine (Baltimore) 94(37):e1272. doi:10.1097/md.0000000000001272
7. Canturk KM, Ozdemir M, Can C, Oner S, Emre R, Aslan H, Cilingir O, Ciftci E, Celayir FM, Aldemir O, Ozen M, Artan S (2014) Investigation of key miRNAs and target genes in bladder cancer using miRNA profiling and bioinformatic tools. Mol Biol Rep 41 (12):8127–8135. doi:10.1007/s11033-014-3713-5
8. Dyrskjot L, Ostenfeld MS, Bramsen JB, Silahtaroglu AN, Lamy P, Ramanathan R, Fristrup N, Jensen JL, Andersen CL, Zieger K, Kauppinen S, Ulhoi BP, Kjems J, Borre M, Orntoft TF (2009) Genomic profiling of microRNAs in bladder cancer: miR-129 is associated with poor outcome and promotes cell death in vitro. Cancer Res 69(11):4851–4860. doi:10.1158/0008-5472.can-08-4043
9. Han Y, Chen J, Zhao X, Liang C, Wang Y, Sun L, Jiang Z, Zhang Z, Yang R, Li Z, Tang A, Li X, Ye J, Guan Z, Gui Y, Cai Z (2011) MicroRNA expression signatures of bladder cancer revealed by deep sequencing. PLoS One 6(3): e18286. doi:10.1371/journal.pone.0018286
10. Ichimi T, Enokida H, Okuno Y, Kunimoto R, Chiyomaru T, Kawamoto K, Kawahara K, Toki K, Kawakami K, Nishiyama K, Tsujimoto G, Nakagawa M, Seki N (2009) Identification of novel microRNA targets based on microRNA signatures in bladder cancer. Int J Cancer 125 (2):345–352. doi:10.1002/ijc.24390
11. Itesako T, Seki N, Yoshino H, Chiyomaru T, Yamasaki T, Hidaka H, Yonezawa T, Nohata N, Kinoshita T, Nakagawa M, Enokida H (2014) The microRNA expression signature of bladder cancer by deep sequencing: the functional significance of the miR-195/497 cluster. PLoS One 9(2):e84311. doi:10.1371/journal.pone.0084311
12. Zaravinos A, Radojicic J, Lambrou GI, Volanis D, Delakas D, Stathopoulos EN, Spandidos DA (2012) Expression of miRNAs involved in angiogenesis, tumor cell proliferation, tumor suppressor inhibition, epithelial-mesenchymal transition and activation of metastasis in bladder cancer. J Urol 188(2):615–623. doi:10.1016/j.juro.2012.03.122
13. Catto JW, Miah S, Owen HC, Bryant H, Myers K, Dudziec E, Larre S, Milo M, Rehman I, Rosario DJ, Di Martino E, Knowles MA, Meuth M, Harris AL, Hamdy FC (2009) Distinct microRNA alterations characterize high- and low-grade bladder cancer. Cancer Res 69 (21):8472–8481. doi:10.1158/0008-5472.can-09-0744
14. Dip N, Reis ST, Timoszczuk LS, Viana NI, Piantino CB, Morais DR, Moura CM, Abe DK, Silva IA, Srougi M, Dall'Oglio MF, Leite KR (2012) Stage, grade and behavior of bladder urothelial carcinoma defined by the microRNA expression profile. J Urol 188 (5):1951–1956. doi:10.1016/j.juro.2012.07.004
15. Pignot G, Cizeron-Clairac G, Vacher S, Susini A, Tozlu S, Vieillefond A, Zerbib M, Lidereau R, Debre B, Amsellem-Ouazana D, Bieche I (2013) microRNA expression profile in a large series of bladder tumors: identification of a 3-miRNA signature associated with aggressiveness of muscle-invasive bladder cancer. Int J Cancer 132(11):2479–2491. doi:10.1002/ijc.27949
16. Sapre N, Macintyre G, Clarkson M, Naeem H, Cmero M, Kowalczyk A, Anderson PD, Costello AJ, Corcoran NM, Hovens CM (2016) A urinary microRNA signature can predict the presence of bladder urothelial carcinoma in patients undergoing surveillance. Br J Cancer 114(4):454–462. doi:10.1038/bjc.2015.472

17. Veerla S, Lindgren D, Kvist A, Frigyesi A, Staaf J, Persson H, Liedberg F, Chebil G, Gudjonsson S, Borg A, Mansson W, Rovira C, Hoglund M (2009) MiRNA expression in urothelial carcinomas: important roles of miR-10a, miR-222, miR-125b, miR-7 and miR-452 for tumor stage and metastasis, and frequent homozygous losses of miR-31. Int J Cancer 124(9):2236–2242. doi:10.1002/ijc.24183
18. Zhou H, Tang K, Xiao H, Zeng J, Guan W, Guo X, Xu H, Ye Z (2015) A panel of eight-miRNA signature as a potential biomarker for predicting survival in bladder cancer. J Exp Clin Cancer Res 34:53. doi:10.1186/s13046-015-0167-0
19. Huang X, Liang M, Dittmar R, Wang L (2013) Extracellular microRNAs in urologic malignancies: chances and challenges. Int J Mol Sci 14(7): 14785–14799. doi:10.3390/ijms140714785
20. Armstrong DA, Green BB, Seigne JD, Schned AR, Marsit CJ (2015) MicroRNA molecular profiling from matched tumor and bio-fluids in bladder cancer. Mol Cancer 14:194. doi:10.1186/s12943-015-0466-2
21. Eissa S, Habib H, Ali E, Kotb Y (2015) Evaluation of urinary miRNA-96 as a potential biomarker for bladder cancer diagnosis. Med Oncol 32(1):413. doi:10.1007/s12032-014-0413-x
22. Eissa S, Matboli M, Essawy NO, Kotb YM (2015) Integrative functional genetic-epigenetic approach for selecting genes as urine biomarkers for bladder cancer diagnosis. Tumour Biol 36(12):9545–9552. doi:10.1007/s13277-015-3722-6
23. Eissa S, Matboli M, Hegazy MG, Kotb YM, Essawy NO (2015) Evaluation of urinary microRNA panel in bladder cancer diagnosis: relation to bilharziasis. Transl Res 165 (6):731–739. doi:10.1016/j.trsl.2014.12.008
24. Hanke M, Hoefig K, Merz H, Feller AC, Kausch I, Jocham D, Warnecke JM, Sczakiel G (2010) A robust methodology to study urine microRNA as tumor marker: microRNA-126 and microRNA-182 are related to urinary bladder cancer. Urol Oncol 28(6):655–661. doi:10.1016/j.urolonc.2009.01.027
25. Mengual L, Lozano JJ, Ingelmo-Torres M, Gazquez C, Ribal MJ, Alcaraz A (2013) Using microRNA profiling in urine samples to develop a non-invasive test for bladder cancer. Int J Cancer 133(11):2631–2641. doi:10.1002/ijc.28274
26. Sasaki H, Yoshiike M, Nozawa S, Usuba W, Katsuoka Y, Aida K, Kitajima K, Kudo H, Hoshikawa M, Yoshioka Y, Kosaka N, Ochiya T, Chikaraishi T (2016) Expression level of urinary microRNA-146a-5p is increased in patients with bladder bancer and decreased in those after transurethral resection. Clin Genitourin Cancer 14(5):e493–e499. doi:10.1016/j.clgc.2016.04.002
27. Snowdon J, Boag S, Feilotter H, Izard J, Siemens DR (2013) A pilot study of urinary microRNA as a biomarker for urothelial cancer. Can Urol Assoc J 7(1–2):28–32. doi:10.5489/cuaj.11115
28. Yamada Y, Enokida H, Kojima S, Kawakami K, Chiyomaru T, Tatarano S, Yoshino H, Kawahara K, Nishiyama K, Seki N, Nakagawa M (2011) MiR-96 and miR-183 detection in urine serve as potential tumor markers of urothelial carcinoma: correlation with stage and grade, and comparison with urinary cytology. Cancer Sci 102(3):522–529. doi:10.1111/j.1349-7006.2010.01816.x
29. Zhang DZ, Lau KM, Chan ES, Wang G, Szeto CC, Wong K, Choy RK, Ng CF (2014) Cell-free urinary microRNA-99a and microRNA-125b are diagnostic markers for the non-invasive screening of bladder cancer. PLoS One 9(7):e100793. doi:10.1371/journal.pone.0100793
30. Mengual L, Ribal MJ, Lozano JJ, Ingelmo-Torres M, Burset M, Fernandez PL, Alcaraz A (2014) Validation study of a noninvasive urine test for diagnosis and prognosis assessment of bladder cancer: evidence for improved models. J Urol 191(1):261–269. doi:10.1016/j.juro.2013.06.083
31. Puerta-Gil P, Garcia-Baquero R, Jia AY, Ocana S, Alvarez-Mugica M, Alvarez-Ossorio JL, Cordon-Cardo C, Cava F, Sanchez-Carbayo M (2012) miR-143, miR-222, and miR-452 are useful as tumor stratification and noninvasive diagnostic biomarkers for bladder cancer. Am J Pathol 180(5):1808–1815. doi:10.1016/j.ajpath.2012.01.034

Chapter 17

Quantitative RNA Analysis from Urine Using Real Time PCR

Lourdes Mengual and Mireia Olivan

Abstract

Urine is emerging as a biological fluid suitable to perform liquid biopsy in a minimally invasive manner, a fundamental attribute for prevention and early detection of cancer. Urine biomarkers can be analyzed in voided urine, in urine sediment, and urine supernatant. In the case of urothelial carcinoma, in which tumor cells are in direct contact with urine, the assessment of the levels of biomarkers in the urinary cell fraction appears to be the most promising approach to identify diagnostic and prognostic biomarkers in a noninvasive way. Here, we describe a protocol to collect and process urine samples to obtain urinary exfoliated cells. Furthermore, we describe the methodology to isolate RNA from urinary cells and to quantify gene expression levels from these urinary cells.

Key words cDNA pre-amplification, Gene expression, Quantitative PCR, Reverse transcription, RNA, Urine

1 Introduction

In recent years interest in new biomarkers obtainable by noninvasive methods has increased significantly. For centuries, physicians have attempted to use urine for the noninvasive assessment of disease. Urine is produced by the kidneys and allows the human body to eliminate waste products from the blood. Ancient clinicians detected glucose in the urine by tasting it or observing whether it attracted ants. The presence of albumin in the urine has been measured as an indicator of renal disease for centuries. Even today clinicians frequently shake a urine sample to determine whether it develops a froth, prima facie evidence for a high level of protein, which often is indicative of glomerular disease [1].

Urine may contain information not only from kidney and urinary tracts, but also from distant organs via plasma obtained through glomerular filtration (Fig. 1). The analysis of this biofluid can, therefore, allow the identification of biomarkers for both urogenital and systemic diseases [2].

Wolfgang A. Schulz et al. (eds.), *Urothelial Carcinoma: Methods and Protocols*, Methods in Molecular Biology, vol. 1655, DOI 10.1007/978-1-4939-7234-0_17, © Springer Science+Business Media LLC 2018

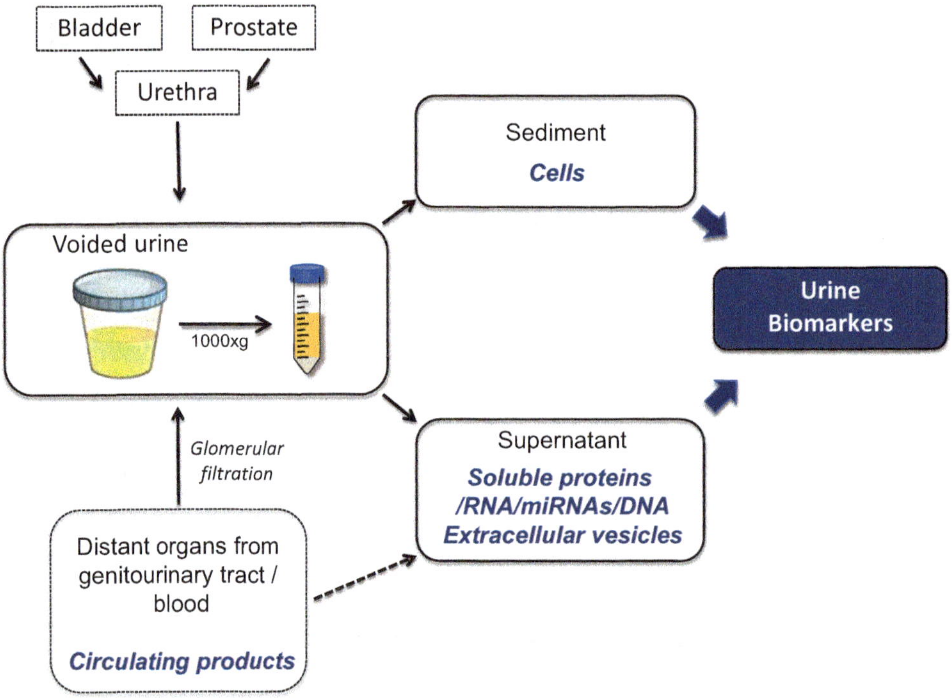

Fig. 1 Urine biomarkers can be analyzed in voided urine, in urine sediment, and urine supernatant. The choice of urine fraction is crucial because the isolated biomarkers are quite different: supernatant contains soluble biomarkers and extracellular vesicles filtered by glomeruli; sediment contains biomarkers released by different cell types contained in this urine fraction; and voided urine contains both fractions. Because of this reason, urine supernatant has a higher accuracy as biomarker of cancer located outside the genitourinary system than cells from the sediment. However, cells from the sediment are more suitable as a source of urinary tract biomarkers

In the last years, urine has received more and more attention for its convenience, as well as for its potential use in identifying new biomarkers [3]. Compared to other body fluids, urine has several characteristics that make it a preferred choice for biomarker discovery: (1) the urine genome can reflect human health status; (2) urine can be obtained in large quantities using noninvasive procedures. This allows repeated sampling of the same individual for disease surveillance; (3) the availability of urine also allows the easy assessment of reproducibility and an improvement in sample preparation protocols; (4) proteins and peptides in urine are quite stable and less complex [4].

Taking into account all these advantages, urine is emerging as a biological fluid suitable to perform liquid biopsy in a minimally invasive manner. For instance, previous studies have shown that RNA from both normal prostate and prostate cancer epithelial cells can be detected in the urine of men and can be used to detect prostate cancer [5]. RNA isolated from urinary cells has been also used to identify patients suffering from urothelial carcinoma and predict aggressiveness of the tumors [6–8].

Once the urine has been collected, it is crucial to determine which fraction of the sample needs to be used depending on the disease of interest. After a first centrifugation, urine is separated into two fractions: (1) the pellet corresponding to the cell content and (2) the supernatant in which can be found soluble proteins, RNA, DNA, and extracellular vesicles such as exosomes. Urinary exosomes have been found to be secreted by every epithelial cell type lining the human urinary tract system. Urinary exosomes are an appealing source for biomarker discovery as they contain molecular constituents of their cell of origin, including proteins and genetic materials, and they can be isolated in a noninvasive manner [9].

This chapter is focused on the most appropriate materials and methodology for the study of RNA content in the urinary cell fraction in order to identify gene expression alterations that could be related to urothelial carcinoma, unveiling novel biomarkers that improve the diagnosis and prognosis of the disease.

2 Materials

In this section the use of a number of specific products have been recommended, however equivalent products from other brands may be perfectly used.

2.1 Urine Sample Collection and Processing

1. 0.5 M EDTA, pH 8.0.
2. TRIzol Reagent (e.g., Invitrogen).
3. 70% ethanol.
4. Isopropyl alcohol.

2.2 RNA Extraction and Quantification

1. Chloroform p.a.
2. Isopropanol (2-propanol) p. a.
3. Nuclease-free H_2O.

2.3 Reverse Transcription (cDNA Synthesis)

1. High Capacity cDNA Reverse Transcription Kit (e.g., Life Technologies).
2. Nuclease-free H_2O.

2.4 cDNA Pre-amplification

1. TaqMan Gene Expression Assays, Life Technologies.
2. TE buffer; 10 mM Tris–HCl (pH 7.5), 02 mM EDTA (pH 8.0), pH final = 7.5.
3. Tris(hydroxymethyl)aminomethane.
4. EDTA (Titriplex).
5. TaqMan®PreAmp Master Mix.

2.5 Quantitative PCR Amplification

1. *GUSB* gene expression assay (Hs 99999908_mL, Life Technologies).
2. TaqMan® Universal PCR Master Mix (Life Technologies).
3. Nuclease-free water.

2.6 Equipment and Supplies

1. Urine collection container.
2. Plastic conical centrifuge tube, 50 mL.
3. Refrigerated centrifuge.
4. Microcentrifuge.
5. Micropipettes.
6. Aerosol-barrier tips.
7. Vortex mixer.
8. Powder-free gloves.
9. Microcentrifuge tubes.

3 Methods

3.1 Sample Collection

1. Add 2–4 mL of RNase-free 0.5 M EDTA, pH 8.0 (1/25 volumes) to each of the urine containers (*see* **Note 1**).
2. Ask the patient to void between 50 and 100 mL of urine (a minimum 50 mL) directly in the urine containers.
3. Once obtained, shake the urine and store it immediately at 4 °C.
4. Process the sample within the following 24 h.

3.2 Sample Processing

1. Split the urine in as many 50 mL Falcon tubes as necessary (Fig. 2) (*see* **Note 2**).
2. Centrifuge for 10 min at 1000 × *g*, and at 4 °C.
3. Drain the supernatant or store it at −80 for other applications.
4. Resuspend the pellets by gentle tapping and join together (collect them with a pipette) all pellets from the same patient into only one Falcon tube. If only one Falcon tube had been used, skip this step and go directly to **step 5**.
5. Centrifuge for 2 min at 1000 × *g*, at 4 °C.
6. Remove the supernatant with a pipette.
7. Add 1 mL TRIzol Reagent (if the pellet is very big, add 2 mL) and mix by passing solution a few times through a pipette until obtaining a homogeneous solution (*see* **Note 3**).
8. Transfer the solution to a 2-mL RNase-free eppendorf tube (or 2 eppendorfs if 2 mL had been used).
9. Continue with RNA extraction or store at −80 °C until further processing.

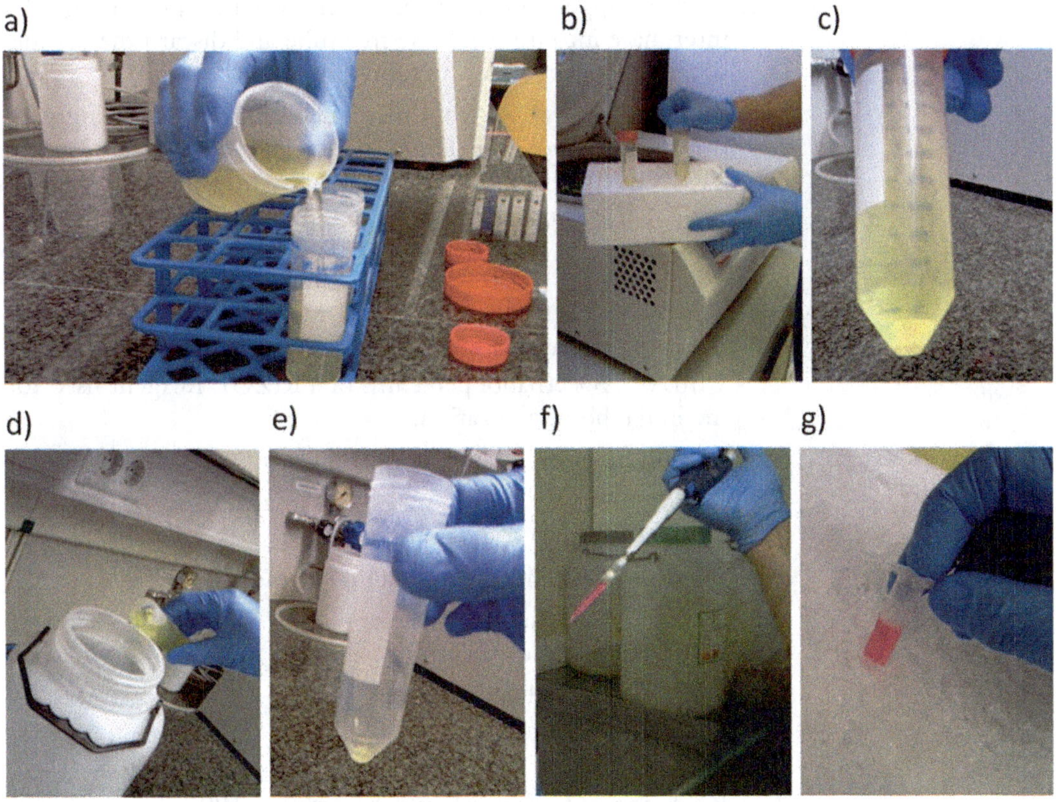

Fig. 2 Processing of urine samples for total RNA isolation. (**a**) Collected urine samples are split in 50 mL Falcon tubes; (**b**) The aliquots are centrifuged at 1000 × *g* for 10 min at 4 °C. Samples are kept on ice during all the processing to avoid RNA degradation; (**c**) Urine cells are separated from supernatant. (**d**) The supernatant is drained; (**e**) All pellets of the same patient have to be put together, resolved briefly (*pipette*), and transferred into 2 mL RNase eppendorf tubes; (**f**) 1 mL of Trizol reagent is added to the sample for RNA extraction and cell pellets have to be resuspended by pipetting; (**i**) Kept on ice or store at −80 °C until further processing

3.3 RNA Extraction from Urine Samples [10] (See Note 4)

1. Incubate the homogenized samples for 5 min at room temperature (*see* **Note 5**).
2. Add 0.2 mL of chloroform per 1 mL of TRIZOL Reagent. Cap sample tubes securely. Vortex samples vigorously for 15 s and incubate them at room temperature for 2–3 min.
3. Centrifuge the samples at 12,000 × *g* for 15 min at 4 °C. Following centrifugation, the mixture separates into a lower red phenol/chloroform phase, an interphase, and a colorless upper aqueous phase. RNA remains exclusively in the aqueous phase (the volume of the aqueous phase is about 60% of the volume of TRIZOL Reagent used for homogenization).

4. Transfer upper aqueous phase carefully without disturbing the interphase into fresh RNAse-free tube and discard the organic phase (lower red phase and interphase).
5. Precipitate the RNA from the aqueous phase by mixing with isopropyl alcohol. Use 0.5 mL of isopropyl alcohol per 1 mL of TRIZOL reagent used for the initial homogenization.
6. Incubate samples at room temperature for 10 min.
7. Centrifuge at 12,000 × *g* for 10 min at 4 °C (*see* **Note 6**).
8. Carefully remove the supernatant completely.
9. Wash the RNA pellet once with 75% ethanol, adding at least 1 mL of 75% ethanol per 1 mL of TRIZOL Reagent used for the initial homogenization.
10. Mix the samples by vortexing and centrifuge at 7500 × *g* for 5 min at 4 °C.
11. Remove all leftover ethanol.
12. Air-dry RNA pellet for 5–10 min (*see* **Note 7**).
13. Dissolve RNA in RNase-free water (5.5–20 μL of water, depending on the amount of pellet) by passing solution a few times through a pipette tip.
14. Leave the RNA in ice.
15. Quantify 1.2 μL of RNA in a NanoDrop spectrophotometer. RNA concentrations should be around 100 ng/μL. If not, adjust with water (*see* **Note 8**). Integrity of RNA can be determined using the 2100 Agilent Bioanalyzer and following the Agilent RNA 6000 Nano Assay Protocol (Fig. 3) (*see* **Note 9**).
16. Continue with cDNA synthesis or freeze RNA at −80 °C until RNA Reverse Transcription.

3.4 Reverse Transcription (cDNA Synthesis) (See Note 10)

1. Calculate the volume of components needed to prepare the required number of reactions. For one reaction: 2.5 μL of 10× RT Buffer, 1 of μL 25× dNTP Mix (100 mM), 2.5 of μL 10× RT Random Primers, 1.25 μL of MultiScribe™ Reverse Transcriptase and 2.25 μL of Nuclease-free H_2O (Total per Reaction 12.5 μL) (*see* **Note 11**).
2. Place the 2× RT master mix on ice and mix gently.
3. Pipette 12.5 μL of 2× RT master mix into each well of a 96-well reaction plate or individual tube.
4. Pipette 12.5 μL of RNA sample into each well (100 ng total RNA if available), pipetting up and down two times to mix (Total per Reaction 25 μL).
5. Seal the plates or tubes.
6. Briefly centrifuge the plate or tubes to spin down the contents and to eliminate any air bubbles.

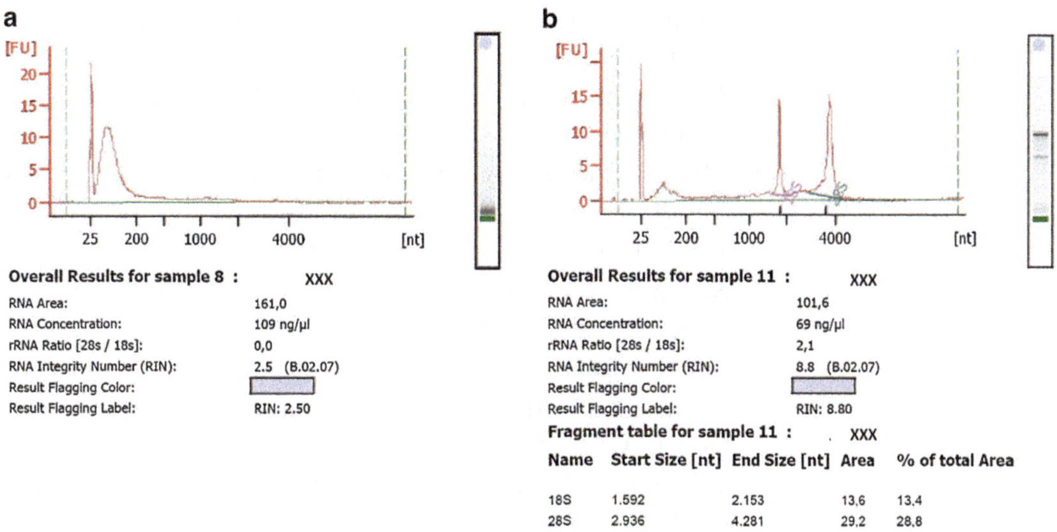

Fig. 3 Bioanalyzer RNA profiles from urine samples (Agilent RNA 6000 Nano Kit). Agilent Bioanalyzer trace and gel image displaying RNA integrity. The two peaks in fluorescence correspond to the 18S and 28S rRNA bands. (**a**) If total RNA is completely degraded 28S and 18S rRNA subunit bands and peaks are not visible. (**b**) On the other hand, if the total RNA sample is undegraded, the 28S rRNA subunit band will appear approximately twice as intense (or has twice the area under the peak in the Bioanalyzer trace) as the 18S rRNA subunit band. In our experience, gene expression analysis from urinary RNA by real-time PCR is possible even when RNA is completely degraded (RIN = 0–2) as long as TaqMan assays have amplicon lengths >150 bp

7. Place the plate or tubes on ice until you are ready to load the thermal cycler.
8. Program the thermal cycler conditions in the thermal cycler: 25 °C for 10 min, 37 °C for 120 min, 85 °C for 5 min and ∞ at 4 °C.
9. Load the reactions into the thermal cycler.
10. Start the reverse transcription run.
11. Upon completion, immediately remove the plate from the thermal cycler and place it on ice to continue with the pre-amplification reaction or store at −20 °C (*see* **Note 12**).

3.5 cDNA Pre-amplification (See Notes 10 and 13)

1. In a microcentrifuge tube, combine equal volumes of each 20× TaqMan® Gene Expression Assay (*see* **Note 14**), up to a total of 100 assays.
2. Dilute the pooled TaqMan assays using 1× TE buffer so that each assay is at a final concentration of 0.2× (*see* **Note 15**).
3. Calculate the volume of components needed to prepare the required number of reactions. For one preamplification reaction: 12.5 µL of 2× TaqMan PreAmp Master Mix, 6.25 µL of 0.2× Pooled assay mix and 6.25 µL of cDNA sample + nuclease-free water (Total per Reaction 25 µL). To increase the

number of reactions, use whole multiples of the specified volumes.

4. Cap the microcentrifuge tube or seal the 96-well plate with adhesive cover.
5. Mix the reactions by gently inverting the tube or plate, then centrifuge briefly.
6. Load the plate or tubes into the thermal cycler.
7. Set up the thermal cycling conditions: 95 °C for 10 min and 14 cycles at 95 °C for 15 s and 60 °C for 4 min.
8. Start the run.
9. Upon completion, immediately remove the plate from the thermal cycler and place it on ice or store at −20 °C.
10. Perform PCR amplification. Alternatively, you may store aliquots of the preamplification product at −20 °C.

3.6 Quantitative PCR Amplification (See Note 10)

3.6.1 Quantity/Quality Control Reaction

1. Thaw any frozen pre-amplified cDNA samples by placing them on ice. When thawed, resuspend the samples by vortexing and then centrifuge the tubes briefly.
2. Prepare the PCR reaction mix for all samples (in duplicate) (*see* **Note 16**). For each reaction add: 1 μL of *GUSB* TaqMan Gene Expression Assay (20×), 10 μL TaqMan Gene Expression Master Mix (2×) and 8 μL Nuclease-free water. (Total Volume 10 μL).
3. Mix the solution by gently pipetting up and down, then cap the tube.
4. Centrifuge the tube briefly to spin down the contents and eliminate air bubbles from the solution.
5. Transfer the appropriate volume (9 μL) of the reaction mixture to wells of an optical plate.
6. Add 1 μL of nondiluted preamplified cDNA products to each well.
7. Cover the plate with an optical adhesive cover or with optical flat caps.
8. Centrifuge the plate briefly to spin down the contents and eliminate air bubbles from the solutions.
9. Place the reaction plate in the instrument.
10. Use the following thermal cycling conditions: 50 °C for 2 min, 95 °C for 10 min and 40 cycles at 95 °C for 15 s and 60 °C for 1 min.
11. Start the run.
12. Check the amplification plots for the entire plate.

13. Setting the baseline and threshold values (Threshold 0.2, automatic baseline).
14. Analyze your data (*see* **Note 17**).
15. Discard from further analysis those samples that provide *GUSB* Ct > 23 (*see* **Note 18**).

3.6.2 Target Genes Amplification

Prepare the PCR reaction mix for each target gene (in duplicate) separately (*see* **Note 16**) following the steps described in Subheading 3.6.1. When analyzing quantitative PCR data, set the baseline and threshold values for each gene independently.

4 Notes

1. Urine samples are to be collected after spontaneous voiding before the patient is submitted to their clinical exploration or surgery.
2. Samples are kept on ice during the entire sample processing to avoid sample degradation. Wear powder-free gloves while processing urine samples to avoid RNA degradation.
3. While working with Trizol reagent always use gloves and eye protection, avoid contact with skin or clothing and use a chemical hood to avoid breathing vapor.
4. The following protocol has been adapted from Life Technologies/Invitrogen's protocol for using TRIzol reagent to isolate total RNA from urine pellet samples.
5. Normal precautions to avoid RNase contamination should be taken, ribonucleases (commonly abbreviated RNases) are everywhere and they are very stable and difficult to inactivate. To ensure success, it is important to maintain an RNase-free environment starting with RNA purification and continuing through analysis.

   Some tips to remember when working with RNA are described below:

   (a) The most common sources of RNase contamination are hands (skin) and bacteria or mold that may be present on airborne dust particles or laboratory glassware. To prevent contamination from these sources, wear gloves at all times.

   (b) Whenever possible, use sterile, disposable plasticware for handling RNA. These materials are generally RNase-free and do not require pretreatment to inactivate RNases.

   (c) Treat nondisposable glassware and plasticware before use to ensure that it is RNase-free. Bake glassware at 250 °C overnight. Thoroughly rinse plasticware with 0.1 N

NaOH/1 mM EDTA and then with diethyl pyrocarbonate (DEPC)-treated water.

(d) Chemicals for use in RNA isolation and analysis should be reserved for RNA applications and kept separate from chemicals for other applications.

(e) Autoclaving alone is not sufficient to inactivate RNases. Solutions prepared in the lab should be treated by adding DEPC to 0.05% and incubating overnight at room temperature. The treated solutions should be autoclaved for 30 min to remove any trace of DEPC.

6. The RNA precipitate, often invisible before centrifugation, forms a gel-like pellet on the side and bottom of the tube.
7. Do not dry the RNA pellet by centrifuge under vacuum. It is important not to let the RNA pellet dry completely as this will greatly decrease its solubility.
8. RNA has an absorption maximum at 260 nm and the ratio of the absorbance at 260 and 280 nm is used to assess the purity of an RNA preparation. Pure RNA has an A260/A280 of 2.1. You will see in many protocols that a value of 1.8–2.0 indicates that the RNA is pure (the A260/A280 ratio should be at least 1.6). This depends, however, on how you performed the measurement and on the source of putative contaminations.
9. We do not suggest checking all RNA samples by the 2100 Agilent Bioanalyzer since we found RIN is not an accurate reflex of the PCR success. We found that samples with a very low RIN number could be successfully analyzed (Fig. 2).

   Agilent RNA 6000 Nano Assay Protocol can be downloaded at: http://rai.unam.mx/manuales/lbg_ARNGuideAgileny.pdf.
10. The Reverse Transcription, cDNA pre-amplification and real-time quantitative PCR protocols have been adapted from https://tools.thermofisher.com/content/sfs/manuals/cms_042557.pdf, https://tools.thermofisher.com/content/sfs/manuals/cms_039316.pdf and https://tools.thermofisher.com/content/sfs/manuals/4304449_TaqManPCRMM_UG.pdf, respectively.
11. Allow the kit components to thaw on ice. Prepare the RT master mix on ice. Include additional reactions in the calculations to provide excess volume for the loss that occurs during reagent transfers.
12. If required, briefly centrifuge the archive plates or tubes before storing to spin down the contents and to eliminate any air bubbles.
13. Keep all TaqMan Gene Expression Assays protected from light, in the freezer, until you are ready to use them. Excessive exposure to light may affect the fluorescent probes. Prior to

use, homogenize the TaqMan PreAmp Master Mix by gently swirling the tube. Thaw any frozen cDNA samples by placing them on ice. When thawed, mix the samples by vortexing and then centrifuge the tubes briefly. Thaw the Gene Expression Assays by placing them on ice. When thawed, mix the assays by vortexing and then centrifuge the tubes briefly.

Do not include the 18S TaqMan assay in the pool because it is so highly expressed. Include *GUSB* TaqMan assay for subsequent cDNA quantity control. Do not include TaqMan assays with amplicons lengths >150 bp. Pool TaqMan assays with a Ct $\leq$ 35 when using 0.3 ng/μL cDNA.

14. For example, to pool 50 TaqMan assays, combine 10 μL of each TaqMan assay
15. For the above example, add 500 μL of 1× TE buffer to the pooled TaqMan assays for a total volume of 1 mL.
16. An additional reaction is included in the calculations to provide excess volume for the loss that occurs during reagent transfers.
17. Data analysis varies depending on the instrument. Refer to the appropriate instrument user guide for instructions on how to analyze your data.
18. Those samples with *GUSB* Ct $\leq$ 18 will be diluted with water to ensure a homogeneous amount of cDNA in all the samples and the correct quantification of targeted mRNAs. *GUSB* Ct ~18 must be expected from the samples when calculating the dilution factor. We have found that most of the tested gene expressions are in the proper range when GUSB Ct ~18 in the sample.

References

1. Pisitkun T, Johnstone R, Knepper MA (2006) Discovery of urinary biomarkers. Mol Cell Proteomics 5:1760–1771
2. Rigau M, Olivan M, Garcia M et al (2013) The present and future of prostate cancer urine biomarkers. Int J Mol Sci 14:12620–12649
3. Decramer S, Gonzalez DP, Breuil B et al (2008) Urine in clinical proteomics. Mol Cell Proteomics 7:1850–1862
4. Wu J, Chen YD, Gu W (2010) Urinary proteomics as a novel tool for biomarker discovery in kidney diseases. J Zhejiang Univ Sci B 11:227–237
5. Rigau M, Ortega I, Mir MC et al (2011) A three-gene panel on urine increases PSA specificity in the detection of prostate cancer. Prostate 71:1736–1745
6. Mengual L, Burset M, Ribal MJ et al (2010) Gene expression signature in urine for diagnosing and assessing aggressiveness of bladder urothelial carcinoma. Clin Cancer Res 16:2624–2633
7. Mengual L, Ribal MJ, Lozano JJ et al (2014) Validation study of a noninvasive urine test for diagnosis and prognosis assessment of bladder cancer: evidence for improved models. J Urol 191:261–269
8. Ribal MJ, Mengual L, Lozano JJ et al (2016) Gene expression test for the non-invasive diagnosis of bladder cancer: a prospective, blinded, international and multicenter validation study. Eur J Cancer 54:131–138
9. Huebner AR, Somparn P, Benjachat T et al (2015) Exosomes in urine biomarker discovery. Adv Exp Med Biol 845:43–58
10. Chomczynski P, Mackey K (1995) Short technical reports. Modification of the TRI reagent procedure for isolation of RNA from polysaccharide- and proteoglycan-rich sources. Biotechniques 19:942–945

Chapter 18

DNA Methylation Analysis from Body Fluids

Dimo Dietrich

Abstract

Circulating cell-free DNA (ccfDNA) can be found in various body fluids, i.e., blood (serum and plasma), urine, pleural effusions, and ascites. While ccfDNA predominantly originates from physiological processes, a fraction might be related to pathological events, e.g., cancer. Aberrant DNA methylation, which is considered a hallmark of cancer, can be assessed accurately in ccfDNA. Consequently, DNA methylation testing in body fluids represents a powerful diagnostic tool in the clinical management of malignant diseases. Frequently, however, the total amount of disease-related ccfDNA in a sample is low and masked by an excess of physiological ccfDNA. Thus, DNA methylation analysis of tumor-derived DNA is challenging, and high volumes of body fluids need to be analyzed in order to ensure a sufficient abundance of the analyte in the test sample. DNA methylation assays are usually based on prior conversion of cytosines to uracils by means of bisulfite. This reaction takes place under harsh chemical conditions leading to DNA degradation and therefore necessitates a proper DNA purification before downstream analyses. This article describes a protocol which allows for the preparation of ultra-pure bisulfite-converted DNA from up to 3 ml blood plasma and serum, which is well suited for subsequent molecular biological techniques, e.g., methylation-specific real-time PCR.

Key words DNA methylation, Circulating cell-free DNA, ccfDNA, Biomarker, Plasma, Serum, Blood, Body fluid, Bodily fluid, Bisulfite, Magnetic beads, Ammonium bisulfite

1 Introduction

Methylation of cytosines within the CpG dinucleotide context is an important epigenetic mechanism fundamental in physiological processes (e.g., cell differentiation and development) as well as pathological processes (most notably carcinogenesis and tumor progression) (for review refs. 1–3). Accordingly, aberrantly methylated genes are promising biomarker candidates in the management of malignant diseases.

Apoptosis and necrosis of malignant cells lead to the release of circulating cell-free DNA (ccfDNA) into the circulation (reviewed in ref. 4), and ccfDNA can be found in in various types of bodily fluids, i.e., blood (plasma and serum), ascites, pleural effusions, and urine. In addition, cells generate and shed extracellular vesicles

Wolfgang A. Schulz et al. (eds.), *Urothelial Carcinoma: Methods and Protocols*, Methods in Molecular Biology, vol. 1655, DOI 10.1007/978-1-4939-7234-0_18, © Springer Science+Business Media LLC 2018

(exosomes and microvesicles) as a form of intercellular communication in the course of physiological and pathological processes (reviewed in ref. 5). Accordingly, DNA methylation analysis of ccfDNA in body fluids is a powerful diagnostic tool in the field of oncology (for review ref. 6).

The base pairing behavior of 5-methylcytosine and cytosine is similar, impairing their discrimination by molecular biological methods, e.g., PCR. In 1992, Frommer and coworkers developed a protocol [7] which allowed for a positive display of 5-methylcytosine. In this protocol, DNA deamination of cytosines to uracils was achieved by contacting single-stranded DNA with bisulfite, whereas methylated cytosines remained unaffected. As a consequence, the epigenetic information of the DNA is transformed into sequence information, which can easily be read out. The principle of the bisulfite reaction is summarized by Hayatsu [8] and Holmes et al. [9]. As bisulfite conversion is a chemical reaction under harsh conditions (high temperature, low pH, and elongated incubation times), it causes significant DNA degradation [10–12]. In the meantime, several technological advances have led to protocols, which are much more convenient, user friendly, and less DNA-degrading compared to the original Frommer protocol [13–18]. However, the choice of a specific protocol for bisulfite conversion is of tremendous importance for the success of downstream DNA methylation analysis.

DNA methylation analyses of body fluids represent a particular technological challenge. The vast majority of ccfDNA molecules derive from leucocytes (reviewed in ref. 19), and the abundance of disease-related ccfDNA is usually low, consequently necessitating the analysis of high volumes of body fluids in order to ensure the presence of a sufficiently high number of DNA molecules of interest. Thus, suitable protocols for the bisulfite conversion of DNA from body fluids start with a reduction of volume to increase the concentration of DNA. This concentration can be achieved by means of magnetic bead-based DNA extraction or polymer-mediated enrichment (PME) of nucleic acids. For the latter, a commercially available kit (innuCONVERT Bisulfite Body Fluids Kit, Analytik Jena, Jena, Germany) facilitates the analysis of up to 3 ml of bodily fluids [9]. The present article introduces an alternative method, which is based on magnetic bead extraction, namely the Dynabeads® SILANE technology (Thermo Fisher Scientific, Waltham, MA, USA).

2 Materials

The protocol comprises nonstandard laboratory reagents and reagents which cannot be prepared by conventional research laboratories, i.e., magnetic beads, silane lysis/binding buffer, ammonium bisulfite. Thus, inexperienced users are encouraged to use commercially available kits [9] or purchase the respective reagents from specialized suppliers. Magnetic beads might be used from alternative suppliers. However, it needs to be considered that magnetic beads highly differ in their specifications (e.g., size, bead material, functionalization). Binding and washing buffers need to be perfectly harmonized with regard to the used magnetic beads. Thus, a simple replacement of the magnetic beads with beads from alternative suppliers necessitates a comprehensive workflow optimization.

Use molecular biology-grade reagents only (i.e., ethanol absolute ≥99.8%, molecular biology grade; water: free of DNase, RNase, and protease, 0.1 μm filtered).

2.1 Plasma and Serum Preparation

1. S-Monovette® 9 ml, K3 EDTA, 92 × 16 mm, or equivalent (*see* **Notes 1** and **2**).
2. S-Monovette® 9 ml, Serum Gel with Clotting Activator, 92 × 16 mm, or equivalent (*see* **Note 3**).
3. Transfer pipets.
4. 15 ml centrifugation tube.
5. Centrifuge with swinging-bucket rotor.

2.2 Lysis

1. Binding buffer: Silane lysis/binding buffer (viral NA) (*see* **Notes 4** and **5**).
2. 15 ml centrifugation tubes.

2.3 DNA Concentration

1. SB3 rotator with SB3/2 test/blood tube holder, 20 × 9 to 20 mm (Stuart Scientific), or equivalent.
2. Magnetic beads: Dynabeads® SILANE (Thermo Fisher Scientific, cat. no. 37005D) (*see* **Note 4**).
3. Binding buffer: Silane lysis/binding buffer (viral NA) (*see* **Note 4**).
4. Wash buffer I: 50% [v/v] silane lysis/binding buffer (viral NA) and 50% [v/v] ethanol abs. (*see* **Note 4**).
5. DynaMag™-15 magnet (Thermo Fisher Scientific), or equivalent.
6. DynaMag™-2 magnet (Thermo Fisher Scientific), or equivalent.
7. Elution buffer; 10 mM Tris–HCl, pH 8.0.
8. Thermomixer.
9. Transfer pipets.
10. Serological pipets (5 ml, sterile).
11. Mini shaker.

12. Table centrifuge.
13. 2 ml safe lock reaction tubes.

2.4 Bisulfite Conversion

1. Ammonium bisulfite (65%) (*see* **Note 4**).
2. Denaturation buffer; 70 mg/ml trolox ((±)-6-Hydroxy-2,5,7,8-tetramethylchromane-2-carboxylic acid) in THFA (tetrahydrofurfuryl alcohol).

2.5 Purification

1. Magnetic beads: Dynabeads® SILANE (*see* **Note 4**).
2. Wash buffer I; 50% [v/v] silane lysis/binding buffer (viral NA) and 50% [v/v] ethanol abs. (*see* **Note 4**).
3. DynaMag™-2 magnet, or equivalent.
4. Thermomixer.
5. Wash buffer II; 15% [v/v] water and 85% [v/v] ethanol abs.
6. Elution buffer; 10 mM Tris–HCl, pH 8.0.
7. 2 ml and 1.5 ml safe lock reaction tubes.
8. Centrifuge.

3 Methods

3.1 Plasma and Serum Preparation

1. Centrifuge the S-Monovette® 9 ml containing the blood for 6 min at 1.350 g. (*see* **Notes 6** and 7).
2. Transfer the supernatant (plasma or serum, respectively) into a 15 ml centrifugation tube.
3. Centrifuge 6 min at 3000 × *g*. Transfer 3 ml plasma or serum, respectively, into a new 15 ml centrifugation tube (*see* **Note 8**).

3.2 Lysis

1. Add 3 ml binding buffer to the 15 ml reaction tube containing the 3 ml plasma or serum. Use a sterile serological pipet (*see* **Note 9**).
2. Mix properly and incubate for 10 min at room temperature.

3.3 DNA Concentration

1. Add 65 μl magnetic beads and 2.2 ml ethanol to the 15 ml centrifugation tube containing the plasma and lysis buffer (*see* **Note 10**).
2. Incubate the mixture for 45 min and 20 rpm in a rotator. Use an inclination angle of 35–45°C.
3. Transfer the reaction tube into the DynaMag™-15 magnet and incubate 5 min at room temperature.
4. Discard the supernatant using a transfer pipet. Make sure that no magnetic beads are discarded (*see* **Note 11**).

5. Add 1.5 ml wash buffer I to the magnetic beads in the 15 ml centrifugation tube.
6. Resuspend the magnetic beads and transfer the magnetic beads/wash buffer I suspension into a 2 ml reaction tube.
7. Transfer the reaction tube into the DynaMag™-2 magnet and incubate 1 min at room temperature.
8. Discard as much of the supernatant as possible. The reaction tube has to remain in the DynaMag™-2 magnet while the supernatant is discarded (*see* **Note 11**).
9. Take the reaction tube out of the DynaMag™-2 magnet and spin down the beads briefly.
10. Transfer the reaction tube into the DynaMag™-2 magnet and incubate 1 min at room temperature.
11. Discard as much of the remaining supernatant as possible. The reaction tube needs to remain in the DynaMag™-2 magnet while the supernatant is discarded (*see* **Note 11**).
12. Add 100 μl elution buffer to the magnetic beads and mix properly.
13. Incubate the suspended magnetic beads 10 min at 85 °C and 1000 rpm in a thermomixer.
14. Spin down briefly in order to remove drops from the tube cap.
15. Transfer the 2 ml reaction tube containing the magnetic beads and the elution buffer into the DynaMag™-2 magnet and incubate for 1 min at room temperature.
16. Transfer the complete supernatant containing the eluted DNA (~100 μl) into a new 2 ml reaction tube.
17. Discard the reaction tube containing the magnetic beads and store the eluted DNA at 6 °C (*see* **Note 15**).

3.4 Bisulfite Conversion

1. Add 150 μl ammonium bisulfite and 25 μl denaturation buffer to the eluted DNA (*see* **Notes 4** and **12**).
2. Mix thoroughly and spin down briefly in order to remove drops from the tube cap (*see* **Note 13**).
3. Incubate 45 min at 85 °C in a waterbath. Start with the subsequent purification immediately after this incubation step (*see* **Note 14**).

3.5 Purification

1. Add 1000 μl wash buffer I and 15 μl magnetic beads to the bisulfite reaction mixture (*see* **Note 10**).
2. Mix thoroughly and spin down briefly. Avoid a sedimentation of the magnetic beads during the centrifugation.
3. Incubate the reaction mixture for 45 min at 1000 rpm and 23 °C in a thermomixer.

4. Spin down briefly.
5. Transfer the reaction tube into the DynaMag™-2 magnet and incubate 2 min at room temperature.
6. Use a 100–1000 μl pipet to discard the supernatant. Make sure that no magnetic beads are discarded (*see* **Note 11**). Leave the tube in the magnet during removal of the supernatant.
7. Add 800 μl wash buffer I. Mix thoroughly and spin down briefly in order to remove drops from the tube cap. Avoid sedimentation of the magnetic beads during the centrifugation.
8. Transfer the reaction tube into the DynaMag™-2 magnet and incubate 2 min at room temperature.
9. Use a 100–1000 μl pipet to discard the supernatant. Make sure that no magnetic beads are discarded (*see* **Note 11**). Leave the tube in the magnet during removal of the supernatant.
10. Add 800 μl wash buffer II to the magnetic beads. Resuspend the magnetic beads thoroughly and spin down briefly to remove drops from the tube cap. Avoid sedimentation of the magnetic beads during the centrifugation.
11. Transfer the reaction tube into the DynaMag™-2 magnet and incubate 2 min at room temperature.
12. Use a 100–1000 μl pipet to discard the supernatant. Make sure that no magnetic beads are discarded (*see* **Note 11**). Leave the tube in the magnet during removal of the supernatant.
13. Add 900 μl wash buffer II to the magnetic beads. Resuspend the magnetic beads thoroughly and spin down briefly to remove drops from the tube cap. Avoid sedimentation of the magnetic beads during the centrifugation.
14. Transfer the reaction tube into the DynaMag™-2 magnet and incubate 2 min at room temperature.
15. Use a 100–1000 μl pipet to discard the supernatant. Make sure that no magnetic beads are discarded (*see* **Note 11**). Leave the tube in the magnet during removal of the supernatant.
16. Add 1000 μl wash buffer II to the magnetic beads. Resuspend the magnetic beads thoroughly and spin down briefly to remove drops from the tube cap. Avoid sedimentation of the magnetic beads during the centrifugation.
17. Transfer the reaction tube into the DynaMag™-2 magnet and incubate 2 min at room temperature.
18. Use a 100–1000 μl pipet to discard the supernatant. Make sure that no magnetic beads are discarded (*see* **Note 11**). Leave the tube in the magnet during removal of the supernatant.
19. Take the tube containing the magnetic beads out of the magnet and spin down the magnetic beads briefly.

20. Transfer the reaction tube again into the DynaMag™-2 magnet and incubate 1 min at room temperature. Use a 2.5–10 μl pipet to discard any remaining supernatant. Make sure that no magnetic beads are discarded (*see* **Note 11**). Leave the tube in the magnet during removal of the remaining supernatant.
21. Dry the magnetic beads for 10 min at 60 °C in a thermomixer. Make sure that the tube caps are open in order to allow for the evaporation of any remaining ethanol.
22. Add 65 μl elution buffer to the magnetic beads. Mix thoroughly. Spin down briefly.
23. Incubate the suspended magnetic beads 10 min at 85 °C and 1000 rpm in a thermomixer.
24. Spin down briefly in order to remove drops from the tube caps.
25. Transfer the 2 ml reaction tube containing the magnetic beads and the elution buffer into the DynaMag™-2 magnet and incubate for 1 min at room temperature.
26. Transfer the complete supernatant containing the eluted DNA (~60 μl) into a new 1.5 ml reaction tube.
27. Discard the reaction tube containing the magnetic beads and store the eluted DNA at 6 °C (*see* **Notes 15** and **16**).

3.6 Analytics

The eluted bisulfite-converted DNA is well suited for methylation-specific real-time PCR. Up to 10 μl eluted DNA should be applied to a single 20 μl PCR reaction because of the low DNA concentration (*see* **Notes 17** and **18**).

4 Notes

1. Blood collection tubes with several different anticoagulants, i.e., potassium EDTA, lithium heparin, and sodium citrate are available. The present protocol is optimized for EDTA K_3 plasma and a winged infusion set (also known as "butterfly") for blood collection. The influence of the different blood collection systems and different anticoagulants should be carefully tested with respect to the desired analytical downstream application.
2. EDTA K_3 plasma needs to be prepared immediately after or within a few hours after blood sampling in order to avoid leucocyte lysis. Streck, Inc. (Omaha, NE, USA) developed blood collection tubes (Cell-Free DNA BCT®) which contain a formalin-releasing reagent leading to a slow fixation of the DNA and the cells in a blood sample. These collection tubes allow for a storage of blood samples for several days at ambient temperature before starting the plasma preparation procedure.

However, the influence of the formalin-releasing agent contained in the Cell-Free DNA BCT® on the downstream analysis needs to be tested thoroughly.

3. Serum contains higher amounts of ccfDNA which is released from leucocytes during coagulation. This leucocyte-derived ccfDNA masks ccfDNA from other origins. Accordingly, depending on the specific scientific question, plasma is preferred over serum.
4. The protocol comprises nonstandard laboratory reagents and reagents which cannot be prepared by conventional research laboratories, i.e., magnetic beads, silane lysis/binding buffer, ammonium bisulfite, and denaturation buffer. Buffers and magnetic beads cannot be exchanged easily without a comprehensive workflow optimization. Ammonium bisulfite is instable in solid form and is only available as solution. Ammonium bisulfite solutions differ with regard to their exact composition. The present protocol is based on ammonium bisulfite purchased from Analytik Jena (Jena, Germany). Inexperienced users are encouraged to use commercially available kits [9].
5. Silane lysis/binding buffer tends to form crystals at low temperatures. This does not influence the performance of the buffer. Crystals can be resolved by a 60 min incubation at 37 °C.
6. Plasma has to be prepared immediately after blood collection in order to avoid a leucocyte lysis leading to a DNA release.
7. The present workflow is also suitable for the analysis of 3 ml ascites and pleural effusion as described elsewhere [9]. In comparison to plasma, the composition of urine from a patient is highly variable, depending on sampling time of day and patients' diet, among others. Furthermore, inhibitory substances might form during storage of urine samples. Thus, the DNA concentration step should be carried out prior to any storage of urine samples.
8. Plasma, serum, ascites, and pleural effusion samples can be stored up to 2 years at −20 °C or −80 °C. Freeze/thaw cycles of samples, however, should be avoided.
9. Samples with less than 3 ml volume can be filled up with phosphate-buffered saline (PBS) before starting the DNA concentration.
10. Magnetic beads tend to sediment quickly, thereby influencing the concentration depending on the time span between resuspension (mixing) and usage. The magnetic beads have to be resuspended freshly and thoroughly directly before usage in order to ensure repeatable amounts of beads per reaction.

11. A high purity of the DNA is mandatory in order to allow for a downstream analysis of the bisulfite-converted DNA. Carry-over of buffers during the different steps of the protocol significantly impairs the purity of the DNA and needs to be avoided. Accordingly, the complete removal of buffers is crucial.
12. Bisulfite is only stable in aqueous solution and not as solid salts and specific properties of bisulfite necessitate a careful handling of this reagent. Bisulfite liberates sulfur dioxide gas under acidic conditions. Consequently, the bisulfite concentration decreases over time. More importantly, bisulfite and sulfite react as reducing agents, and oxygen in the air slowly oxidizes the solution to sulfuric acid and sulfate. This oxidation is indicated by a decreasing pH, a decreasing viscosity, ammonia odor, and lightly lucid yellow color. The bisulfite conversion of DNA is impaired, once the oxidation of bisulfite exceeds a critical level. In addition, sulfate might form solid crystals especially in contact to ethanol containing wash buffers. These sulfates will be dissolved when eluting the converted DNA and will act as potent PCR inhibitors. Accordingly, bisulfite has to be stored in the absence of oxygen. Bisulfite solutions should not be used once the expiry date is reached. Preferably, bisulfite solution should be purchased from vendors (e.g., Analytik Jena, Jena, Germany) that provide bisulfite in gas-tight vials without oxygen. The single-use vials should not be used for more than 1 month after they have been opened. The pH value of the bisulfite should be tested with pH-paper. Do not use the bisulfite if pH is lower than pH 5.1.
13. Bisulfite is used as an aqueous solution with a high salt concentration that has to be mixed thoroughly with the organic solvent (denaturation buffer) and the sample in order to avoid any concentration gradients during the bisulfite-conversion step. An improper mixing will lead to an incomplete conversion.
14. Increasing the bisulfite-conversion incubation time or temperature will lead to an increased DNA degradation and an increased undesired conversion of methylated cytosines to thymines. Decreasing the bisulfite-conversion incubation time or temperature will lead to an incomplete conversion of unmethylated cytosines to uracils. A lower temperature cannot be compensated by extended incubation times since the DNA needs to be single-stranded in order to allow for the bisulfite-conversion. The usage of a waterbath is preferred because the temperature can be controlled easily. If a thermomixer is used, it should be checked if the instrument runs within its specification. Furthermore, in order to ensure an efficient heat exchange, the usage of appropriate reaction tubes is needed.

15. The concentrated genomic and the bisulfite-converted DNA contains only low DNA concentrations. Thus, storage of these samples is not recommended since a loss of DNA due to unspecific binding to the tube walls might occur. Carrier RNA or DNA (poly-A, poly-dA) might be added to the plasma sample in order to reduce DNA loss due to unspecific binding.
16. A quantification of bisulfite-converted or concentrated genomic DNA via UV spectrophotometry is not possible due to the low concentration of ccfDNA in plasma and other body fluids. However, UV spectrophotometry is a suitable tool to determine the carryover of impurities [9]. Quantitative real-time PCR using bisulfite-specific but methylation-unspecific primers which do not contain CpG sites in their target sequence is a suitable tool to quantify the total DNA concentration. An established assay for this purpose amplifies a CpG-free sequence within the *ACTB* gene locus. This assay has been successfully multiplexed with methylation-specific real-time PCR assays thereby allowing for a simultaneous quantification of total and methylated alleles in a single-tube reaction [20].
17. The carryover of impurities due to an improper purification, carryover of wash buffers in addition to a too high input volume into the PCR can lead to a direct PCR inhibition. Furthermore, an indirect inhibition might occur due to a degradation of Cy-dyes under acidic or redox conditions. Thus more stable dyes compared to Cy-dyes should be used in real-time PCR applications.
18. The concentration of bisulfite-converted DNA obtained from body fluids is usually low. On average, approximately 15 ng bisulfite-converted DNA (equivalent to approximately 2200 haploid genome copies) are obtained from 3 ml plasma. Accordingly, high volumes of the eluted DNA have to be applied to a downstream analytical procedure.

Acknowledgment

Conflict of Interest: Dimo Dietrich is a consultant for AJ Innuscreen GmbH (Berlin, Germany) and receives royalties from product sales (innuCONVERT kits).

References

1. Taby R, Issa JP (2010) Cancer epigenetics. CA Cancer J Clin 60:376–392. doi:10.3322/caac.20085
2. Jones PA (2012) Functions of DNA methylation: islands, start sites, gene bodies and beyond. Nat Rev Genet 13:484–492. doi:10.1038/nrg3230
3. Shen H, Laird PW (2013) Interplay between the cancer genome and epigenome. Cell 153:38–55. doi:10.1016/j.cell.2013.03.008

4. Diaz LA Jr, Bardelli A (2014) Liquid biopsies: genotyping circulating tumor DNA. J Clin Oncol 32:579–586. doi:10.1200/JCO.2012.45.2011
5. Desrochers LM, Antonyak MA, Cerione RA (2016) Extracellular vesicles: satellites of information transfer in cancer and stem cell biology. Dev Cell 37:301–309. doi:10.1016/j.devcel.2016.04.019
6. Dietrich D (2016) Current status and future perspectives of circulating cell-free DNA methylation in clinical diagnostics. Laboratoriums-Medizin 40:335–343. doi:10.1515/labmed-2016-0039
7. Frommer M, McDonald LE, Millar DS et al (1992) A genomic sequencing protocol that yields a positive display of 5-methylcytosine residues in individual DNA strands. Proc Natl Acad Sci U S A 89:1827–1831
8. Hayatsu H (2008) The bisulfite genomic sequencing used in the analysis of epigenetic states, a technique in the emerging environmental genotoxicology research. Mutat Res 659:77–82. doi:10.1016/j.mrrev.2008.04.003
9. Holmes EE, Jung M, Meller S et al (2014) Performance evaluation of kits for bisulfite-conversion of DNA from tissues, cell lines, FFPE tissues, aspirates, lavages, effusions, plasma, serum, and urine. PLoS One 9:e93933. doi:10.1371/journal.pone.0093933
10. Raizis AM, Schmitt F, Jost JP (1995) A bisulfite method of 5-methylcytosine mapping that minimizes template degradation. Anal Biochem 226:161–166. doi:10.1006/abio.1995.1204
11. Grunau C, Clark SJ, Rosenthal A (2001) Bisulfite genomic sequencing: systematic investigation of critical experimental parameters. Nucleic Acids Res 29(13):E65–E65
12. Tanaka K, Okamoto A (2007) Degradation of DNA by bisulfite treatment. Bioorg Med Chem Lett 17:1912–1915. doi:10.1016/j.bmcl.2007.01.040
13. Darst RP, Pardo CE, Ai L, et al (2010) Bisulfite sequencing of DNA. Curr Protoc Mol Biol. Chapter 7:Unit 7.9.1–17. doi: 10.1002/0471142727.mb0709s91.
14. Millar DS, Warnecke PM, Melki JR et al (2002) Methylation sequencing from limiting DNA: embryonic, fixed, and microdissected cells. Methods 27(2):108–113
15. Boyd VL, Zon G (2004) Bisulfite conversion of genomic DNA for methylation analysis: protocol simplification with higher recovery applicable to limited samples and increased throughput. Anal Biochem 326:278–280. doi:10.1016/j.ab.2003.11.020
16. Hayatsu H, Negishi K, Shiraishi M (2004) Accelerated bisulfite-deamination of cytosine in the genomic sequencing procedure for DNA methylation analysis. Nucleic Acids Symp Ser (Oxf) 48:261–262. doi:10.1093/nass/48.1.261
17. Hayatsu H, Shiraishi M, Negishi K (2008) Bisulfite modification for analysis of DNA methylation. Curr Protoc Nucleic Acid Chem. Chapter 6:Unit 6.10. doi: 10.1002/0471142700.nc0610s33.
18. Shiraishi M, Hayatsu H (2004) High-speed conversion of cytosine to uracil in bisulfite genomic sequencing analysis of DNA methylation. DNA Res 11:409–415
19. Warton K, Samimi G (2015) Methylation of cell-free circulating DNA in the diagnosis of cancer. Front Mol Biosci 2:13. doi:10.3389/fmolb.2015.00013
20. Dietrich D, Jung M, Puetzer S et al (2013) Diagnostic and prognostic value of SHOX2 and SEPT9 DNA methylation and cytology in benign, paramalignant and malignant pleural effusions. PLoS One 8(12):e84225. doi:10.1371/journal.pone.0084225

Chapter 19

Urinary Protein Markers for the Detection and Prognostication of Urothelial Carcinoma

Tibor Szarvas, Péter Nyirády, Osamu Ogawa, Hideki Furuya, Charles J. Rosser, and Takashi Kobayashi

Abstract

Bladder cancer diagnosis and surveillance is mainly based on cystoscopy and urine cytology. However, both methods have significant limitations; urine cytology has a low sensitivity for low-grade tumors, while cystoscopy is uncomfortable for the patients. Therefore, in the last decade urine analysis was the subject of intensive research resulting in the identification of many potential biomarkers for the detection, surveillance, or prognostic stratification of bladder cancer. Current trends move toward the development of multiparametric models to improve the diagnostic accuracy compared with single molecular markers. Recent technical advances for high-throughput and more sensitive measurements have led to the development of multiplex assays showing potential for more efficient tools toward future clinical application. In this review, we focus on the findings of urinary protein research in the context of detection and prognostication of bladder cancer. Furthermore, we provide an up-to-date overview on the recommendations for the quality evaluation of published studies as well as for the conduction of future urinary biomarker studies.

Key words Urine, Bladder cancer, Biomarker, Diagnosis, Prognosis

1 Introduction

Cystoscopy is the gold standard tool to diagnose the presence of BC, while histological diagnosis is made by transurethral resection (TUR) or biopsy. Although imaging studies including computerized tomography, magnetic resonance imaging, and positron emission tomography are useful for the evaluation of disease extent, cystoscopy and TUR cannot be replaced by these less invasive modalities.

Urothelial carcinoma (UC) is the most common histological type of BC. Although the natural history of UC has not been fully elucidated, it is classically considered to involve two pathways,

The original version of this chapter was revised. An erratum to this chapter can be found at DOI 10.1007/978-1-4939-7234-0_25

Wolfgang A. Schulz et al. (eds.), *Urothelial Carcinoma: Methods and Protocols*, Methods in Molecular Biology, vol. 1655, DOI 10.1007/978-1-4939-7234-0_19, © Springer Science+Business Media LLC 2018

namely one for non-muscle invasive papillary tumors, and another one leading via carcinoma in situ (CIS) to non-papillary muscle invasive tumors [1–3]. This concept is clinically important as the former can be generally treated less invasively with TUR alone or with intravesical therapy with excellent survival outcomes whereas the latter typically requires radical cystectomy for cure. Several clinical observations suggest that the two pathways are not perfectly distinct or mutually exclusive. Papillary non-muscle invasive bladder cancer (NMIBC) is often accompanied by CIS lesions, which are considered as a precursor for non-papillary muscle invasive bladder cancer (MIBC). Approximately 10% of patients with papillary NMIBC develop MIBC during postoperative follow-up after transurethral resection. Recent genetic analyses showed that a subset of MIBC harbor *FGFR3* activating mutations that are considered as one of the drivers of papillary NMIBC [4, 5].

According to the general principle in oncology to diagnose and treat tumors as early as possible, urine analysis has been tested for the early diagnosis of bladder cancer with the aim to screen asymptomatic individuals at high risk of BC. Because of the low prevalence of BC in the general population, population-based screening for BC would be not feasible. Therefore, pre-selection of patients at risk of bladder cancer seems to be necessary for the performance of screening analyses. Nonspecific symptoms including hematuria and voiding symptoms may be helpful for the selection of potential patients for urine biomarker analysis. In addition, as significant environmental risk factors for BC associated with lifestyle and professions are well documented, these may also be used for the identification of risk groups for which BC screening may be indicated and feasible.

NMIBC is characterized by high multiplicity and frequent intraluminal recurrence even after complete resection by TUR. This phenomenon is explained by the field defect and tumor cell seeding hypotheses, both of which seem to contribute to this clinically very important characteristic of NMIBC. Due to the high intravesical recurrence rate, patients are advised to have periodic cystoscopy examination for tumor surveillance [6]. With such vigilant post-TUR surveillance, most intravesical recurrences are detected as a NMIBC but approximately 10% of the patients with NMIBC eventually develop MIBC during the follow-up. Thus, patients with NMIBC very rarely die of the disease, but they need to tolerate almost life-long repetitions of unpleasant cystoscopy exams, which also makes BC the most costly cancer to care on a per patient basis [7–9].

Therefore, it is a clinical challenge to reduce patients' perceived and social economical burdens in the management of BC. As a potential alternative to cystoscopy, researchers have long attempted to identify and utilize urinary markers for the detection of BC [10]. Several urine-based assays are clinically available (Table 1), including urinary cytology, molecular markers such as BTA tests and NMP22, FISH-based cytogenetic assays such as UroVysion® and ImmunoCyt® (extensively discussed in excellent reviews [10–12]).

Table 1
Diagnostic performances of FDA-approved urinary markers for the detection and surveillance of bladder cancer

	Overall		Newly diagnosed		Recurrent	
	Sens.	Spec.	Sens.	Spec.	Sens.	Spec.
Cytology	12–85	58–100	16–85	78–100	12–70	93–99
BTA Stat (qualitative)	64	77	76	78	60	76
BTA Trak (quantitative)	65	74	76	53	58	79
NMP22 BladderCheck (qualitative)	58	88	47	93	70	83
NMP22 Bladder cancer test (quantitative)	69	77	67	84	61	71
ImmunoCyst/uCyt+	78	78	85	83	75	76
UroVysion	63	87	73	95	55	80

Sens. sensitivity, *Spec.* specificity, *N/A* Not available, Modified from refs. [6, 11]

Among them, urine cytology has become the standard test despite some weaknesses. Most of all, it is highly dependent on skills and experience of cytopathologists. Additionally, it yields high specificity but the sensitivity is generally low, particularly for low-grade tumors. Other commercially available markers have been reported to complement urine cytology, but they have other limitations or shortcomings. For example, NMP22 is prone to false positive results because of concomitant urinary tract infection. Thus, mainly due to their modest performance, presently available urine-based assays have a limited role for the detection or surveillance of BC.

Accordingly, there remains an urgent need for discovery of noninvasive urine-based tests with clinical utility for BC management. Urine analysis includes the assessment of both the cellular and the cell-free fraction of urine. The adherence between tumor cells is known to be decreased leading to an increased number of tumor cells in the urine sediment. These shed cells can be analyzed morphologically by urine cytology or by molecular biological techniques. The cellular fraction of the urine can be immunohistochemically stained (immune cytology, uCyt), its DNA content can be assessed by fluorescent in situ hybridization (FISH) or by microsatellite analysis in order to improve diagnostic sensitivity. Furthermore, the cell-free fraction of the urine contains DNA, RNA and proteins originating from the tumor cells which can also be tested.

In addition to BC detection, several biomarkers were shown to have potential as prognostic markers that are correlated with future risks of intravesical recurrence, muscle-invasive/metastatic progression, or cancer-specific mortality. There is a trend toward the development of multiparametric models to improve the diagnostic accuracy over that of single molecular markers. Recent technical advances for high-throughput and more sensitive measurements have led to the development of multiplex assays which show potential for becoming more efficient tools toward future clinical application. Here, we focus on urine-based protein biomarkers of the urine supernatant for the detection and prognostication of BC, introducing processes for the discovery of novel markers and discussing how to apply them to daily clinical practice. As standardization is essential in biomarker analyses, we give a brief overview on current recommendations for study design and data interpretation. In a further section, we provide an overview on single diagnostic protein markers illustrated by some of our own results in the identification of potential diagnostic markers. Then, we show an example for an integrative genomic and proteomic approach for the determination of a diagnostic urinary protein panel. Finally, we give a comprehensive overview on prognostic urine biomarkers in BC and discuss their possible clinical implementation.

2 Quality of Urine-Based Protein Biomarker Studies

2.1 Issues in Urine Based Protein Biomarkers for BC Detection

Due to the unique clinical course of BC patients as described above, the settings for their application should be clearly defined when we consider urine-based biomarkers for BC detection. The diagnostic significance is expected to vary according to the subject population such as healthy (primary) screening setting, secondary screening population after a positive primary result, patients presenting with macroscopic hematuria, or surveillance for recurrence in patients with a history of BC [13–16]. Most of the previous reports on urine-based protein markers employed a case-control design, in which known BC cases and non-BC controls were studied. The majority of them lack information whether BC patients had prior history of BC or not. This information is very important since BC patients with or without prior history are usually diagnosed through completely different diagnostic processes. Many diagnostic studies are biased by enrichment of advanced cases and by the use of healthy volunteers as controls, leading to false high specificity and sensitivity of the tested assay. Therefore, for diagnostic/surveillance studies both cases and controls should be patients undergoing investigation for suspected BC.

2.2 Classifications in Diagnostic Accuracy Studies

As we have rapidly increasing numbers of publications on urine-based protein biomarkers, assessments of (a) classification of studies, (b) study quality, and (c) reporting quality have become key issues in weighing the relevance of new information reported.

Classification of studies should be clearly defined according to their level of evidence or developmental stage. In terms of level of evidence, the Oxford Center of Evidence-Based Medicine (OCEBM) 2009 criteria for diagnostic and prognostic marker trials

Table 2
Criteria, recommendations, designs for improved quality of biomarker studies

Criteria	Context	Refs.
IBCN criteria	Study phases in BC biomarker development	[14, 18, 19]
OCEBM LoE criteria 2001/2009/2011	Level of evidence according to study design and quality	[17]
NOS	Quality assessment of case-control and cohort studies for biomarker development	[20]
QUADAS	Quality assessment of diagnostic accuracy studies	[21]
QUADAS-2	Quality assessment of diagnostic accuracy studies	[22]
STARD	Quality assessment of reporting of diagnostic accuracy studies	[23, 24]
REMARK	Quality assessment of reporting of prognostic marker studies	[25]
BRISQ	Recommendations for reporting biospecimen handling	[26]
PRoBE	Design of biospecimen collection for rapid and unbiased evaluation	[27]

IBCN International Bladder Cancer Network, *OCEBM* Oxford Center of Evidence-Based Medicine, *LoE* Level of Evidence, *NOS* Newcastle-Ottawa Scale, *QUADAS* Quality Assessment of Studies of Diagnostic Accuracy, *STARD* Standards for Reporting of Diagnostic Accuracy, *REMARK* REporting recommendations for tumor MARKer prognostic studies, *PRoBE* Prospective Specimen Collection Retrospective Blinded Evaluation

provides five levels of evidence based on the study design [17]. As for developmental stage, the International Bladder Cancer Network (IBCN) classified marker studies into four phases [14, 18]; (1) feasibility, (2) evaluation, (3) confirmation, and (4) application phases. In phase 1, a reproducible and optimized assay should be developed. In phase 2, the assay should be evaluated for clinical utility. In phase 3, a prospective study should be designed to confirm or validate the previous findings in an independent cohort. In phase 4, a multi-institutional study is desirable to transfer the established techniques and methods into clinical practice (Table 2).

2.3 Quality Assessment of Diagnostic Accuracy Studies

Unstandardized study quality is considered to cause discrepant or controversial results between diagnostic marker studies. Indeed, Dreier et al. identified 147 distinct quality assessment tools for assessing the study quality in the literature [28]. The IBCN described frequent methodological shortcomings and parameters varying between diagnostic accuracy trials [19]. Currently, several quality assessment tools are widely accepted; Newcastle-Ottawa Scale (NOS) [20], Quality Assessment of Studies of Diagnostic Accuracy (QUADAS) [21], and the QUADAS-2 tools [22]. NOS has been widely accepted as a tool to evaluate nonrandomized studies for systemic reviews or meta-analyses. Indeed, it was used for systemic reviews or meta-analyses on urine biomarkers [29] and others [30, 31]. However, several investigators have questioned its reliability due to a high inter-rater variability [32–34].

QUADAS is comprised of 14 items and designed to examine bias, internal and external validity and reporting of diagnostic accuracy studies [29]. It has been used in systematic reviews on urine-based BC markers [35, 36]. The inter-rater agreements in the final consensus rating were reported to be high but there were inter-rater disagreements in the results of some individual items [37, 38]. The revised version (QUDAS 2) is comprised of 4 domains; patient selection, index test(s), references standard and flow and timing [22]. Although the external validation process is underway, it has been already used in several systemic reviews and pooled analyses on urinary biomarkers (Table 2) [39, 40].

2.4 Quality Assessment of Reporting

In terms of reporting quality, diagnostic accuracy studies should adhere to Standards for Reporting of Diagnostic Accuracy (STARD) [23], while prognostic marker studies should adhere to REporting recommendations for tumur MARKer prognostic studies (REMARK) criteria [25]. STARD is comprised of 25 items that correspond to each section of the article including title, keywords, abstract, introduction, methods, results, and discussion. It has been validated with a high inter-rater agreement (85%), but some individual items showed low agreement rates (Table 2) [41].

It is critically important in biomarker studies to describe the types of biospecimens analyzed and the details of biospecimen collection and storage conditions. Biospecimen Reporting for Improved Study Quality (BRISQ) criteria [26] is comprised of three tiers of recommendation; items necessary to report (Tier 1), items advisable to report (Tier 2), and additional items (Tier 3).

Collectively, good biomarker studies should adhere to the above-described criteria or recommendations. This would facilitate development of novel biomarkers, reproduction of the biomarker studies, critical comparisons of various biomarkers, development of novel assay systems on given biomarkers, and clinical application of biomarker platforms.

3 Single Urine-Based Diagnostic Protein Markers

A variety of urine-based protein markers have been studied for potential use in BC detection in clinical practice (Tables 3 and 4). The reported sensitivities range from 52% to 97%, and the specificities range from 43% to 100%. Recent advancements in proteomics technology have drastically promoted discovery of novel protein markers and the number of urine-based biomarkers has explosively increased.

In our own study, we employed a shotgun proteomics technology approach in an attempt to identify urine-based protein

Table 3
Sensitivity and specificity of urine-based single protein biomarkers for the detection of bladder cancer

Protein name	*Gene symbol*	Sens.	Spec.	Cancer (n)	Control (n)	ND/ Rec	Control	Refs.
Alpha-1-anti-trypsin	*SERPINA1*	74	80	54	46	ND	Benign	[42]
Alpha-1-anti-trypsin	*SERPINA1*	71	72	102	206	ND	Benign	[43]
Angiogenin	*ANG*	66	75	50	40	N/A	Benign & HV	[44]
Apolipoprotein A1	*APOA1*	95	92	49	37	N/A	Benign	[45]
Apolipoprotein A4	*APOA4*	79	100	110	66	N/A	HV	[46]
AMFR	*AMFR*	84	75	45	62	N/A	Benign	[47]
BIGH3	*TGFB1*	93	80	30	15	N/A	Benign	[48]
Calprotectin	*S100A8 & A9*	80	93	46	40	N/A	HV	[49]
Cathepsin B	*CTSB*	56	56	122	107	Rec	Benign & HV	[50]
Cathepsin L	*CTSL*	71	75	122	107	Rec	Benign & HV	[50]
CCL18	*CCL18*	70	68	102	206	ND	Benign	[43]
CD147	*BCG*	97	100	30	15	N/A	Benign	[48]
CEACAM1	*CEACAM1*	74	95	95	82	N/A	Benign & HV	[51]
Clusterin	*CLU*	68	61	68	61	N/A	Benign	[52]
Clusterin	*CLU*	70	83	50	40	N/A	Benign & HV	[44]
Coronin-1A	*CORO1A*	67	100	110	66	N/A	HV	[46]
CXCL1	*CXCL1*	72	95	95	30	ND	HV	[53]
CXCL1	*CXCL1*	57	95	79	30	Rec	HV	[53]
CXCL1	*CXCL1*	56	84	43	43	ND	Benign	[54]
CYFRA21-1	*KRT19*	79	89	82	70	ND	Benign	[55]
CYFRA21-1	*KRT19*	76	73	37	70	Rec	Benign	[55]
CYFRA21-1	*KRT19*	81	97	86	76	N/A	Benign	[56]
CYFRA21-1	*KRT19*	70	43	125	321	Rec	Benign & HV	[57]

(continued)

Table 3 (continued)

Protein name	*Gene symbol*	Sens.	Spec.	Cancer (n)	Control (n)	ND/ Rec	Control	Refs.
CYFRA21-1	*KRT19*	97	67	48	80	N/A	Benign & HV	[58]
DJ1	*PARK7*	83	100	110	66	N/A	HV	[46]
EN2	*EN2*	82	75	466	55	N/A	Benign	[59]
FDP	*FGA & FGB*	52	91	57	139	N/A	Benign	[60]
Fibronectin	*FN1*	91	88	75	55	N/A	Benign & HV	[61]
Fibronectin	*FN1*	72	82	126	41	N/A	Benign	[62]
Prothrombin	*F2*	71	75	76	80	N/A	Benign	[63]
Reg-1	*REG1A*	81	81	23	48	N/A	Benign	[64]
Semenogelin-2	*SEMG2*	67	80	110	66	N/A	HV	[46]
Stathmin-1	*STMN1*	90	87	30	15	N/A	Benign	[48]
Teromerase	*TERT*	83	89	73	37	N/A	Benign & HV	[65]
UBC antigen	*KRT8 & KRT18*	*See* Table 3						
gamma-Synuclein	*SNCG*	88	90	110	66	N/A	HV	[46]

Sens. Sensitivity, *Spec.* Specificity, *ND* Newly diagnosed, *Rec* Recurrent, *N/A* Not available, *HV* Healthy volunteers

biomarker candidates from urinary supernatants of human urothelial cancer cells [77]. Among proteins detected by mass spectrometry (MS), we focused on secreted proteins and identified CXCL1 as a potential biomarker positively correlating with tumor grade and stage. We established an ELISA-based assay system and demonstrated that urine CXCL1 levels are useful for the detection of BC in both populations with and without prior history of BC [53, 54]. Moreover, we showed that urine CXCL1 levels predicted post-TUR intravesical recurrence-free survival.

Due to the continued technologic advancements, proteomic approaches using voided urine have become more widespread [78–80], and indeed, several investigators have identified urine-based protein biomarker profiles for the detection and prognostication of BC using the proteomics approach [42, 43, 45, 81–88]. For example, one group adopted isobaric tag for relative and absolute quantitation (iTRAQ) technique to identify 55 candidate protein biomarkers [82]. Among these, APOA1 was significantly

Table 4
Sensitivity and specificity of qualitative (UBC Rapid) and quantitative (UBC ELISA) urinary bladder cancer (UBC) tests for the detection of bladder cancer

Sensitivity	Specificity	Cancer (n)	Control (n)	ND/Rec	Control	Refs.
UBC Rapid						
64.4	63.6	90	22	N/A	Benign	[66]
66.0	90.0	53	127	ND/Rec	Benign	[67]
78.4	97.4	111	76	ND/Rec	No BC on surveillance	[68]
68.0	91.0	92	33	N/A	HV	[69]
48.7	79.3	78	140	N/A	Benign & HV	[70]
UBC ELISA						
80.5	80.2	118	95	Overall	Benign	[71]
80.9	N/A	68	50	ND	Benign	[71]
80.0	N/A	50	45	Rec	Benign	[71]
46.6	86.3	90	22	N/A	Benign	[66]
40.3	75.0	62	104	ND/Rec	Benign	[72]
64.8	92.0	54	186	ND/Rec	Benign	[73]
60.0	75.0	66	64	ND	Benign	[74]
72.0	40.0	93	81	Rec	No BC on surveillance	[74]
70.5	64.5	78	140	N/A	Benign & HV	[70]
61.0	73.0	59	48	ND	Benign	[75]
20.7	84.7	29	72	Rec	Benign	[76]

ND Newly diagnosed, *Rec* Recurrent, *N/A* Not available, *HV* Healthy volunteers

elevated in urine samples from BC patients. The follow-up study using an commercial ELISA assay confirmed that APOA1 is potentially useful as a diagnostic marker [45]. Furthermore, Yang and colleagues identified a panel of urine glycoproteins associated with BC [42]. They showed that SERPINA1 is the most informative protein and demonstrated diagnostic potential using an independent validation cohort [42, 43].

Despite these efforts, present urinary biomarkers are considered to have insufficient accuracy to replace cystoscopy for primary diagnosis or surveillance setting. A recently published guideline strongly recommends that a clinician should NOT use urinary biomarkers in place of cystoscopic evaluation in NMIBC surveillance (Evidence strength: B) [6].

4 Multiparametric Urine-Based Protein Markers

Thus, the presence or absence, or even abundance of any single biomarker yields very limited diagnostic ability. Accordingly, recently, a growing number of studies has been published proposing panels of protein biomarkers for the detection of BC (Table 5).

In our studies, we identified protein signatures with the potential to accurately detect BC from voided urine samples. We first performed gene expression profiling employing urine pellets collected from 46 subjects (26 controls and 20 BC) by Affymetrix U133 Plus 2.0 arrays followed by quantitative PCR verification to evaluate the urine from healthy volunteers and patients with BC in order to define a unique gene-expression profile [83]. The genomics analysis found that 319 genes have different expression levels between the two cohorts. Utilizing a selection/classification algorithm, we aimed to identify the gene signature that could most accurately diagnose the presence of BC among the 46 subjects. With this modeling classification approach, a 14-gene model achieved 76% overall accuracy in predicting class label during leave-one-out cross-validation. Next, we performed glycoprotein profiling in naturally voided urine collected from 10 subjects (5 controls and 5 BC) by dual-lectin affinity chromatography and liquid chromatography/tandem mass spectrometry followed by Western blot and ELISA [42, 84]. A total of 186 urinary proteins were identified including 40% categorized as secreted proteins, 18% as membrane proteins, and 14% as extracellular proteins. As mentioned in Subheading 2, further studies identified SERPINA1 (A1AT) as a potential protein biomarker [42, 43]. Bioinformatics analysis integrated the information from genomics and proteomics analyses and identified a panel of 14 protein biomarkers [85]. Subsequent studies confirmed the promise of 10 biomarkers for noninvasive detection of BC (IL8, MMP9, MMP10, ANG, APOE, SDC1, A1AT, PAI1, CA9, and VEGFA) [86–88, 90]. Most recently, we have developed a custom electrochemiluminescent multiplex assay (Meso Scale Diagnostics, LLC, Rockville, MD, USA). The multiplex measurement platform permits to simultaneously monitor the 10-protein biomarker panel in a single assay without loss of performance, thereby allowing a quick and high-throughput analysis on single voided urine samples [90]. In addition, we also investigated the potential utility of the multiplex assay in a Japanese cohort [92]. The study demonstrated that the multiplex urinary diagnostic assay has the potential to be developed for the noninvasive detection of BC in at-risk Japanese patients and eventually multiethnic patients.

An additional study showed that the diagnostic performance of multiplex urinary protein profiling was further improved when combined with clinical information such as age, race, and smoking

Table 5
Examples of multiparametric urine-based biomarkers for bladder cancer detection

Protein name	Sensitivity	Specificity	Cancer (n)	Control (n)	ND/ Rec	Control	AUROC	Refs.
Afamin, Adiponectin, Complement C4 gamma chain, Apolipoprotein A-II precursor, Ceruloplasmin, and Prothrombin	76	78	76	80	N/A	Benign	0.81	[63]
Coronin-1A, Apolipoprotein A4, Semenogelin-2, Gamma synuclein and DJ-1/PARK7	79	100	110 (Ta/1)	66	N/A	HV	0.92	[46]
Same as above	86	100	63 (T2/3)	66	N/A	HV	0.94	[46]
MMP9, MMP10, IL8, VEGFA, SERPINE1, SERPINA1, CA9, APOE, ANG, and SCD1 + Demographic information (Age, Race, and Smoking)	78	86	394	292	N/A	Benign & HV	0.89	[89]
IL8, MMP9, PAI1, VEGF, ANG, CA9, APOE, and MMP10	92	97	64	63	ND	HV	0.98	[85]
IL8, MMP9 and 10, PAI1, VEGF, ANG, and APOE	74	90	102	206	ND	Benign & HV	0.88	[86]
IL8, MMP9, MMP10, SERPINA1, VEGFA, ANG, CA9, APOE, SERPINE1, and SDC1	79	79	183	137	ND	Benign & HV	0.85	[87]
IL8, MMP9, MMP10, SERPINA1, VEGFA, ANG, CA9, APOE, SERPINE1, and SDC1	79	88	53	72	Rec	Benign	0.90	[88]
IL8, MMP9, MMP10, ANG, APOE, SDC1, A1AT, PAI1, CA9 and VEGFA	85	81	129	133	ND	Benign & HV	0.93	[90]
116 Peptides	91	68	168	102	ND	Benign	0.87	[91]
106 Peptides	88	51	55	156	Rec	Benign	0.75	[91]

ND Newly diagnosed, *Rec* Recurrent, *N/A* Not available, *HV* Healthy volunteers, *AUROC* Area under receiver operating characteristics curve

status [89]. The new multiplex protein panel will be rapidly commercialized and introduced to our clinical practice in the near future.

5 Prognostic Urinary Protein Biomarkers

Prognostic heterogeneity of bladder cancer represents a significant problem in the management of both NMIBC and MIBC. In NMIBC frequent (~80%) the two main risks are disease recurrence and the relative rarely occurring (~15%) but potentially life-threatening stage progression. In contrast, in MIBC metastatic progression represents the main risk for the patients. About 50% of MIBC patients benefit from radical surgical therapy by a long disease-free survival, while the other patients do have or will develop metastases and will die of bladder cancer [93]. Current prognostic methods are not effective to reliably predict the behavior of individual bladder cancers. The unmet clinical need for better prognostication has attracted much effort in the last years which resulted in the identification of several promising biomarkers [12]. However, none of these were implemented in the clinical practice yet.

Some of the assessed proteins were selected in a hypothesis-driven fashion, whereas other research groups performed screening using a proteomic approach. Most of the identified proteins were secreted cytokines, degraded extracellular matrix proteins, endogenous proteases, and their inhibitors, underlining the importance of proteolytic processes in the progression of bladder cancer. In addition a few oncofetal proteins were identified (Table 6).

5.1 Commercially Available Tests

BTA and NMP22 tests are both commercially available and FDA-approved immunoassays developed for bladder cancer detection. BTA test detects the antigen human complement factor H-related protein (hCFHrp), also called bladder tumor antigen (BTA), which is produced by bladder cancer cells. NMP22 test detects an antigen called nuclear mitotic apparatus (NuMa) protein which is a part of the mitotic spindle complex and thereby is involved in chromosome separation to daughter cells during cell division [110]. The BTA test has been shown to have superior sensitivity to that of voided urine cytology in detecting and monitoring recurrent bladder cancer. However, because BTA is present at high concentrations in blood, a false positive BTA test will occur when hematuria is present, regardless of the presence or absence of urothelial tumors. The function of hCFHrp/BTA protein is to interrupt the complement cascade and thereby help to escape tumor cells from the lytic degradation by host immune cells. This function suggested that the BTA test may possess not only diagnostic but also prognostic value. In accordance, Raitanen et al. found BTA test positivity to be

Table 6
Prognostic urinary biomarkers

Biomarker		Subjects pat.	ctr.	Methods analysis	Correlations T/N	T	G	Prognosis	Refs.
Cytokines and cytokine receptors									
BTA	Bladder tumor antigen	333	ND	IC	ND	yes	yes	no corr. with RFS	[94]
BTA	Bladder tumor antigen	97	ND	IC	ND	ND	ND	poor RFS	[95]
EGFR	Epidermal growth factor receptor	436	60	ELISA	no	yes	yes	poor DSS[a]	[96]
PDGFRβ	Platelet-derived growth factor receptor β	185	0	ELISA	ND	no	no	poor RFS	[97]
sFas		188	41	ELISA	C < T	yes	no	poor RFS[a]	[98]
sFas		128	88	ELISA	C < T	yes	yes	RFS[a]	[99]
Cell adhesion/Matrix proteins									
EpCAM	Epithelial cell adhesion molecule	607	53	ELISA	C < T	yes	yes	poor DSS[a]	[100]
TNC	Tenascin-C	66	42	ELISA	C < T	yes	yes	poor OS	[101]
NMP22	Nuclear matrix protein No.22	333	ND	IC	ND	yes	yes	poor RFS	[94]
Proteases/Protease inhibitors									
MMP-1	Matrix metalloproteinase-1	131	69	ELISA	C < T	yes	yes	poor PFS and DSS	[102]
MMP-9	Matrix metalloproteinase-9	188	29	ELISA	C < T	yes	yes	poor OS[a]	[103]
MMP-9	Matrix metalloproteinase-9	134	69	ELISA	C < T	yes	no	no corr. with DSS	[104]
TIMP1	Tissue inhibitor of metalloproteinase-1	131	69	ELISA	ND	yes	no	poor RFS	[104]
TIMP1	Tissue inhibitor of metalloproteinase-1	131	69	ELISA	C < T	yes	no	poor PFS	[102]
PAI-1	Plasminogen activator inhibitor type 1	244	74	ELISA	no	no	yes	no corr. with DSS	[105]
TATI	Tumor-associated trypsin inhibitor	157	0	RIA	ND	yes	yes	no corr. with DSS	[106]
CSTB	Cystatin B	47	0	WB	ND	yes	yes	poor RFS and PFS[a]	[107]

(continued)

Table 6 (continued)

Biomarker		Subjects pat.	Subjects ctr.	Methods analysis	Correlations T/N	Correlations T	Correlations G	Prognosis	Refs.
Oncofetal proteins									
CEA	Carcinoembryonic antigen	297	50	RIA	C < T	yes	no	poor OS[a]	[108]
ED-A FN	ED-A fibronectin	110	35	ELISA	no	no	no	poor OS[a]	[109]

[a]independent prognostic effect

ELISA Enzyme-linked immunosorbent assay, *RIA* Radioimmunassay, *IC* Immunochromatography, *WB* Western blot, *DSS* Disease-specific survival, *RFS* Recurrence-free survival, *PFS* Progression-free survival, *OS* Overall survival, *ND* Not determined

associated with shorter recurrence-free intervals in NMIBCs [95], most obviously in the subgroup of G2 tumors. Based on these results the number of follow-up cystoscopies might be reduced in patients with negative BTA test and G2 bladder cancer. However, these promising results were contrasted by the data of Poulakis et al. who found no significant value for BTA test in the prediction of tumor recurrence [94]. In their study the NMP22 test, instead, proved to be prognostic for increased risk of bladder cancer recurrence.

5.2 Cytokines

Epidermal growth factor receptor (EGFR) has been identified as a potential urinary biomarker by proteomic analysis of cell culture media of bladder cancer cell lines in order to identify proteins released by bladder cancer cells [96]. The ectodomain of the transmembrane receptor EGFR is released by proteolytic cleavage and this shedded ectodomain can be measured in the urine. Urinary EGFR levels were similar between controls and NMIBC patients suggesting no diagnostic value for urinary EGFR. On the other hand, high EGFR ectodomain concentrations were associated with poor disease-specific survival. This correlation remained significant in the multivariate analysis revealing an independent prognostic value for urinary EGFR concentrations. In accordance with these results, EGFR overexpression in MIBC was found to be characteristic for the "basal-like" molecular subtype of bladder cancer which represents a clinically highly aggressive type of this disease.

Platelet-derived growth factor receptor β (PDGFRβ) is a further cytokine that has been identified by proteomic analysis as a potential prognostic urinary biomarker of tumor recurrence. Its preoperative and postoperative levels were similar in NMIBC patients suggesting no diagnostic significance for this protein in bladder cancer [97].

The Fas-FasL pathway plays a key role in apoptosis. Fas is a transmembrane receptor which upon activation by FasL triggers apoptosis. An alternative splice variant of Fas encodes a soluble form of Fas which prevents the activation of an apoptotic signal by trapping FasL. This mechanism may help tumor cells to escape apoptosis. Both serum and urine levels of sFas were associated with poor prognosis in bladder cancer [98, 111]. A further independent analysis confirmed the value of urinary sFas in the prediction of tumor recurrence in the subgroup of NMIBC [99].

5.3 Proteases, Protease Inhibitors and ECM Proteins

Degradation of the extracellular matrix (ECM) is essential for invasive tumor growth. Tumor cells are able to secrete proteases or enhance the protease expression of neighboring nonmalignant stromal cells in a paracrine manner, leading to ECM degradation. This tumor-induced protease activity is a prerequisite for intravasation and extravasation of tumor cells and invasion of distant organs during metastatic progression. Matrix metalloproteinases (MMPs) are the main enzymes involved in ECM degradation. Therefore, MMPs have attracted much interest as potential prognostic factors in a number of human malignancies including bladder cancer [112]. MMP-9 degrades type IV collagen, an important component of the basement membrane, thereby supporting the invasive potential of tumor cells. Of the over 25 members of the MMP family, only MMP-1 and MMP-9 have been analyzed so far for their prognostic relevance in urine [102–104]. Durkan et al. measuring MMP-9 levels in urine samples of 134 patients with various tumor stages found no prognostic significance for MMP-9 [104]. However, the same study identified a clear and unfavorable prognostic relevance for positive MMP-9 tissue expression. In a more recent study Offersen et al., assessing both active and pro-enzymatic form of MMP-9 in urine samples of 188 bladder cancer patients, found MMP-9 to be a significant and independent prognostic factor for poor patient survival [103]. Based on the larger study group and the longer follow-up period in the study by Offersen, in addition to the positive prognostic association with expression in tissues observed by Durkan et al. MMP-9 seems to be a potential urinary marker for bladder cancer prognosis. Urinary MMP-1 could be detected in 16% of bladder cancer cases [102] and was associated with higher tumor stage, grade, and shorter progression-free and disease-specific survival [102]. A further promising prognostic factor in bladder cancer is MMP-7. Its elevated serum and plasma levels were found to be associated with the presence of lymph node metastasis and proved to be independent prognostic factors for disease-specific survival [113, 114]. Similarly, urinary MMP-7 levels were strongly increased in preoperatively collected urine samples of bladder cancer patients with lymph node metastasis [114]. These findings have a significant clinical potential considering that current imaging techniques are unable to sensitively detect especially low volume lymph node metastases. As a consequence, about 30% of patients with MIBC have undetected metastasis at the time of surgical treatment [115].

An important regulatory mechanism of MMP activity is achieved by their endogenous inhibitors, the tissue inhibitors of metalloproteinases (TIMPs). At present, four TIMPs have been identified, with largely overlapping MMP inhibitory activities [116]. Surprisingly, high TIMP-1 and TIMP-2 expression correlated with poor prognosis in a range of malignant diseases, and overexpressing TIMP-1 and TIMP-2 was found to enhance tumorigenicity in transgenic mice [117, 118]. In accordance with these findings, high urinary TIMP1 levels were associated with poor recurrence-free survival also in bladder cancer [102]. Two further protease inhibitors were tested for their prognostic value in urine of bladder cancer patients; the plasminogen activator inhibitor type I (PAI-I) and the tumor associated trypsin inhibitor (TATI). None of them proved to have any prognostic value in bladder cancer [105, 106]. Using a proteomic approach, a cathepsin protease inhibitor, cystatin B has been identified as a differentially expressed protein between urine samples from normal controls, bladder cancer patients with Ta and with high-grade tumors [107]. In the subsequent analysis by semi-quantitative Western blot analysis the authors identified cystatin B as an independent prognostic urinary marker of poor recurrence-free and progression-free survival [107].

The epithelial cell adhesion molecule (EpCAM, CD326) is a glycoprotein that was originally identified as a carcinoma marker, attributable to its high expression on rapidly proliferating tumors of epithelial origin including bladder cancer [119]. Its extracellular domain, similar to EGFR, is released into the urine by proteolytic shedding. Urinary EpCAM levels were strongly correlated with muscle-invasive tumor stages and in addition, independently associated with cancer-specific survival [100].

Tenascin-C (TNC) is also a glycoprotein and a component of extracellular matrix which is expressed more strongly in many epithelial tumors including bladder cancer. Higher TNC tissue expression was correlated with poor prognosis in MIBC but not in NIMBC [120]. Determined in the urine, TNC levels were higher in healthy controls than in bladder cancer patients, while higher TNC levels were observed in high-stage and high-grade tumors compared to low-stage, low-grade cancers [101]. In addition, elevated TNC levels were independently associated with poor patient survival [101]. Whether the elevated urinary TNC level in bladder cancer patients is the consequence of its higher tissue expression or the enhanced proteolytic activity of tumor cells remains to be evaluated.

5.4 Oncofetal Proteins

The carcinoembryonic antigen (CEA) is a well-established oncofetal protein which has proven useful for the detection and monitoring of colorectal carcinoma. CEA can also be determined in the urine and an early study assessing its urine levels in a large group of patients who were radiologically treated for MIBC reported CEA as an independent prognosticator of patient survival [108]. In addition, slowly decreasing or increasing CEA levels during the treatment were associated with poor prognosis. These results suggest potential roles of CEA not only in prognostication but also in disease monitoring.

Fibronectin (FN) is an abundant glycoprotein of the extracellular matrix. In the urine, the presence of FN appears to be related to proteolytic degradation by enzymes produced by tumor cells and due to leakage from blood. The urinary levels of FN were found to be elevated in bladder cancer, but showed no prognostic value [109]. Some alternatively spliced FN isoforms such as FN ED-A and FN ED-B are expressed during embryonic development but are absent in normal adult tissues. FN ED-A and ED-B isoforms were found to be re-expressed in tumor and tumor surrounding stromal cells [109]. Both FN splice variants were tested for their prognostic value in the urine of patients with mostly high-grade and muscle-invasive bladder cancer [109]. The presence of FN ED-A was independently associated with shorter overall survival of patients especially in lymph node negative cases. Based on these findings, ED-A seems to be a promising urinary marker in the risk stratification of MIBC.

6 Conclusion and Possible Clinical Consequences

In the era of high-throughput proteomics, comprehensive, unbiased approaches to the discovery of novel urine-based protein biomarkers are technically and economically feasible. We are encouraged by the promising results with multiplex protein assays based on combinations of candidate proteins that yield a more robust performance. Currently an increased number of proteins are added to a panel moving forward to the next phase toward clinical diagnostic application.

The National Cancer Institute's Early Detection Research Network (EDRN) established specimen reference sets including urine samples under Prospective Specimen Collection Retrospective Blinded Evaluation (PRoBE) design criteria [121]. This system is expected to enable quick triaging of biomarker to the full validation phase, for rapid evaluation of biomarkers with high potential. The highly systematic approach with standardized quality described above will hopefully result in rapid development of novel biomarkers yielding high diagnostic performance.

Prognostic protein biomarkers of disease recurrence and progression may be used as indicators for earlier aggressive treatment of NMIBC or alter the algorithm for surveillance of patients. Those NMIBC patients at risk for a rapid recurrence could be followed with a more frequent schedule of surveillance, whereas those with biomarker evidence of low risk could be surveyed less frequently. High BTA, NMP22, PDGFRβ, CSTNB, and sFas urine levels were found to be predictive for disease recurrence in NMIBC. Of these, NMP22, CSTNB, and PDGFRβ have not been confirmed in independent patient cohorts yet, while the data on BTA are rather controversial. The most promising urinary marker seems to be sFas as its prognostic relevance has been confirmed by two large studies and both of these revealed sFas as an independent prognostic factor in the multivariable analysis. Patients with low risk of recurrence, proven by low urinary sFas levels, may benefit from the extension of follow-up intervals thereby reducing the number of the uncomfortable and invasive cystoscopic control examinations.

Additionally, a dependable urinary biomarker of invasive disease might be a valuable complementary tool to cytology and cystoscopy in the surveillance of bladder cancer. In this regard EpCAM, EGFR, MMP-1, and TIMP1 urinary analyses look especially promising as these markers were able to yield predictive information on the risk of present or future muscle-invasion. As a consequence, NMIBC at greater risk of progression identified by validated biomarkers may be more appropriately managed with an early aggressive surgical resection.

In MIBC patients, high urinary EpCAM, EGFR, MMP-9, CEA, and ED-A fibronectin levels were found to be independently associated with patient disease-specific or overall survival. The identification of high-risk MIBC patients may benefit from an early systemic treatment. In addition, these markers hold the potential to select high-risk patients for clinical trials of current or novel therapies.

Acknowledgements

This study was supported by National Research, Development and Innovation Office; Grant number: NKFIH/PD 115616 and by János Bolyai Research Scholarship of the Hungarian Academy of Sciences.

References

1. Pasin E, Josephson DY, Mitra AP et al (2008) Superficial bladder cancer: an update on etiology, molecular development, classification, and natural history. Rev Urol 10:31–43
2. Castillo-Martin M, Domingo-Domenech J, Karni-Schmidt O et al (2010) Molecular pathways of urothelial development and bladder tumorigenesis. Urol Oncol 28:401–408
3. Knowles MA, Hurst CD (2015) Molecular biology of bladder cancer: new insights into pathogenesis and clinical diversity. Nat Rev Cancer 15:25–41

4. Cancer Genome Atlas Research Network (2014) Comprehensive molecular characterization of urothelial bladder carcinoma. Nature 507:315–322
5. McConkey DJ, Lee S, Choi W et al (2010) Molecular genetics of bladder cancer: emerging mechanisms of tumor initiation and progression. Urol Oncol 28:429–440
6. Chang SS, Boorjian SA, Chou R et al (2016) Diagnosis and treatment of non-muscle invasive bladder cancer: AUA/SUO guideline. J Urol 196:1021–1029
7. Kaplan AL, Litwin MS, Chamie K (2014) The future of bladder cancer care in the USA. Nat Rev Urol 11:59–62
8. Mossanen M, Gore JL (2014) The burden of bladder cancer care: direct and indirect costs. Curr Opin Urol 24:487–491
9. Yeung C, Dinh T, Lee J (2014) The health economics of bladder cancer: an updated review of the published literature. Pharmacoeconomics 32:1093–1104
10. Rosser CJ, Urquidi V, Goodison S et al (2013) Urinary biomarkers of bladder cancer: an update and future perspectives. Biomark Med 7:779–790
11. Budman LI, Kassouf W, Steinberg JR et al (2008) Biomarkers for detection and surveillance of bladder cancer. Can Urol Assoc J 2:212–221
12. D'Costa JJ, Goldsmith JC, Wilson JS et al (2016) A systematic review of the diagnostic and prognostic value of urinary protein biomarkers in Urothelial bladder cancer. Bladder Cancer 2:301–317
13. Chatziharalambous D, Lygirou V, Latosinska A et al (2016) Analytical performance of ELISA assays in urine: one more bottleneck towards biomarker validation and clinical implementation. PLoS One 11:e0149471
14. Goebell PJ, Groshen SL, Schmitz-Dräger BJ (2008) Guidelines for development of diagnostic markers in bladder cancer. World J Urol 26:5–11
15. Lotan Y, Shariat SF, Schmitz-Dräger BJ et al (2010) Considerations on implementing diagnostic markers into clinical decision making in bladder cancer. Urol Oncol 28:441–448
16. Kobayashi T, Owczarek TB, McKiernan JM et al (2015) Modelling bladder cancer in mice: opportunities and challenges. Nat Rev Cancer 15:42–54
17. Oxford Centre for Evidence-based Medicine Levels of Evidence (2016). Available from: http://www.cebm.net
18. Goebell PJ, Groshen S, Schmitz-Dräger BJ et al (2014) The International bladder cancer Bank: proposal for a new study concept. Urol Oncol 22:277–284
19. Goebell PJ, Kamat AM, Sylvester RJ et al (2014) Assessing the quality of studies on the diagnostic accuracy of tumor markers. Urol Oncol 32:1051–1060
20. Wells G et al (2014) Newcastle-Otawa scale. Available from: http://www.ohri.ca/programs/clinical_epidemiology/oxford.asp
21. Whiting P, Rutjes AW, Reitsma JB et al (2003) The development of QUADAS: a tool for the quality assessment of studies of diagnostic accuracy included in systematic reviews. BMC Med Res Methodol 3:25
22. Whiting PF, Rutjes AW, Westwood ME et al (2011) QUADAS-2 Group.QUADAS-2: a revised tool for the quality assessment of diagnostic accuracy studies. Ann Intern Med 155:529–536
23. Bossuyt PM, Reitsma JB, Bruns DE et al (2003) Standards for reporting of diagnostic accuracy the STARD statement for reporting studies of diagnostic accuracy: explanation and elaboration. Clin Chem 49:7–18
24. Bossuyt PM, Reitsma JB, Bruns DE et al (2004) Towards complete and accurate reporting of studies of diagnostic accuracy: the STARD initiative. Fam Pract 21:4–10
25. McShane LM, Altman DG, Sauerbrei W et al (2005) Statistics subcommittee of the NCI-EORTC working group on cancer diagnostics. REporting recommendations for tumour MARKer prognostic studies (REMARK). Br J Cancer 93:387–391
26. Moore HM, Kelly A, McShane LM et al (2013) Biospecimen reporting for improved study quality (BRISQ). Transfusion 53:e1
27. Simeon-Dubach D, Moore HM (2014) BIO comes into the cold to adopt BRISQ. Biopreserv Biobank 12:223–224
28. Dreier M, Borutta B, Stahmeyer J et al (2010) Comparison of tools for assessing the methodological quality of primary and secondary studies in health technology assessment reports in Germany. GMS Health Technol 6:Doc07
29. Qi D, Li J, Jiang M et al (2015) The relationship between promoter methylation of p16 gene and bladder cancer risk: a meta-analysis. Int J Clin Exp Med 8:20701–20711
30. Lopez LM, Chen M, Mullins Long S et al (2015) Steroidal contraceptives and bone fractures in women: evidence from observational studies. Cochrane Database Syst Rev 21 (7):CD009849

31. Thelma Beatriz GC, Isela JR, Alma G et al (2014) Association between HTR2C gene variants and suicidal behaviour: a protocol for the systematic review and meta-analysis of genetic studies. BMJ Open 4:e005423
32. Hartling L, Milne A, Hamm MP et al (2013) Testing the Newcastle Ottawa scale showed low reliability between individual reviewers. J Clin Epidemiol 66:982–993
33. Oremus M, Oremus C, Hall GB et al (2012) ECT & Cognition Systematic Review Team. Inter-rater and test-retest reliability of quality assessments by novice student raters using the Jadad and Newcastle-Ottawa scales. BMJ Open 2:e001368
34. Stang A (2010) Critical evaluation of the Newcastle-Ottawa scale for the assessment of the quality of nonrandomized studies in meta-analyses. Eur J Epidemiol 25:603–605
35. Xia Y, Liu YL, Yang KH (2010) The diagnostic value of urine-based survivin mRNA test using reverse transcription-polymerase chain reaction for bladder cancer: a systematic review. Chin J Cancer 29:441–446
36. Yang X, Huang H, Zeng Z et al (2013) Diagnostic value of bladder tumor fibronectin in patients with bladder tumor: a systematic review with meta-analysis. Clin Biochem 46:1377–1382
37. Hollingworth W, Medina LS, Lenkinski RE et al (2006) Interrater reliability in assessing quality of diagnostic accuracy studies using the QUADAS tool. A preliminary assessment. Acad Radiol 13:803–810
38. Whiting PF, Weswood ME, Rutjes AW et al (2006) Evaluation of QUADAS, a tool for the quality assessment of diagnostic accuracy studies. BMC Med Res Methodol 6:9
39. Cai Q, Wu Y, Guo Z et al (2015) Urine BLCA-4 exerts potential role in detecting patients with bladder cancers: a pooled analysis of individual studies. Oncotarget 6:37500–37510
40. Huang YL, Chen J, Yan W et al (2015) Diagnostic accuracy of cytokeratin-19 fragment (CYFRA 21-1) for bladder cancer: a systematic review and meta-analysis. Tumour Biol 36:3137–3145
41. Smidt N, Rutjes AW, van der Windt DA et al (2006) Reproducibility of the STARD checklist: an instrument to assess the quality of reporting of diagnostic accuracy studies. BMC Med Res Methodol 6:12
42. Yang N, Feng S, Shedden K et al (2011) Urinary glycoprotein biomarker discovery for bladder cancer detection using LC/MS-MS and label-free quantification. Clin Cancer Res 17:3349–3359
43. Miyake M, Ross S, Lawton A et al (2013) Investigation of CCL18 and A1AT as potential urinary biomarkers for bladder cancer detection. BMC Urol 13:42
44. Shabayek MI, Sayed OM, Attaia HA et al (2014) Diagnostic evaluation of urinary angiogenin (ANG) and clusterin (CLU) as biomarker for bladder cancer. Pathol Oncol Res 20:859–866
45. Chen YT, Chen CL, Chen HW et al (2010) Discovery of novel bladder cancer biomarkers by comparative urine proteomics using iTRAQ technology. J Proteome Res 9:5803–5815
46. Kumar P, Nandi S, Tan TZ et al (2015) Highly sensitive and specific novel biomarkers for the diagnosis of transitional bladder carcinoma. Oncotarget 6:13539–13549
47. Korman HJ, Peabody JO, Cerny JC et al (1996) Autocrine motility factor receptor as a possible urine marker for transitional cell carcinoma of the bladder. J Urol 155:347–349
48. Bhagirath D, Abrol N, Khan R et al (2012) Expression of CD147, BIGH3 and Stathmin and their potential role as diagnostic marker in patients with urothelial carcinoma of the bladder. Clin Chim Acta 413:1641–1646
49. Ebbing J, Mathia S, Seibert FS et al (2014) Urinary calprotectin: a new diagnostic marker in urothelial carcinoma of the bladder. World J Urol 32:1485–1492
50. Svatek RS, Karam J, Karakiewicz PI et al (2008) Role of urinary cathepsin B and L in the detection of bladder urothelial cell carcinoma. J Urol 179:478–484
51. Tilki D, Singer BB, Shariat SF et al (2010) CEACAM1: a novel urinary marker for bladder cancer detection. Eur Urol 5:648–654
52. Hazzaa SM, Elashry OM, Afifi IK (2010) Clusterin as a diagnostic and prognostic marker for transitional cell carcinoma of the bladder. Pathol Oncol Res 16:101–109
53. Nakashima M, Matsui Y, Kobayashi T et al (2015) Urine CXCL1 as a biomarker for tumor detection and outcome prediction in bladder cancer. Cancer Biomark 15:357–364
54. Burnier A, Shimizu Y, Dai Y et al (2015) CXCL1 is elevated in the urine of bladder cancer patients. Springerplus 4:610
55. Nisman B, Barak V, Shapiro A et al (2002) Evaluation of urine CYFRA 21-1 for the detection of primary and recurrent bladder carcinoma. Cancer 94:2914–2922

56. Sánchez-Carbayo M, Espasa A, Chinchilla V et al (1999) New electrochemiluminescent immunoassay for the determination of CYFRA 21-1: analytical evaluation and clinical diagnostic performance in urine samples of patients with bladder cancer. Clin Chem 45:1944–1953
57. Fernandez-Gomez J, Rodríguez-Martínez JJ, Barmadah SE et al (2007) Urinary CYFRA 21.1 is not a useful marker for the detection of recurrences in the follow-up of superficial bladder cancer. Eur Urol 51:1267–1274
58. Pariente JL, Bordenave L, Michel P et al (1997) Initial evaluation of CYFRA 21-1 diagnostic performances as a urinary marker in bladder transitional cell carcinoma. J Urol 158:338–341
59. Morgan R, Bryan RT, Javed S et al (2013) Expression of engrailed-2 (EN2) protein in bladder cancer and its potential utility as a urinary diagnostic biomarker. Eur J Cancer 49:2214–2222
60. Ramakumar S, Bhuiyan J, Besse JA et al (1999) Comparison of screening methods in the detection of bladder cancer. J Urol 161:388–394
61. Mutlu N, Turkeri L, Emerk K (2003) Analytical and clinical evaluation of a new urinary tumor marker: bladder tumor fibronectin in diagnosis and follow-up of bladder cancer. Clin Chem Lab Med 41:1069–1074
62. Li LY, Yang M, Zhang HB et al (2008) Urinary fibronectin as a predictor of a residual tumour load after transurethral resection of bladder transitional cell carcinoma. BJU Int 102:566–571
63. Chen YT, Chen HW, Domanski D et al (2012) Multiplexed quantification of 63 proteins in human urine by multiple reaction monitoring-based mass spectrometry for discovery of potential bladder cancer biomarkers. J Proteomics 75:3529–3545
64. Orenes-Piñero E, Cortón M, González-Peramato P et al (2007) Searching urinary tumor markers for bladder cancer using a two-dimensional differential gel electrophoresis (2D-DIGE) approach. J Proteome Res 6:4440–4448
65. Eissa S, Labib RA, Mourad MS et al (2003) Comparison of telomerase activity and matrix metalloproteinase-9 in voided urine and bladder wash samples as a useful diagnostic tool for bladder cancer. Eur Urol 44:687–694
66. Hakenberg OW, Fuessel S, Richter K et al (2004) Qualitative and quantitative assessment of urinary cytokeratin 8 and 18 fragments compared with voided urine cytology in diagnosis of bladder carcinoma. Urology 64:1121–1126
67. Mian C, Lodde M, Haitel A (2000) Comparison of two qualitative assays, the UBC rapid test and the BTA stat test, in the diagnosis of urothelial cell carcinoma of the bladder. Urology 56:228–231
68. Sánchez-Carbayo M, Herrero E, Megías J et al (1999) Initial evaluation of the new urinary bladder cancer rapid test in the detection of transitional cell carcinoma of the bladder. Urology 54:656–661
69. Ecke TH, Arndt C, Stephan C et al (2015) Preliminary results of a multicentre study of the UBC rapid test for detection of urinary bladder cancer. Anticancer Res 35:2651–2655
70. Babjuk M, Kostírová M, Mudra K et al (2002) Qualitative and quantitative detection of urinary human complement factor H-related protein (BTA stat and BTA TRAK) and fragments of cytokeratins 8, 18 (UBC rapid and UBC IRMA) as markers for transitional cell carcinoma of the bladder. Eur Urol 41:34–39
71. Giannopoulos A, Manousakas T, Gounari A et al (2001) Comparative evaluation of the diagnostic performance of the BTA stat test, NMP22 and urinary bladder cancer antigen for primary and recurrent bladder tumors. J Urol 166:470–475
72. May M, Hakenberg OW, Gunia S, Pohling P, Helke C, Lübbe L, Nowack R, Siegsmund M, Hoschke B (2007) Comparative diagnostic value of urine cytology, UBC-ELISA, and fluorescence in situ hybridization for detection of transitional cell carcinoma of urinary bladder in routine clinical practice. Urology 70(3):449–453
73. Mian C, Lodde M, Haitel A et al (2000) Comparison of the monoclonal UBC-ELISA test and the NMP22 ELISA test for the detection of urothelial cell carcinoma of the bladder. Urology 55:223–226
74. Boman H, Hedelin H, Holmäng S (2002) Four bladder tumor markers have a disappointingly low sensitivity for small size and low grade recurrence. J Urol 167:80–83
75. Boman H, Hedelin H, Jacobsson S et al (2002) Newly diagnosed bladder cancer: the relationship of initial symptoms, degree of microhematuria and tumor marker status. J Urol 168:1955–1959
76. Mungan NA, Vriesema JL, Thomas CM et al (2002) Urinary bladder cancer test: a new urinary tumor marker in the follow-up of superficial bladder cancer. Urology 56:787–792

77. Kawanishi H, Matsui Y, Ito M et al (2008) Secreted CXCL1 is a potential mediator and marker of the tumor invasion of bladder cancer. Clin Cancer Res 14:2579–2587
78. Su L, Cao L, Zhou R et al (2013) Identification of novel biomarkers for sepsis prognosis via urinary proteomic analysis using iTRAQ labeling and 2D-LC-MS/MS. PLoS One 8: e54237
79. Bakun M, Niemczyk M, Domanski D et al (2012) Urine proteome of autosomal dominant polycystic kidney disease patients. Clin Proteomics 9:13
80. Lei T, Zhao X, Jin S et al (2013) Discovery of potential bladder cancer biomarkers by comparative urine proteomics and analysis. Clin Genitourin Cancer 11:56–62
81. Lindén M, Lind SB, Mayrhofer C et al (2012) Proteomic analysis of urinary biomarker candidates for nonmuscle invasive bladder cancer. Proteomics 12:135–144
82. Majewski T, Spiess PE, Bondaruk J et al (2012) Detection of bladder cancer using proteomic profiling of urine sediments. PLoS One 7:e42452
83. Urquidi V, Goodison S, Cai Y et al (2012) A candidate molecular biomarker panel for the detection of bladder cancer. Cancer Epidemiol Biomarkers Prev 21:2149–2158
84. Kreunin P, Zhao J, Rosser C et al (2007) Bladder cancer associated glycoprotein signatures revealed by urinary proteomic profiling. J Proteome Res 6:2631–2639
85. Goodison S, Chang M, Dai Y et al (2012) A multi-analyte assay for the non-invasive detection of bladder cancer. PLoS One 7:e47469
86. Rosser CJ, Ross S, Chang M et al (2013) Multiplex protein signature for the detection of bladder cancer in voided urine samples. J Urol 190:2257–2262
87. Chen LM, Chang M, Dai Y et al (2014) External validation of a multiplex urinary protein panel for the detection of bladder cancer in a multicenter cohort. Cancer Epidemiol Biomarkers Prev 23:1804–1812
88. Rosser CJ, Chang M, Dai Y et al (2014) Urinary protein biomarker panel for the detection of recurrent bladder cancer. Cancer Epidemiol Biomarkers Prev 23:1340–1345
89. Huang S, Kou L, Furuya H et al (2016) A Nomogram derived by combination of demographic and biomarker data improves the non-invasive evaluation of patients at risk for bladder cancer. Cancer Epidemiol Biomarkers Prev 25:1361–1366
90. Shimizu Y, Furuya H, Bryant Greenwood P et al (2016) A multiplex immunoassay for the non-invasive detection of bladder cancer. J Transl Med 14:31
91. Frantzi M, van Kessel KE, Zwarthoff EC et al (2016) Development and validation of urine-based peptide biomarker panels for detecting bladder cancer in a multi-center study. Clin Cancer Res 22:4077–4086
92. Goodison S, Ogawa O, Matsui Y et al (2016) A multiplex urinary immunoassay for bladder cancer detection: analysis of a Japanese cohort. J Transl Med 14:287
93. Stein JP, Skinner DG (2006) Radical cystectomy for invasive bladder cancer: long-term results of a standard procedure. World J Urol 24:296–304
94. Poulakis V, Witzsch U, De Vries R (2001) A comparison of urinary nuclear matrix protein-22 and bladder tumour antigen tests with voided urinary cytology in detecting and following bladder cancer: the prognostic value of false-positive results. BJU Int 88:692–701
95. Raitanen MP, Kaasinen E, Rintala E et al (2001) Prognostic utility of human complement factor H related protein test (the BTA stat test). Br J Cancer 85:552–556
96. Bryan RT, Regan HL, Pirrie SJ et al (2015) Protein shedding in urothelial bladder cancer: prognostic implications of soluble urinary EGFR and EpCAM. Br J Cancer 112:1052–1058
97. Feng J, He W, Song Y et al (2014) Platelet-derived growth factor receptor beta: a novel urinary biomarker for recurrence of non-muscle-invasive bladder cancer. PLoS One 9: e96671
98. Svatek RS, Herman MP, Lotan Y et al (2006) Soluble Fas–a promising novel urinary marker for the detection of recurrent superficial bladder cancer. Cancer 106:1701–1707
99. Yang H, Li H, Wang Z et al (2013) Is urinary soluble Fas an independent predictor of non-muscle-invasive bladder cancer? A prospective chart study. Urol Int 91:456–461
100. Bryan RT, Shimwell NJ, Wei W et al (2014) Urinary EpCAM in urothelial bladder cancer patients: characterisation and evaluation of biomarker potential. Br J Cancer 110:679–685
101. Guan Z, Zeng J, Wang Z et al (2014) Urine tenascin-C is an independent risk factor for bladder cancer patients. Mol Med Rep 9:961–966
102. Durkan GC, Nutt JE, Rajjayabun PH et al (2001) Prognostic significance of matrix metalloproteinase-1 and tissue inhibitor of metalloproteinase-1 in voided urine samples from patients with transitional cell carcinoma of the bladder. Clin Cancer Res 7:3450–3456

103. Offersen BV, Knap MM, Horsman MR et al (2010) Matrix metalloproteinase-9 measured in urine from bladder cancer patients is an independent prognostic marker of poor survival. Acta Oncol 49:1283–1287
104. Durkan GC, Nutt JE, Marsh C et al (2003) Alteration in urinary matrix metalloproteinase-9 to tissue inhibitor of metalloproteinase-1 ratio predicts recurrence in nonmuscle-invasive bladder cancer. Clin Cancer Res 9:2576–2582
105. Becker M, Szarvas T, Wittschier M et al (2010) Prognostic impact of plasminogen activator inhibitor type 1 expression in bladder cancer. Cancer 116:4502–4512
106. Kelloniemi E, Rintala E, Finne P et al (2003) Tumor-associated trypsin inhibitor as a prognostic factor during follow-up of bladder cancer. Urology 62:249–253
107. Feldman AS, Banyard J, Wu CL et al (2009) Cystatin B as a tissue and urinary biomarker of bladder cancer recurrence and disease progression. Clin Cancer Res 15:1024–1031
108. Zimmerman R, Wahren B, Edsmyr F (1980) Assessment of serial CEA determinations in urine of patients with bladder carcinoma. Cancer 46:1802–1809
109. Arnold SA, Loomans HA, Ketova T et al (2016) Urinary oncofetal ED-A fibronectin correlates with poor prognosis in patients with bladder cancer. Clin Exp Metastasis 33:29–44
110. Compton DA, Cleveland DW (1993) NuMA is required for the proper completion of mitosis. J Cell Biol 120:947–957
111. Mizutani Y, Yoshida O, Ukimura O et al (2002) Prognostic significance of a combination of soluble Fas and soluble Fas ligand in the serum of patients with ta bladder cancer. Cancer Biother Radiopharm 17:563–567
112. Szarvas T, vom Dorp F, Ergün S et al (2011) Matrix metalloproteinases and their clinical relevance in urinary bladder cancer. Nat Rev Urol 8:241–254
113. Szarvas T, Becker M, vom Dorp F et al (2010) Matrix metalloproteinase-7 as a marker of metastasis and predictor of poor survival in bladder cancer. Cancer Sci 101:1300–1308
114. Szarvas T, Jäger T, Becker M et al (2011) Validation of circulating MMP-7 level as an independent prognostic marker of poor survival in urinary bladder cancer. Pathol Oncol Res 17:325–332
115. Szarvas T, Singer BB, Becker M et al (2011) Urinary matrix metalloproteinase-7 level is associated with the presence of metastasis in bladder cancer. BJU Int 107:1069–1073
116. Cruz-Munoz W, Khokha R (2008) The role of tissue inhibitors of metalloproteinases in tumorigenesis and metastasis. Crit Rev Clin Lab Sci 45:291–338
117. Thomas P, Khokha R, Shepherd FA et al (2000) Differential expression of matrix metalloproteinases and their inhibitors in non-small cell lung cancer. J Pathol 190:150–156
118. Rhee JS, Diaz R, Korets L et al (2004) TIMP-1 alters susceptibility to carcinogenesis. Cancer Res 64:952–961
119. Brunner A, Prelog M, Verdorfer I et al (2008) EpCAM is predominantly expressed in high grade and advanced stage urothelial carcinoma of the bladder. J Clin Pathol 61:307–310
120. Brunner A, Mayerl C, Tzankov A et al (2004) Prognostic significance of tenascin-C expression in superficial and invasive bladder cancer. J Clin Pathol 57:927–931
121. Feng Z, Kagan J, Pepe M et al (2013) The early detection research Network's specimen reference sets: paving the way for rapid evaluation of potential biomarkers. Clin Chem 59:68–74

Chapter 20

Isolation and Characterization of CTCs from Patients with Cancer of a Urothelial Origin

Vladimir Bobek and Katarina Kolostova

Abstract

Monitoring of circulating tumor cells' (CTCs) presence has the potential to improve therapeutic management of oncological diseases at an early stage and also to identify patients with increased risk of tumor progression or recurrence before the onset of clinically detected metastasis. Here we describe a new simplified efficient methodology for the separation and in vitro culturing of viable CTCs from peripheral blood by size-based filtration (MetaCell®). The isolation protocol yields preferentially cells bigger than 8 μm enabling further cytomorphological and molecular analysis.

Key words CTCs, Circulating tumor cells, Prostate cancer, Renal, Bladder cancer, Cultivation, In vitro, Gene expression

1 Introduction

CTCs may represent an opportunity to assess cancer spread directly and earlier than established/traditional methods, which classify tumor growth in general. A functional methodology to harvest separated tumor cells from blood provides researchers with a population of viable and proliferating cells to examine gene expression profiles or gene mutations in cancer [1–3].

The examination for CTCs could be useful as well as a complementary cancer screening test, especially for excluding cancer, and including patients with indications for repeated biopsies, e.g. in case of prostate cancer. Serial examination of CTCs enriched from peripheral blood after radical prostatectomy could help in prognosis determination, prospectively [4]. CTCs examination offers an alternative, minimally invasive approach to characterize cancer cell and to study early-stage disease [5, 6].

CTCs are frequently detected in cancer of urothelial origin (CUO) and are also found in patients with clinically localized CUO [6–8]. The analysis of the survival of patients with metastatic CUO suggested that CTCs might have prognostic significance in

Wolfgang A. Schulz et al. (eds.), *Urothelial Carcinoma: Methods and Protocols*, Methods in Molecular Biology, vol. 1655, DOI 10.1007/978-1-4939-7234-0_20, © Springer Science+Business Media LLC 2018

those with advanced disease. There are multiple approaches to detect CTCs. CTC counts in patients with metastatic CUO could, therefore, be useful for monitoring the response to cancer therapy.

The methodology described here targets viable CTCs captured on a membrane, enriched in a good fitness with a remarkable proliferation potential. Filtration flow of the peripheral blood through the separation membrane is driven by capillarity. The speed of the filtration process depends on the natural blood viscosity. These properties enable setting up in vitro cell cultures from the viable CTCs unaffected by any fixatives, antibodies, or lysing solutions.

In vitro culturing of CTCs is a prerequisite for proliferation tests assessing chemosensitivity of tumors [9]. The protocol described below allows successful culturing of CTCs by use of filtration device (MetaCell®), which enables direct transfer of CTCs captured on the separation membrane to culturing plates (*see* Fig. 1). In the future, CTCs in culture could be used for personalizing oncological treatment and diagnostics.

2 Materials

2.1 Peripheral Blood Collection

1. Monovette tubes (Sarstedt AG & Co., Numbrecht, Germany) containing 1.6 mg EDTA/mL blood as an anticoagulant. Alternatively, Vacuette tubes (Greiner Bio-One) coated with 1.2–2 mg EDTA/mL blood or any similar EDTA—treated tubes can be used.

2.2 Isolation of CTCs

1. Size-based separation device MetaCell® (MetaCell, Ostrava, Czech Republic) (*see* Fig. 2 Meta Cell® filtration tube).
2. Washing fluid: RPMI 1640 medium.

2.3 Incubation and Cultivation of CTCs

1. 6-well plates.
2. RPMI 1640 medium complete (assigned as R+); additives Fetal bovine serum, antibiotics, and Amphotericin B solution.
3. EL-buffer (79217, Qiagen).
4. TrypLE™ Select Enzyme (1X) (Thermofisher Scientific).
5. Cell culture CO_2 incubator.

2.4 CTCs Visualization

1. NucBlue® Live ReadyProbes® Reagent (R37605, Thermofisher Scientific).
2. CellTracker™ Green CMFDA Dye (C2925, Thermofisher Scientific).

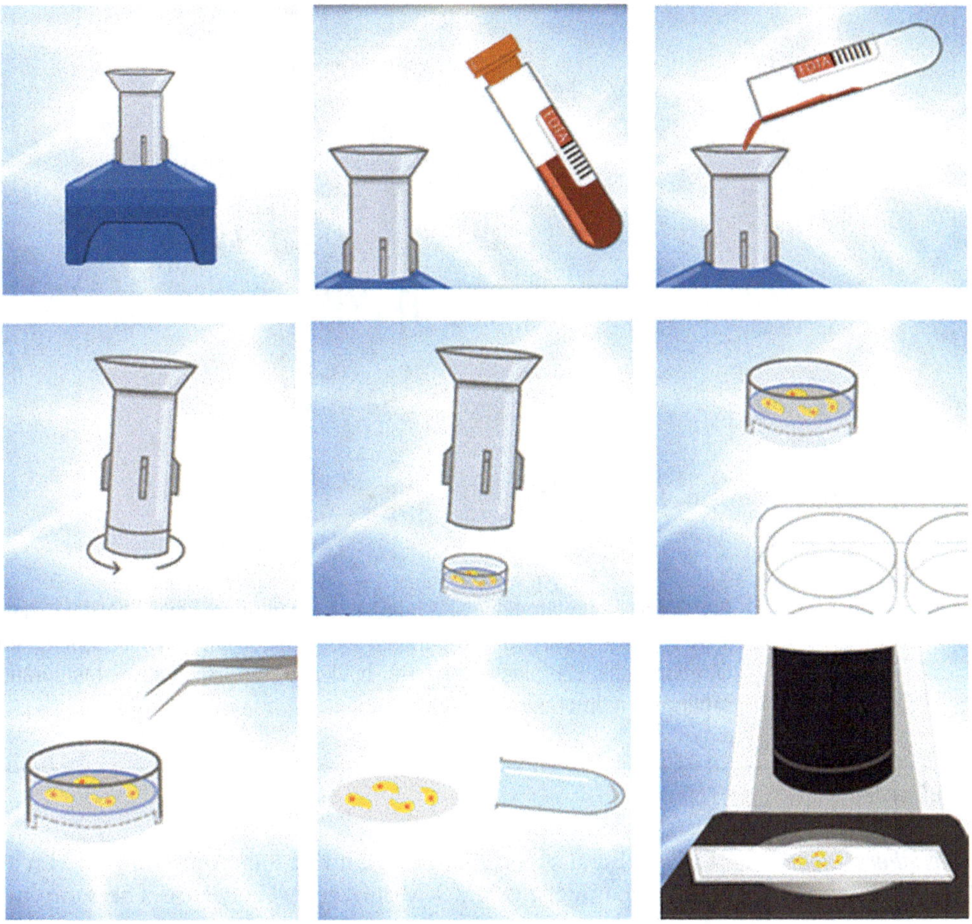

Fig. 1 Filtration procedure as presented by MetaCell is shown in short. Blood is transferred into the separation tube. The filtration starts as soon as the separation membrane touches the absorbent mass placed in the *blue* separation tube holder. After the filtration process the plastic ring with the separation membrane can be removed and placed directly into the culturing wells. After the short incubation period (min. 72 h) the membrane can be taken out of the plastic ring, the cells on the membrane are cytomorphologically evaluated and/or stored for later RNA/DNA analysis in Eppendorf tubes

2.5 Cytomorphological Analysis of CTCs

1. Fluorescence microscope or Inverted fluorescence microscope.

2.6 Isolation of RNA and DNA from CTCs

1. RLT buffer (Qiagen).
2. β-mercaptoethanol; add 100 μL per 10 mL RLT buffer.

2.7 Gene Expression Analysis and Mutational Analysis of CTCs

1. High-Capacity RNA-to-cDNA™ Kit (Thermofisher Scientific) 2. TaqMan® Fast Advanced Master Mix (Thermofisher Scientific)TaqMan® hydrolysis probes (Thermofisher Scientific).

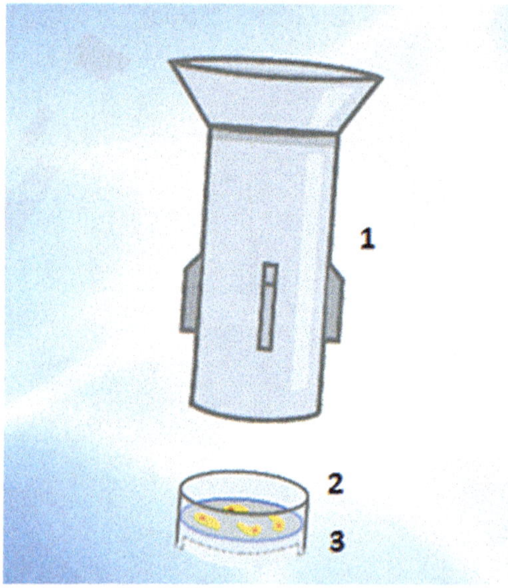

Fig. 2 Part of the filtration set (MetaCell®)—a filtration tube is shown in detail to identify specific parts of the filtration tube used in the protocol description. (1) filtration tube (2) plastic ring—a holder of the separation membrane (3) separation membrane

3 Methods

3.1 Peripheral Blood Collection

1. Peripheral blood is collected into tubes containing EDTA as an anticoagulant (e.g., S-Monovette/Vacuette). The samples are stored at a temperature of 4–8 °C. The isolation procedure should be completed within 24–48 h after the blood withdrawal.

3.2 CTC-Isolation

1. Size-based separation method for viable CTCs-enrichment from unclotted peripheral blood uses MetaCell® filtration tubes within filtration procedure (*see* Fig. 1).
2. MetaCell® tube (*see* Fig. 2) should be treated with UV–light for at least 15 min before use to prevent external contamination.
3. As a standard, 8 mL of blood is transferred into filtration tube. The minimum and maximum volume of the filtered peripheral blood may be adjusted with washing fluid up to 50 mL.
4. After completing the blood transfer, slightly push the plastic column (*see* Fig. 2–No. 1) to create a direct contact between the separation membrane and the absorbent.
5. Control the blood filtration flow, check if the whole blood volume has been filtered (*see* **Note 1**).
6. After blood filtration, the separation membrane (*see* Fig. 2–No. 3) placed in a plastic holder (*see* Fig. 2–No. 3) with captured

cells is washed with RPMI. Use 50% of the starting blood volume for RPMI washing.

7. Repeat the washing step at least twice (*see* **Note 2**).

3.3 CTCs Incubation and Cultivation

1. Remove the tube from the blue holder (*see* Fig. 2) (*see* **Note 3).**
2. Slightly turn and loosen the plastic ring (*see* Fig. 2–No.2) with the membrane (*see* Fig. 2–No. 3).
3. Place the plastic ring (*see* Fig. 2–No. 2–3) with the membrane into the 6-well plate.
4. Add growing medium to the well (*see* **Note 4**).
5. Place the 6-well plate into a CO_2 incubator under standard cell culture conditions (37 °C, 5% atmospheric CO_2) for a minimum of 72 h (incubation) or longer (cultivation) (*see* **Note 5**).
6. If an intermediate CTCs-analysis is intended/necessary, the CTC-fraction can be transferred from the separation membrane (*see* Fig. 2–No. 3) by splashing the plastic ring with the membrane (*see* Fig. 2–No. 2–3) with PBS (1.5 mL) to a cytospin slide (2 slides).

3.4 CTCs Visualization

1. The cells are analyzed by means of vital fluorescent microscopy using unspecific nuclear (NucBlue™) and cytoplasmatic (Celltracker™) stain. Basic cytomorphological parameters (*see* Fig. 3) are evaluated by an experienced cytologist/pathologist. As alternative standard hematological staining may be used (May-Grunwald) (*see* **Note 6**).

3.5 Cytomorphological Analysis

1. The cells captured on the separation membrane are fluorescently stained after the short incubation period (72 h minimum). After the short staining period (15 min) the membrane (*see* Fig. 2–No. 3) with adherent cells is taken out from the plastic ring holder (*see* Fig. 2–No. 2) and the membrane is placed on the microscopic slide.
2. The fluorescently stained cells on the membrane are examined using fluorescence microscopy in two steps: (1) screening at ×20 magnification to locate the cells; (2) observation at ×40/×60 magnification for detailed cytomorphological analysis. Isolated cells and/or clusters of cells of interest are selected, digitized, and the images are then examined by an experienced researcher and/or pathologist.
3. Basic cytomorphological parameters are evaluated by experienced cytologist/pathologist. CTCs are defined as cells with the following characteristics (Fig. 3): (1) with a nuclear size ≥10 μm); (2) irregular nuclear contour; (3) visible cytoplasm, cells size over 15 μm; (4) prominent nucleoli; numerous nucleoli (5) high nuclear-cytoplasmic ratio; (6) observed proliferation, (7) cells invading the membrane pores creating 2D or 3D cell groups.

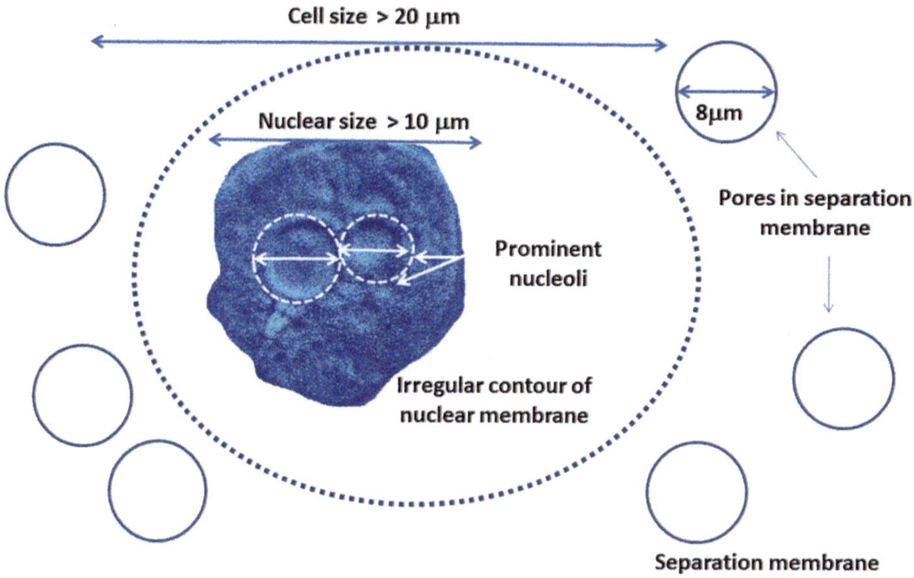

Fig. 3 Cytomorphological parameters of the cancer cells captured on the separation membrane are evaluated based on standard cytomorphological parameters. As the standard parameters were not set for the CTCs officially, we apply cytomorphological criteria reported by MetaCell. Based on these CTCs are defined as cells with the following characteristics: (1) with a nuclear size ≥10 μm); (2) irregular nuclear contour; (3) visible cytoplasm, cells size over 15 μm; (4) prominent nucleoli; numerous nucleoli; (5) high nuclear-cytoplasmic ratio; (6) observed proliferation, (7) cells invading the membrane pores creating 2D or 3D cell groups

CTCs separated, cultured, and visualized by fluorescence are shown on Fig. 4–9 (examples are shown for prostate carcinoma (*see* Figs. 4 and 5), bladder carcinoma (*see* Figs. 6 and 7), and renal carcinoma (*see* Figs. 8 and 9)). In all of the cases single CTCs observed are shown in comparison to the proliferating and growing CTC cultures.

3.6 Isolation of RNA and DNA

1. For RNA/DNA isolation, transfer captured cells (including the separation membrane) directly into the RLT buffer with β-mercaptoethanol (600 μL) and store at −20 °C. Standard protocols for RNA or DNA isolation can then be applied. As a rule up to 10–20 ng of RNA are isolated from one membrane.
2. RNA/DNA isolated from the CTC-fraction can be used for molecular analysis according to standard protocols (*see* **Note** 7).

4 Notes

1. In case of blood clotting, please add TrypLE solution, applying ratio Blood: TrypLE = 1:1, maximum volume of TrypLE is 5 mL.

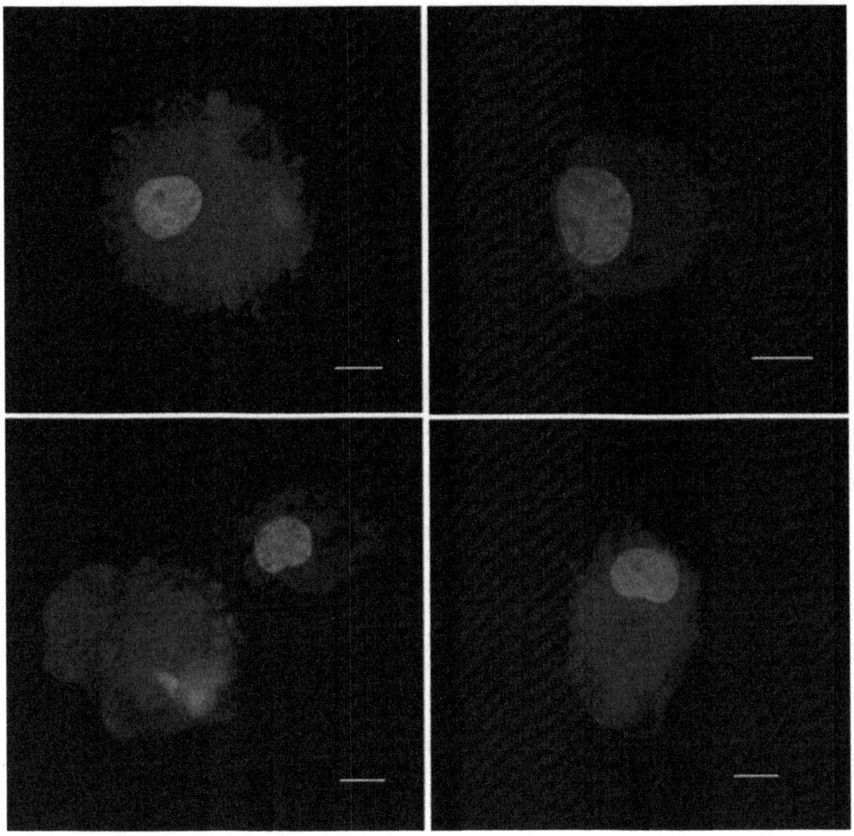

Fig. 4 Single circulating tumor cells isolated from peripheral blood of prostate cancer patient. Bar represents 10 μm

2. If some blood remains on the membrane after the filtration is completed, you may increase the washing solution volume and repeat the washing.
3. You may collect the filtered blood absorbed into the absorbent mass and preserve it for subsequent DNA isolation in dry place.
4. FBS-enriched RPMI medium (10%). Add 1 mL of the media to the bottom of the well first. Add 1 mL of the media to the membrane space over the plastic ring. Add 1 mL of the media to the bottom of the well again. Add 1 mL of the media into the membrane space in the plastic Alternatively, the enriched CTCs fraction can be transferred from the membrane and cultured directly on any plastic surface or a microscopic slide, or the separation membrane may be translocated on a microscopic slide.
5. CellTracker™ solution prepared according to the manufacturer's protocol (max 500 μL) is added to the cultivation well, additionally one drop of NucBlue™ is added directly to

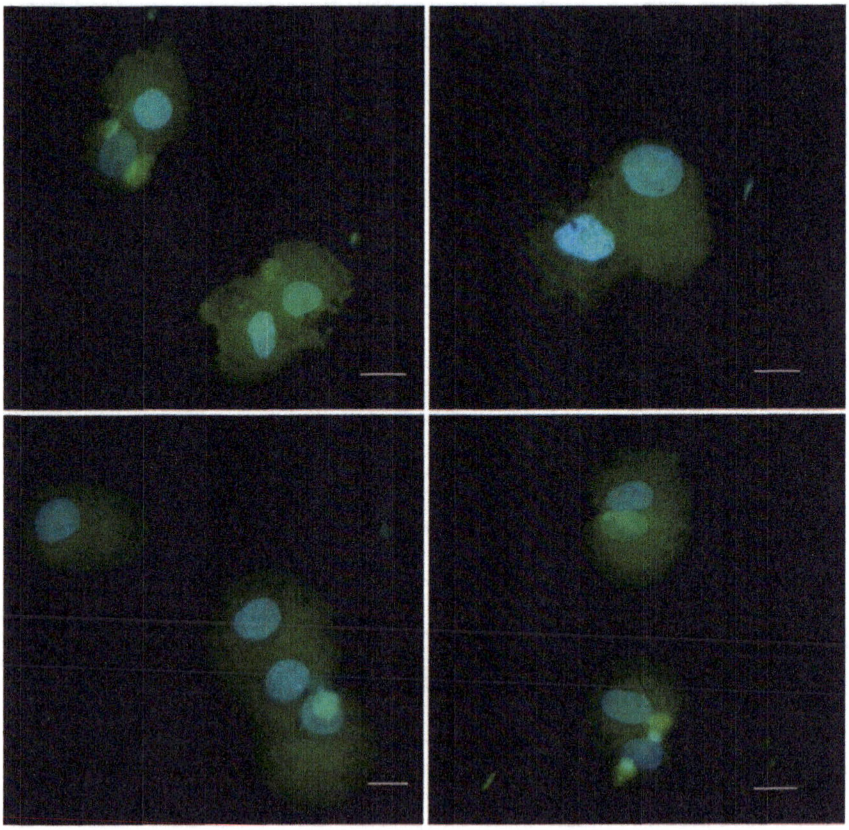

Fig. 5 Circulating tumor cells isolated from peripheral blood of prostate cancer patient are shown as proliferating in a culture. Bar represents 10 μm

the well with captured cells (plastic ring). Cells are stained for a minimun of 15 min.

6. Any commercial test using DNA isolated from the separated cell fraction
7. We usually perform qPCR using probes for highest sensitivity.

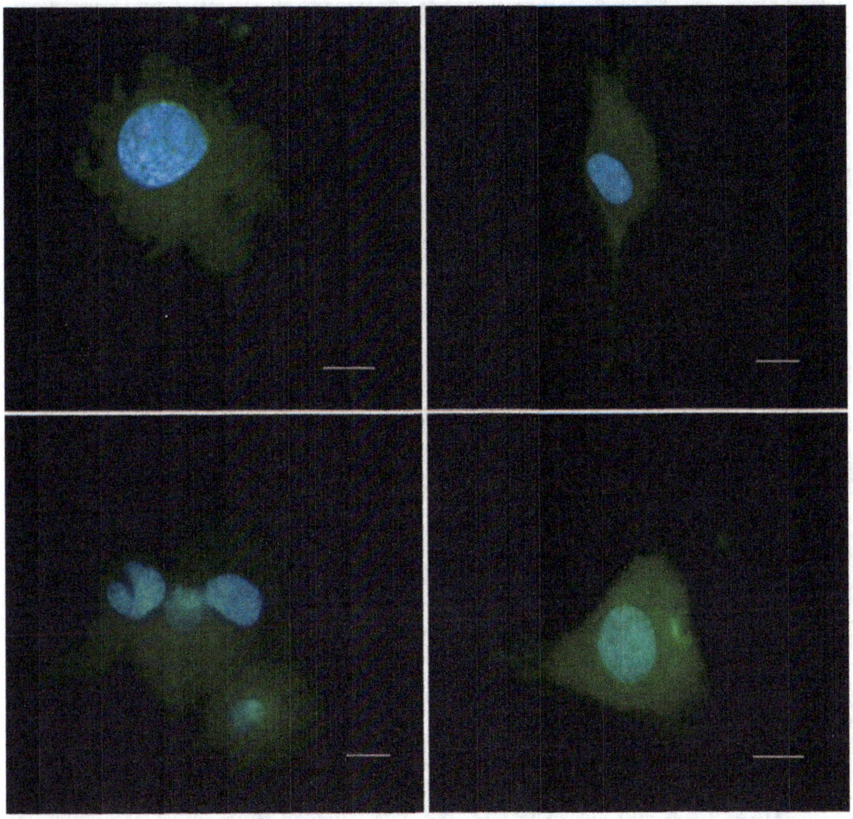

Fig. 6 Single circulating tumor cells isolated from peripheral blood of bladder cancer patient. Bar represents 10 μm

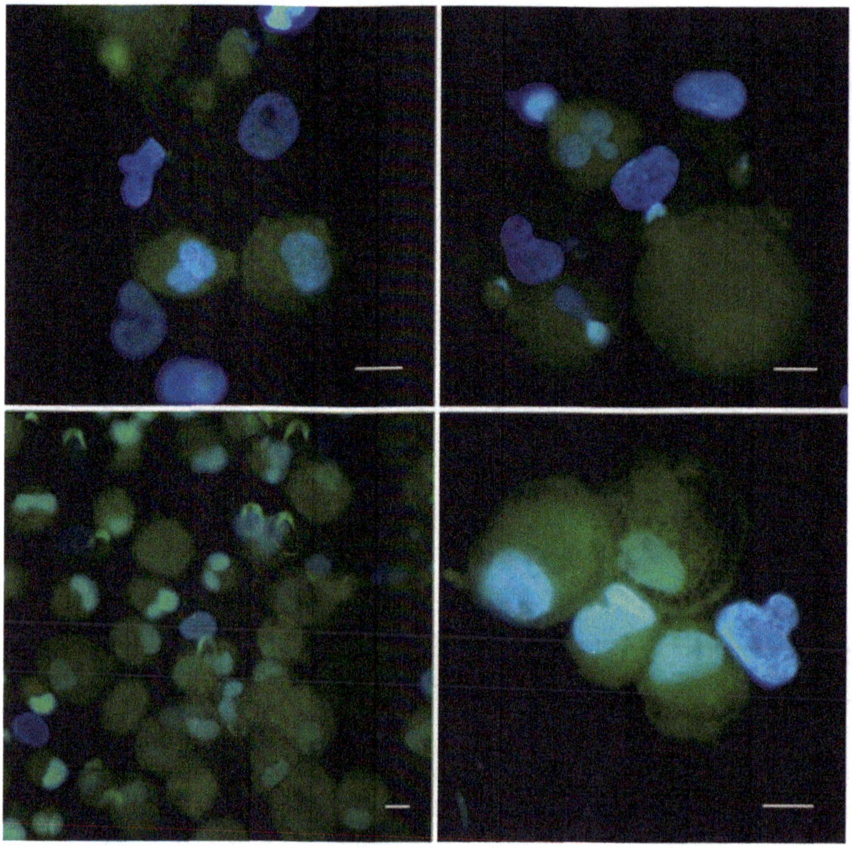

Fig. 7 Circulating tumor cells isolated from peripheral blood of bladder cancer patient are shown as proliferating in a culture. Bar represents 10 μm

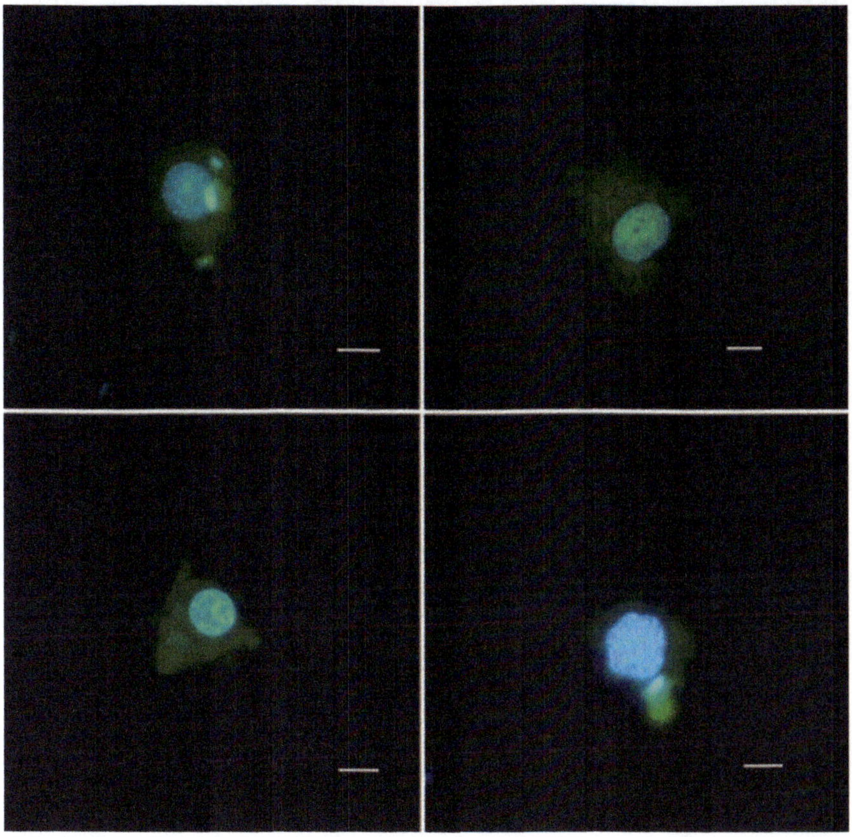

Fig. 8 Single circulating tumor cells isolated from peripheral blood of renal cancer patient. Renal carcinoma CTCs usually exhibit the biggest size (>20 μm) in the comparison with prostate and bladder cancer. Bar represents 10 μm

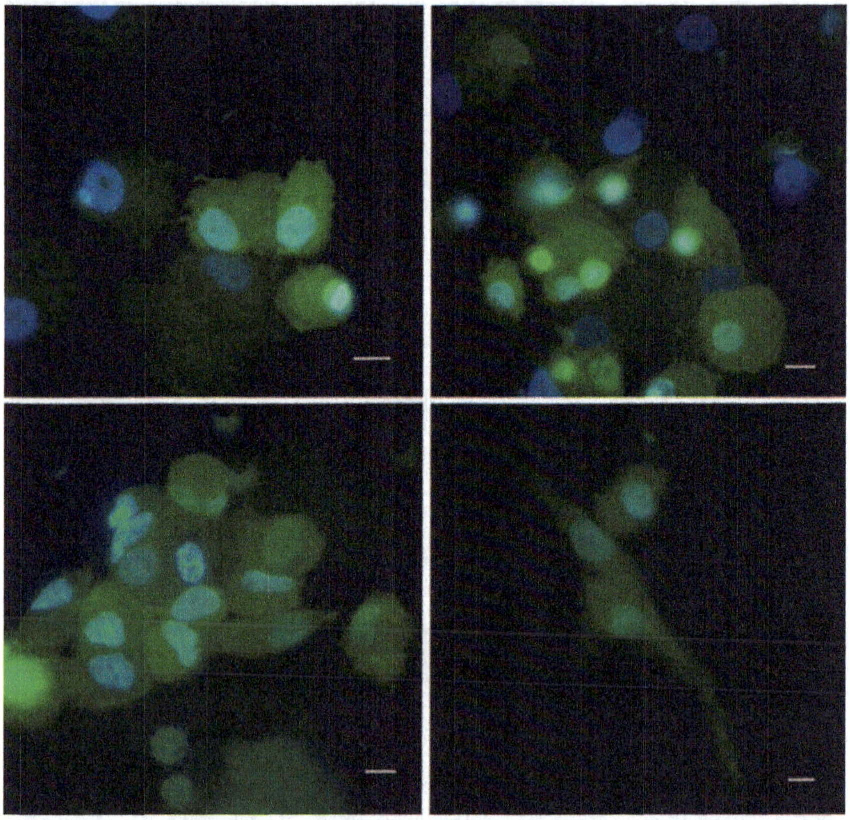

Fig. 9 Circulating tumor cells isolated from peripheral blood of renal cancer patients are shown as proliferating in a culture. The captured cells do exhibit both epithelial and mesenchymal (spindle cell like) morphology. Bar represents 10 μm

References

1. Liberko M, Kolostova K, Bobek V (2013) Essentials of circulating tumor cells for clinical research and practice. Crit Rev Hematol Oncol 88(2):338–356
2. Zheng Y, Zhang C, Wu J, Cheng G, Yang H, Hua L, Wang Z (2016) Prognostic value of circulating tumor cells in castration resistant prostate cancer: a meta-analysis. Urol J 13 (6):2881–2888
3. Gorin MA, Verdone JE, van der Toom E, Bivalacqua TJ, Allaf ME, Pienta KJ (2017) Circulating tumour cells as biomarkers of prostate, bladder, and kidney cancer. Nat Rev Urol 14 (2):90–97
4. Hu B, Rochefort H, Goldkorn A (2013) Circulating tumor cells in prostate cancer. Cancers (Basel) 5(4):1676–1690
5. Hegemann M, Stenzl A, Bedke J, Chi KN, Black PC, Todenhöfer T (2016) Liquid biopsy: ready to guide therapy in advanced prostate cancer? BJU Int 118:855–863
6. Kolostova K, Broul M, Schraml J, Cegan M, Matkowski R, Fiutowski M, Bobek V (2014) Circulating tumor cells in localized prostate cancer: isolation, cultivation in vitro and relationship to T-stage and Gleason score. Anticancer Res 34:3641–3646
7. Cegan M, Kolostova K, Matkowski R, Broul M, Schraml J, Fiutowski M, Bobek V (2014) In vitro culturing of viable circulating tumor cells of urinary bladder cancer. Int J Clin Exp Pathol 7(10):7164–7171
8. Kolostova K, Cegan M, Bobek V (2014) Circulating tumor cells in patients with urothelial tumors: enrichment and in vitro culture. Can Urol Assoc J 8(9–10):E715–E720
9. Bobek V, Hoffman RM, Kolostova K (2013) Site-specific cytomorphology of disseminated PC-3 prostate cancer cells visualized in vivo with fluorescent proteins. Diagn Cytopathol 41 (5):413–417

Part V

Therapy Development

Chapter 21

Epigenetic Treatment Options in Urothelial Carcinoma

Maria Pinkerneil, Michèle J. Hoffmann, and Günter Niegisch

Abstract

Mutations, dysregulation, and dysbalance of epigenetic regulators are especially frequent in urothelial carcinoma (UC) compared to other malignancies. Accordingly, targeting epigenetic regulators may provide a window of opportunity particularly in anticancer therapy of UC. In general, these epigenetic regulators comprise DNA methyltransferases and DNA demethylases (for DNA methylation), histone methyltransferases, and histone demethylases (for histone methylation) as well as acetyl transferases and histone deacetylases (for histone and non-histone acetylation).

As epigenetic regulators target a plethora of cellular functions and available inhibitors often inhibit enzymatic activity of more than one isoenzyme or may have further off-target effects, analysis of their functions in UC pathogenesis as well as of the antineoplastic capacity of according inhibitors should follow a multidimensional approach.

Here, we present our standard approach for the analysis of the cellular and molecular functions of individual HDAC enzymes, their suitability as treatment targets and for the evaluation of isoenzyme-specific HDAC inhibitors regarding their antineoplastic efficacy. This approach may also serve as prototype for the preclinical evaluation of other epigenetic treatment approaches.

Key words Urothelial carcinoma, Targeted therapy, Epigenetics, Histone deacetylases, Histone deacetylase inhibitors

1 Introduction

Only recently, a comprehensive genetic characterization of invasive UCs has been published by The Cancer Genome Atlas project. In this analysis, several presumably "drugable" genetic alterations were confirmed and a number of additional ones were newly identified [1]. Thus, in principle, UCs should be susceptible to targeted treatment approaches. However, clinical trials investigating the use of "targeted therapies" (e.g., Sunitinib, Sorafenib, Everolimus, Gefitinib, Trastuzumab) for treatment of UC have so far revealed only modest efficacy [2–6].

The failure of targeted approaches in UC can be attributed to a multitude of molecular "treatment escape mechanisms." For example, applying tyrosine kinase or mTOR inhibitors in UC triggers a

Wolfgang A. Schulz et al. (eds.), *Urothelial Carcinoma: Methods and Protocols*, Methods in Molecular Biology, vol. 1655, DOI 10.1007/978-1-4939-7234-0_21, © Springer Science+Business Media LLC 2018

variety of molecular mechanisms counteracting the antineoplastic effects of these inhibitors at various steps of the targeted signaling pathways [7, 8]. Therefore, focusing treatment directly on the genomic targets of signaling pathways might be more sensible. This assumption is underlined by recent findings of high-throughput sequencing analyses showing that mutations, dysregulation, and dysbalance of epigenetic regulators are especially frequent in UC compared to other malignancies [1, 9]. These epigenetic regulators generally target DNA methylation (DNA methyltransferases, DNA demethylases), histone methylation (histone methyltransferases, histone demethylases), and protein acetylation (histone acetyl transferases, histone deacetylases) [10].

In the last years, our group has focused particularly on investigating the function of histone deacetylases (HDACs), which maintain homeostasis of chromatin acetylation together with histone acetyltransferases, regarding their suitability as antineoplastic target in the treatment of UC [11–15]. An overview on current knowledge on HDACs and HDAC inhibitors (HDACi) in UC is given in [16].

"Classical" histone deacetylases are usually subdivided in four classes (class I, class IIA, class IIB, and class IV). In summary, class I HDACs (HDAC1, 2, 3, and 8) are essential for global acetylation patterns in the nucleus and epigenetic regulation of gene expression, thereby promoting cellular proliferation and inhibiting differentiation as well as apoptosis. Class IIA HDACs (HDAC4, 5, 7, and 9) act as transcriptional co-repressors at specific genes, assembling into multiprotein complexes with other transcriptional co-repressors [17, 18]. Furthermore, they can act as transcriptional co-activators, as SUMO-E3 ligases and as components of DNA repair complexes and in the regulation of the cell cycle [19]. HDAC6 and HDAC10 are the isoenzymes comprised in HDAC class IIB. HDAC6 is involved mostly in cytoplasmic processes, e.g., post-translational protein modifications. However, some studies point towards a direct epigenetic function of HDAC6 as well [20, 21]. In various cancers, critical involvement of HDAC6 in tumorigenesis, metastatic spread and invasion has been shown [22]. Little information is available about the function of HDAC10 except in neuroblastoma, where it activates autophagy rendering cells resistant to chemotherapy [23]. It is unknown whether this mechanism is relevant in other cancers. Not much is likewise known on the physiological functions of HDAC11, the sole member of HDAC class IV. It is best studied as a regulator of immune cell function [24]. Only recently, HDAC11 has been proposed as a target for antineoplastic treatment in several solid tumors [25].

Like other epigenetic regulators, these enzymes target a plethora of cellular functions. In addition, available HDACi often do not inhibit enzymatic activity of only one isoenzyme and may exhibit a variety of off-target effects on other nuclear and/or cytosolic enzymes [26]. Therefore, analysis of both the role of individual HDACs in pathogenesis of urothelial carcinoma and the antineoplastic capacity of HDACi should follow a multidimensional approach. On the following pages, we present a workflow of our standard approach for the analysis of the molecular functions of individual HDAC enzymes, their suitability as treatment targets and for evaluating isoenzyme-specific HDACi for their antineoplastic efficacy (*see* Fig. 1). Analogous approaches may be used in the preclinical evaluation of other epigenetic treatment approaches.

In order to obtain a comprehensive characterization of the effects of targeting HDACs in UC cells (UCCs), we generally select

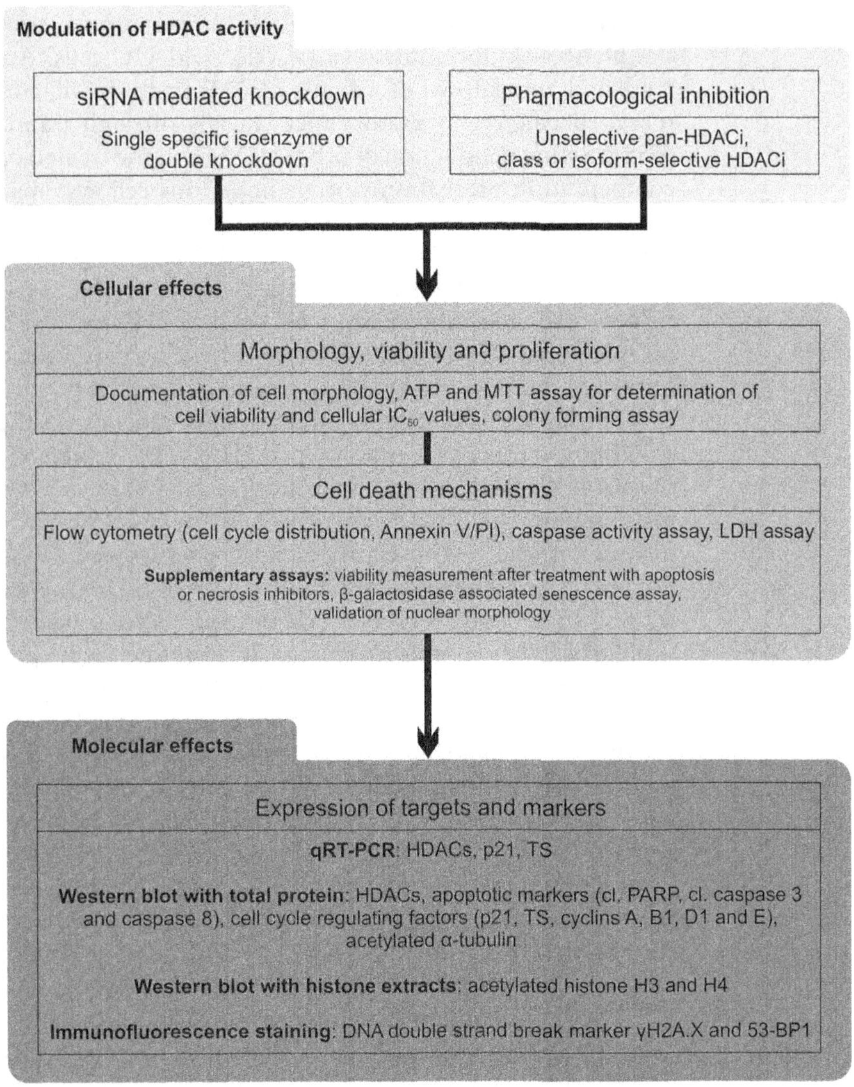

Fig. 1 Workflow of standard approach for the analysis of cellular and molecular functions of different HDACs after siRNA-mediated knockdown or pharmacological inhibition of single HDAC isoenzymes or in combination

a set of cell lines which represents a heterogeneous spectrum of UCs with different stages of differentiation and morphology and different HDAC expression patterns. HDAC expression patterns of different classes in UCCs and UC tissues are described in various publications [12–15, 27–31], and HDAC expression in UCCs and tissues is comprehensively reviewed elsewhere [16]. To assess the specificity of HDAC inhibition on UCCs, we perform selected experiments additionally in different nonmalignant urothelial and non-urothelial control cells.

We target HDAC activity (single specific isoenzymes or in combination) either by small interfering RNA (siRNA)-mediated knockdown or by pharmacological inhibition with various HDACi (*see* Fig. 1). In our experience, it is useful to initially perform an siRNA-based screen of individual HDACs or up to two isoforms simultaneously for antineoplastic effects in UC cells. An siRNA-mediated knockdown of a single HDAC isoform will additionally reveal specific compensatory mechanisms through transcriptional or translational induction of other HDACs in the treated cells. Such compensation mechanisms occur in various cell systems between isoenzymes within one class. The best-known example is the compensatory HDAC2 induction after HDAC1 targeting and vice versa [32–35], which is also highly active in UCCs following siRNA-mediated inhibition of HDAC1 or HDAC2 [12]. Based on this initial screen, HDACi with suitable inhibitory activity can be more efficiently chosen for subsequent investigation.

The choice of a suitable inhibitor also depends on the specific scientific question. One may use pan-HDACis to inhibit all isoforms of mammalian HDACs nonspecifically, e.g., SAHA or, alternatively, may employ isoform-selective HDACi to target selected specific members of the HDAC family, e.g., the class I-specific Romidepsin. For the in-cell evaluation of the selectivity of HDACi, specific substrates can be studied by Western blotting. For instance, we use α-tubulin acetylation as a convenient, albeit not perfectly specific indicator of class IIB HDAC6 inhibition [36–38], whereas global histone hyperacetylation ensues following efficient inhibition of class I enzymes. Development of truly isoform-selective HDACi is difficult due to the high homology within the HDAC classes, but progress has been made [39, 40]. To date, single isoform-selective HDACi are available for HDAC3, HDAC6 and HDAC8 [41, 42]. In addition to selectivity, HDACi can be classified by their chemical structure (hydroxamic acids, benzamides, short-chain fatty acid (carboxylic acids), cyclic peptides (thiols)) [40, 43] and by their inhibitory concentrations ranging from low nM to mM [41]. HDACi can be consigned to three groups according to their specific target selectivity: unselective pan-HDACi, class selective HDACi and isoform-selective HDACi (*see* Fig. 1 and Subheading 2.2.2). We use SAHA as a prototypic pan-HDACi control in almost all of our HDAC experiments [11–13, 15].

For detailed analysis of the cellular changes induced by siRNA-mediated or pharmacological inhibition of HDACs we determine several cellular parameters including morphology, viability, proliferation and induction of cell death by different methods (*see* Fig. 1). Cell cycle distribution of UCCs and control cells is measured by flow cytometry. The relative content of apoptotic and necrotic cells is determined by Annexin V/PI-staining. To further study cell death mechanisms in addition to flow cytometry, luminescence-based caspase activity for apoptosis and lactate dehydrogenase (LDH) assays for necrosis are performed. Apoptosis induction is confirmed by western blot detection of the apoptotic markers cleaved PARP (poly(ADP-ribose) polymerase) and cleaved Caspase 3. Controls for apoptotic and necrotic cell death are generated by treatment with Bortezomib and Actinomycin D, respectively. Depending on the results obtained with these measurements, additional experiments for the exact determination of cell death mechanisms may be conducted. These supplementary methods include viability measurements after additional treatment with apoptosis and necrosis inhibitors, β-galactosidase associated senescence assay and qualitative and quantitative evaluation of nuclear morphology (*see* Fig. 1). For example, detailed viability experiments with apoptosis/pan-Caspase (e.g., Q-VD-OPh) or necrosis (e.g., Necrox-2) inhibitors are indicated to confirm hints at apoptotic or necrotic mechanisms from the previous assays. Assays for senescence-associated β-galactosidase are advisable if an increased G1 fraction in cell cycle measurements or the morphology of cells suggest cellular senescence. Staining of microfilaments (by rhodamine-phalloidin) and nuclei (by DAPI) of treated and fixed cells for validation of nuclear morphology is used to follow up indications for cell cycle disruption and mitotic defects via a distinctly elevated G2/M cell cycle peak or an irregular cell cycle profile. To quantify changes of nuclear morphology, we define and count different nuclear phenotypes including mitosis, pro-apoptotic nuclei and micronuclei as a percentage of interphase nuclei.

Of note, after siRNA-mediated or pharmacological modulation of HDAC activity, we often perform different experiments simultaneously from a single treated well in order to more directly compare different cellular parameters. These combined experiments may thus include documentation of morphology, an ATP assay for determination of cell viability, a caspase activity assay, a measurement of cell cycle distribution and a colony forming assay.

Molecular parameters include expression of HDACs, relevant target genes, apoptotic markers and acetylation status of specific substrates using extracted mRNA and protein by qRT-PCR, western blotting of total protein and histone extracts or immunofluorescence staining (*see* Fig. 1). Assessed markers include, in addition

Table 1
QuantiTect primer assays (Qiagen) and self-designed primers (Eurofins) for qRT-PCR (T_A = annealing temperature)

Target		Primer	Size (bp)	T_A (°C)	Order number/sequence
10× QuantiTect assays and self-designed primers					
HDACs	HDAC1	Hs_HDAC1_1_SG	140	55	QT00015239, exons 3/4/5
	HDAC2	Hs_HDAC2_1_SG	127	55	QT00001890, exons 12/13
	HDAC3	Hs_HDAC3_1_SG	100	55	QT00093730, exons 2/3
	HDAC8	Hs_HDAC8_1_SG	91	55	QT00049630, exons 10/11
	HDAC4	Hs_HDAC4_1_SG	86	55	QT00005810, exons 12/13
	HDAC5	HDAC5_qPCR	108	56	Fwd. ATGTCAGGTCGGGAACCATC Rev. GGAACTGGGCATGGCTCTT
	HDAC7	Hs_HDAC7_1_SG	121	55	QT00031822, exons 15/16/17
	HDAC9	HDAC9_qPCR	133	56	Fwd. AAGTAGAGAGGCATCGCAGAGA Rev. TTCGTTGCTGATTTACTCAGT AGG
	HDAC6	Hs_HDAC6_1_SG	64	55	QT00002709, exons 22/23
	HDAC10	Hs_HDAC10_1_SG	161	55	QT00007252, Exons 15/16/17
	HDAC11	HDAC11_qPCR	189	59	Fwd. ACTCGCCGCGCTACAACA Rev. GCTCATTAAGATAGCGCCTCGTG
p21	p21_qPCR		146	55	Fwd. GGAAGACCATGTGGACCTGT Rev. GGCGTTTGGAGTGGTAGAAA
TS	TS_qPCR		102	57	Fwd. ATCACGGGCCTGAAGCCA Rev. GGGTTCTCGCTGAAGCTGAATT
TBP	TBP_qPCR		119	55	Fwd. ACAACAGCCTGCCACCTTA Rev. GAATAGGCTGTGGGTCAGT

to HDACs themselves, apoptotic markers (cleaved PARP1, cleaved Caspase 3 and Caspase 8), cell cycle regulating factors such as $p21^{CIP1}$, thymidylate synthase (TS), and informative cyclins (A, B1, D1, and E), acetylated substrates (ac. histone H3, ac. histone H4, and ac. α-tubulin), and markers of DNA double-strand breaks (γH2A.X and 53-BP1; *see* Tables 1 and 2). In this chapter we describe histone extraction [44] and immunofluorescence staining in detail. RNA isolation, cDNA synthesis, qRT-PCR, total protein extraction, and western blot analysis are performed by standard protocols that are not elaborated here. However, Tables 1 and 2 contain detailed lists of primers and antibodies used for these techniques. Of note, for HDACs with marginal expression in UCCs, suitable positive controls should be used in Western blot analyses. For example, human neuroblastoma cells overexpress HDAC8 [45] and can be used as positive controls for HDAC8 measurements.

Table 2
Antibodies for western blot analyses and immunofluorescence staining

Antigen		Antibody	Size (kDa)	Dilution	Order number, source
Antibodies for western blot analyses					
HDACs	HDAC1	HDAC1 C-19	69	1/1000	sc-6298, Santa Cruz Biotechnology
	HDAC2	HDAC2 H-54	59	1/5000	sc-7899, Santa Cruz Biotechnology
	HDAC3	HDAC3 H-99	49	1/1000	sc-11417, Santa Cruz Biotechnology
	HDAC8	HDAC8	42	1/400	A-4008, Epigentek
	HDAC4	HDAC4 A-4	140	1/500	sc-46672, Santa Cruz Biotechnology
	HDAC7	HDAC7 A-7	105	1/1000	sc-74563, Santa Cruz Biotechnology
	HDAC6	HDAC6 H-300	160	1/5000	sc-11420, Santa Cruz Biotechnology
	HDAC10	HDAC10 D-9	70	1/500	sc-365270 Santa Cruz Biotechnology
	HDAC11	HDAC11 EPR11342(B)	39	1/1000	ab166907, Abcam
p21		p21 Sx118	21	1/1000	556430, BD Biosciences
TS		TS106	36	1/400	MAB4130, Merck Millipore
Cyclins	Cyclin A	Cyclin A H-432	54	1/1000	sc-751, Santa Cruz Biotechnology
	Cyclin B1	Cyclin B1 H-433	60	1/1000	sc-752, Santa Cruz Biotechnology
	Cyclin D1	Cyclin D1 H-295	37	1/1000	sc-753, Santa Cruz Biotechnology
	Cyclin E	Cyclin E HE-12	53	1/500	sc-247, Santa Cruz Biotechnology
Cleaved PARP		Cl. PARP Asp214	89	1/1000	9541, Cell Signaling Technology
Cleaved Caspase3		Cl. Caspase 3 Asp175	17	1/1000	9664, Cell Signaling Technology
Caspase 8		Caspase-8 (1C12)	18, 41/43, 57	1/1000	9746, Cell Signaling Technology
Histones	Ac. His. H3	Histone H3ac pAB	17	1/2000	39139, Active Motif
	Ac. His. H4	Histone H4ac pAB	8	1/1000	39243, Active Motif
	Total His. H3	Histone H3 96C10	17	1/2000	3638, Cell Signaling Technology
	Total His. H4	Histone H4 pAB	8	1/1000	39269, Active Motif
Ac. α-Tubulin		Ac. Tubulin 6-11B-1	55	1/15000	T-7451, Sigma Aldrich

(continued)

Table 2
(continued)

Antigen	Antibody	Size (kDa)	Dilution	Order number, source
Antibodies for immunofluorescence staining				
γH2A.X	H2A.X Ser139	4 °C, overnight	1/100	2577, Cell Signaling Technology
53-BP1	53-BP1 BP18	4 °C, overnight	1/250	05–725, Merck Millipore

2 Materials

2.1 Urothelial Carcinoma Cell Lines, Control Cell Lines, Cell Culture Media and Materials

1. UCCs of various differentiation states and distinct HDAC expression: epithelial phenotype (RT-112, 5637, VM-CUB1, SW-1710) and mesenchymal phenotype (639-V, UM-UC-3 and T24).
2. Nonmalignant control cell lines (*see* **Note 1**): normal urothelial control cell lines HBLAK (spontaneously immortalized from primary culture of uroepithelial cells (CELLnTEC)) [46], (*see* **Note 2**) and TERT-NHUC (TERT-immortalized normal human urothelial cells), non-urothelial control cell lines HEK-293 (immortalized human embryonic kidney cells) and HFF (human foreskin fibroblasts), and primary cultures of NUC (normal urothelial control) cells [47, 48] isolated from ureters after nephrectomy (*see* **Note 3**).
3. UCCs, HEK-293, and HFF cell culture medium: DMEM (Dulbecco's modified eagle medium) GlutaMAX-I supplemented with 10% heat-inactivated FCS (fetal calf serum).
4. HBLAK cell culture medium: serum-free CnT-Prime Epithelial Culture Medium (CELLnTEC, *see* **Note 2**).
5. TERT-NHUC cell culture medium: keratinocyte serum-free medium (KSFM) supplemented with 0.125 ng/m EGF (epidermal growth factor), 30 μg/mL BPE (bovine pituitary extract), 1% ITS (insulin-transferrin-selenium), 0.35 μg/mL (−)N-epinephrine and 0.33 mg/mL hydrocortisone (*see* **Note 4**).
6. NUC cell culture medium: calcium-free KSFM supplemented with 5 ng/mL EGF, 50 μg/mL BPE and 100 μg/mL penicillin/streptomycin (pen/strep, [47, 48], *see* **Note 4**).
7. PBS (phosphate buffered saline) buffer for washing cells before detachment (*see* **Note 5**).
8. Trypsin-EDTA (ethylenediaminetetraacetate) cell detachment solution for UCCs, HEK-293, HFF, TERT-NHUC, and NUC cells.

9. Trypsin inhibitor for TERT-NHUC and NUC cells: Dissolve trypsin inhibitor in PBS buffer as a 1 mg/mL solution and store at −20 °C.
10. Accutase cell detachment solution for HBLAK cells.
11. Versene/EDTA solution (0.02% EDTA) for NUC cells.
12. Collagen IV solution: 50 μg/mL collagen IV dissolved in 0.1% acetic acid (*see* **Note 1**).
13. Pen/strep stock: Dissolve pen/strep as a stock of 10 mg/mL and store at −20 °C.
14. Cell culture vessels: flasks (T25, T75), dishes (6 cm) and plates (96 and 6 well).
15. Sterile cover slips for seeding of cells for immunofluorescence staining.

2.2 Modulation of HDAC Activity

2.2.1 SiRNA Transfection

1. siRNAs: HDAC-specific siRNAs and nonspecific or scrambled siRNA controls (e.g., Silencer Select validated siRNA and Silencer Select negative control, Ambion, Life Technologies) dissolved in medium or ultrapure water at recommended concentration, e.g., 20 μM.
2. Transfection reagent suitable for siRNAs, e.g., Lipofectamine RNAi MAX (Life Technologies).
3. Reduced serum medium, e.g., Opti-MEM suitable for cationic lipid transfections.

2.2.2 Inhibitor Treatment

1. Unselective pan-HDACi, e.g., SAHA (suberoylanilide hydroxamic acid, Vorinostat).
2. Class-selective HDACi, e.g., class I selective HDACi Romidepsin (FK228, Depsipeptide), Givinostat (ITF2357), Entinostat (MS-275), Mocetinostat (MGCD0103), 4SC-202.
3. Isoform-selective HDACi, e.g., targeting HDAC3 (RGFP966 and BG45) or HDAC6 (tubacin, tubastatin A, and ST-80).
4. Inhibitor DMSO (dimethyl sulfoxide) stock: Dissolve HDACi in DMSO as stocks of 10 or 50 mM, aliquot and store at −20 °C (*see* **Note 6**).

2.3 Assessing Effects of HDAC Targeting in UCCs and Control Cells

2.3.1 Documentation of Cell Morphology

1. Microscope and software for documentation of cell morphology.

2.3.2 ATP Assay for Determination of Cell Viability Following siRNA-Transfection and HDACi Treatment (6-Well Format)

1. Reagent to measure number of viable cells on basis of ATP determination e.g., CellTiter-Glo® Luminescent Cell Viability Assay (Promega): after equilibration to room temperature dissolve 1 vial of lyophilized CellTiter-Glo® substrate in appropriate amount of CellTiter-Glo® buffer and store protected from light at −20 °C (*see* **Note 7**).
2. PBS buffer for washing cells before detachment.
3. Specific cell detachment solution (*see* Subheading 2.1).
4. Cell culture medium for specific cell type (*see* Subheading 2.1).
5. Collecting tubes.
6. 96-well microplates (*see* **Note 8**).
7. Stepper pipette and pipette tips.
8. Orbital plate shaker.
9. Luminescence microplate reader (0.25–1 s integration time per well (*see* **Note 7**)).

2.3.3 MTT Assay for Determination of Cellular IC_{50} Values of HDACi

1. MTT reagent 3-(4,5-dimethylthiazol-2-yl)-2,5-diphenyltetrazolium bromide: dissolve MTT in PBS buffer as a stock of 5 mg/mL and store at −20 °C.
2. DMSO for denaturation of cells.
3. Stepper pipette and pipette tips.
4. Incubator: 37 °C, 5% CO_2.
5. UV/Vis microplate reader (570 nm against reference wavelength of 620 nm).
6. Software for approximation of IC_{50} values and dose response curves by nonlinear regression analysis.

2.3.4 Colony Forming Assay

1. Cell culture medium for specific cell type with 100 μg/mL pen/strep (*see* Subheading 2.1).
2. 6 cm dishes (UCCs and HEK-293) or 6-well plates (urothelial control cells) (*see* **Note 9**).
3. PBS buffer for washing cells before detachment and for Giemsa staining.
4. Specific cell detachment solution (*see* Subheading 2.1).
5. Collecting tubes.
6. 50 μg/mL collagen IV dissolved in 0.1% acetic acid for coating of control cell culture plates (*see* **Note 10**).
7. 50% methanol in PBS buffer.
8. 100% methanol.
9. Giemsa staining solution.

10. Tap water.
11. Plastic tray for washing Giemsa plates.
12. Scanner for documentation (*see* **Note 11**).

2.3.5 Flow Cytometry

The following listed materials are those that are required for both applications, analysis of cell cycle and apoptosis.

1. Propidium iodide (PI) stock: dissolve PI in PBS as a stock of 2 mg/mL and store in the dark at 4 °C (*see* **Note 12**).
2. PBS buffer for washing cells before detachment and cell pellet.
3. Specific cell detachment solution (*see* Subheading 2.1).
4. Cell culture medium for specific cell type (*see* Subheading 2.1).
5. Flow cytometer tubes.
6. Rack for flow cytometer tubes.
7. Aluminum foil for wrapping tubes with stained cells.
8. Flow cytometer and software.
9. Vortex mixer.
10. Centrifuge with tube inserts up to 15 mL.

    Additionally required for cell cycle analysis.

11. Nicoletti buffer: 0.1% sodium citrate ($Na_3C_6H_5O_7$), 0.1% Triton X-100, 50 μg/mL PI (*see* **Note 13**) [49].

    Additionally required for Annexin staining.

12. Annexin V FITC (fluorescein isothiocyanate) conjugate, e.g., (FITC)-conjugated recombinant chicken Annexin V (Immunotools)
13. Annexin V binding buffer: 10 mM HEPES (4-(2-hydroxyethyl)-1-piperazineethanesulfonic acid; $C_8H_{18}N_2O_4S$) pH 7.4, 150 mM sodium chloride (NaCl), 5 mM potassium chloride (KCl), 5 mM magnesium chloride ($MgCl_2$), 1.6 mM calcium chloride ($CaCl_2$).

2.3.6 Caspase Activity Assay

1. Reagent to measure caspase activity on basis of a specific luminogenic Caspase substrate generating luminescence signal after Caspase cleavage, e.g., Caspase-Glo® 3/7 assay (Promega), which assesses Caspase 3 and 7 activity with the specific tetrapeptide sequence DEVD (Asp/Glu/Val/Asp) substrate: after equilibration to room temperature dissolve lyophilized Caspase-Glo® 3/7 substrate in the appropriate amount of Caspase-Glo® 3/7 buffer and store protected from light at −20 °C (*see* **Note 14**).
2. PBS buffer for washing cells before detachment.
3. Specific cell detachment solution (*see* Subheading 2.1).

4. Cell culture medium for specific cell type (*see* Subheading 2.1).
5. Collecting tube.
6. 96-well microplates (*see* **Note 8**).
7. Stepper pipette and pipette tips.
8. Orbital plate shaker.
9. Luminescence microplate reader.

2.3.7 LDH Assay

1. 10 mL BSA (bovine serum albumin) solution: dissolve BSA in PBS buffer as a 1% stock.
2. Colorimetric kit to measure LDH release from damaged cells as a marker for cellular cytotoxicity and necrosis induction, e.g., Pierce™ LDH Cytotoxicity Assay Kit (Thermo Fisher Scientific) containing substrate mix, assay buffer, 10× lysis buffer, stop solution, and LDH positive control: dissolve 1 vial of lyophilized substrate mix in 11.4 mL ultrapure water and add 0.6 mL assay buffer. Store this reaction mix protected from light at −20 °C. Mix 1 μL LDH positive control with 10 mL 1% BSA solution (*see* **Note 15**).
3. Cell culture medium with a minimum serum amount previously ascertained for each cell line, e.g., DMEM GlutaMAX-I supplemented with 1–5% heat-inactivated FCS for UCCs (*see* **Note 16**).
4. Bortezomib (apoptosis control): dissolve Bortezomib in DMSO as a stock of 10 mM and store at −20 °C.
5. Actinomycin D (necrosis control): dissolve Actinomycin D in DMSO as a stock of 2 mg/mL and store at −20 °C.
6. Incubator: 37 °C, 5% CO_2.
7. 96-well microplates.
8. Stepper pipette and pipette tips.
9. UV/Vis microplate reader (490 nm against reference wavelength of 680 nm).

2.3.8 Histone Extraction and Determination of Concentration by BCA Protein Assay

We perform histone extraction according to a published Nature protocol by Shechter et al. 2007 based on sulfuric acid extraction and trichloroacetic acid (TCA)-precipitation [44].

1. PBS buffer for washing cells before detachment and cell pellet.
2. Specific cell detachment solution (*see* Subheading 2.1).
3. Cell culture medium for specific cell type (*see* Subheading 2.1).
4. Collection tubes up to 15 mL.
5. Centrifuge with tube inserts up to 15 mL.
6. Vortex mixer.
7. 1.5 mL microliter tubes.

8. Cooling centrifuge for microliter tubes up to 1.5 mL.
9. 100× protease inhibitor cocktail.
10. 100× phosphatase inhibitor cocktail.
11. Hypotonic lysis buffer (ice-cold, *see* **Note 17**): 10 mM TRIS Cl pH 8.0, 1 mM KCl, 1.5 mM $MgCl_2$, 1 mM dithiothreitol (DTT), 1 mM phenylmethanesulfonylfluoride (PMSF), 1× protease inhibitor cocktail (1/100), 1× phosphatase inhibitor cocktail (1/100).
12. 0.2 M sulfuric acid (H_2SO_4).
13. 100% TCA (4 °C): 2.2 g TCA plus 1 mL ultrapure water.
14. 100% acetone (ice-cold).
15. Ultrapure water for dilution of histone pellet, BSA standard, and as a blank (*see* **Note 18**).
16. Rotating shaker for incubation at 4 °C.
17. Bicinchoninic acid (BCA) protein assay for determination of protein concentration e.g., Pierce BCA Protein Assay Kit (Thermo Fisher Scientific) containing BCA reagent A (sodium carbonate (Na_2CO_3), sodium bicarbonate ($NaHCO_3$), BCA, sodium tartrate ($C_4H_4O_6Na_2$) in 0.1 M sodium hydroxide (NaOH)), BCA reagent B (4% cupric sulfate), and 2 mg/mL BSA standard ampules (*see* **Note 19**). All components of the kit can be stored at room temperature.
18. Staining solution: mix 50 volumes of BCA reagent A with 1 volume of BCA reagent B in required quantity (200 μL per probe: BSA standards (7×), samples, and blanks (2×) in 2 replicates). Staining solution can be stored at room temperature for some days.
19. BSA standard dilution set: 2000, 1000, 500, 250, 125, 62.5, and 31.25 μg/mL final BSA concentrations (*see* **Note 18**).
20. 96-well microplates.
21. Orbital plate shaker.
22. Incubator: 37 °C.
23. Stepper pipette and pipette tips.
24. UV/Vis microplate reader (562 nm).

2.3.9 Immunofluorescence Staining

1. Microscope slides and cover slips.
2. Ultraviolet (UV) crosslinker instrument for generation of DNA double-strand breaks as positive control.
3. PBS buffer for washing cells.
4. Fixation solution: 4% formaldehyde in PBS buffer.
5. PBST washing buffer: 0.3% BSA, 0.1% Triton X-100 in PBS buffer.

6. Permeabilization solution: 0.3% Triton X-100 in PBS buffer.
7. Blocking solution: 10% goat serum, 0.3 M glycine, 0.1% Triton X-100 in PBS buffer.
8. Primary antibodies pH2A.X and 53-BP1 (*see* Table 2).
9. Secondary antibodies e.g., Alexa Fluor 488 Goat Anti-Rabbit IgG and TRITC-Goat Anti-Mouse IgG (H + L) Conjugate (Life Technologies).
10. Antibody dilution buffer: 1% BSA, 0.1% Triton X-100 in PBS buffer.
11. Elastic plastic paraffin film.
12. Big glass container and towels.
13. Aluminum foil for covering slips.
14. DAPI (4′,6-diamidino-2-phenylindole) stock: Dissolve DAPI in PBS buffer as a stock of 0.5 mg/mL and store protected from light at −20 °C.
15. 70% ethanol.
16. Fluorescence mounting medium.
17. Orbital plate shaker.
18. Microscope and software for documentation of fluorescence signals.

3 Methods

3.1 Cell Culture and Seeding for Experiments

1. Cell seeding in 96-well plates for determination of HDACi cellular IC_{50} values by MTT assay (*see* Subheading 3.3.3): Seed UCCs and control cells (*see* **Note 1**) 24 h before treatment in quadruplicates per treatment option (72 h). Include medium control, DMSO solvent control and defined concentration ranges of HDACi (*see* **Note 20**). Prepare four medium-containing wells without cells for a blank. Depending on the cell line plate 1000–5000 cells per well in 100 μL cell culture medium.
2. Cell seeding in 96-well plates for LDH assay (*see* Subheading 3.3.7): Seed UCCs and control cells (*see* **Note 1**) 24 h before treatment in quadruplicates per treatment option (24 and 48 h, medium control, DMSO solvent control, up to two defined concentrations of specific HDACi, pan HDACi SAHA control, Bortezomib (apoptosis), and Actinomycin D (necrosis) control). Further prepare wells in quadruplicates for kit internal controls consisting of medium without serum and medium with minimum serum amount (both without cells) and for spontaneous LDH activity control and maximum LDH activity control (both with cells). Before preparing and running the

first HDACi-mediated cytotoxicity assay determine the suitable minimum serum amount in medium (*see* **Note 16**) and optimal cell number for each specific cell line for the LDH assay.

3. Cell seeding in 6-well plates for siRNA transfection (*see* Subheading 3.2.1) and inhibitor treatment (*see* Subheading 3.2.2): Seed UCCs and control cells (*see* **Note 1**) 24 h before treatment in duplicates per treatment option (siRNA transfection: 72 h, medium control, transfection control, nonspecific or scrambled siRNA control, and HDAC-specific siRNA; inhibitor treatment: 24 and 48 h, medium control, DMSO solvent control, up to two defined concentrations of specific HDACi, and pan HDACi SAHA control). Depending on the cell line plate 100,000–250,000 cells per well in 2 mL cell culture medium. For immunofluorescence staining (*see* Subheading 3.3.9) following inhibitor treatment place sterile cover slips in 6-well plates before seeding cells. Additionally, for inhibitor treatment options prepare extra wells for generation of DNA double-strand break positive controls and wells with untreated cells for primary antibody negative control (*see* **Note 21**).
4. Cell seeding in T25 or T75 flasks for histone extraction (*see* Subheading 3.3.8): Depending on the cell line seed UCCs and control cells (*see* **Note 1**) in T25 or T75 flasks 24 h before treatment. Prepare one flask for each treatment option and time point (24–120 h, medium control, DMSO solvent control, up to two defined concentrations of specific HDACi and pan HDACi SAHA control).

3.2 Modulation of HDAC Activity

For siRNA transfection and inhibitor treatment cells should be 50–80% confluent.

3.2.1 SiRNA Transfection

1. Add 2 mL fresh medium without antibiotics to the cells.
2. Transfection solution A: Prepare 249 μL reduced serum medium plus 1 μL siRNA stock [20 μM] per transfection reaction and mix thoroughly. For transfection control use reduced serum medium without siRNA.
3. Transfection solution B: Prepare 245 μL reduced serum medium plus 5 μL transfection reagent per transfection and mix thoroughly.
4. Add transfection solution A to transfection solution B at a 1:1 ratio, mix gently and incubate for 15 min at room temperature.
5. Add 500 μL of the transfection solution drop by drop to each well (6-well plate). End concentration is 10 nM siRNA (in 2.5 mL total medium volume).
6. Culture cells for 72 h, as a rule, before using them for further experiments.

3.2.2 Inhibitor Treatment

In steps 2–4 the concentration of the specific HDACi should correspond to the approximate IC_{50} values of the inhibitors.

1. Treatment in 96-well plates for MTT assay for determination of cellular IC_{50} values of HDACi (*see* Subheading 3.3.3): Treat cells with defined concentration ranges of the HDACi in quadruplicates for 72 h with a treatment volume of 100 μL medium per well. For control and normalization treat cells with medium and DMSO solvent control (max. 0.1%) and use medium wells only as a blank. Perform at least three independent experiments (*see* **Note 20**).
2. Treatment in 96-well plates for LDH assay (*see* Subheading 3.3.7): Treat cells with up to two defined concentrations of specific HDACi, 2.5 μM SAHA, DMSO solvent control (max. 0.1%), and medium in quadruplicates for 24 and 48 h with a treatment volume of 100 μL medium per well (*see* **Note 16**). As additional control for apoptotic and necrotic cell death treat cells with 30 nM Bortezomib (apoptosis) and 4 μg/mL Actinomycin D (necrosis) and add 10 μL of ultrapure water to the spontaneous LDH activity control. Do not treat the remaining wells with the kit internal controls since they are required only when performing the assay.
3. Treatment in 6-well plates for documentation of morphology (*see* Subheading 3.3.1), determination of viability via ATP assay (*see* Subheading 3.3.2), colony forming assay (*see* Subheading 3.3.4), flow cytometry (*see* Subheading 3.3.5), caspase activity assay (*see* Subheading 3.3.6) and immunofluorescence staining (*see* Subheading 3.3.9): Treat cells with up to two defined concentrations of specific HDACi, 2.5 μM pan-HDACi SAHA, DMSO solvent control (max. 0.1%) and medium in duplicates for 24 and 48 h with a treatment volume of 2 mL per well.
4. Treatment in T25 or T75 flasks for histone extraction (*see* Subheading 3.3.8): Treat cells with up to two defined concentrations of specific HDACi, 2.5 μM pan HDACi SAHA, DMSO solvent control (max. 0.1%) and medium for 24 and 48 h or additionally for 72, 96 and 120 h in a total volume of 5 (T25) or 12 (T75) mL per flask. For an additional histone acetylation positive control cells treated with 3 nM Romidepsin for 48 h may be used.

3.3 Assessing Effects of HDAC Targeting in UCCs and Control Cells

3.3.1 Documentation of Cell Morphology

1. Document shape and appearance of untreated and siRNA-transfected or inhibitor-treated cells with a microscope at different magnifications and time points, e.g., 24, 48, or 72 h after modulation of HDAC activity (*see* **Note 22**).

3.3.2 ATP Assay for Determination of Cell Viability Following siRNA-Transfection and HDACi Treatment (6-Well Format)

1. Wash cells with PBS buffer and detach cells with 300 μL specific detachment solution (*see* Subheading 2.1).
2. Resuspend detached cells in 1 mL cell culture medium and collect cell suspension in collecting tubes.
3. Transfer 50 μL of each cell suspension in quadruplicates to a new 96-well microplate. Additionally, prepare 50 μL of medium in quadruplicates as a blank for background luminescence (*see* **Note 23**).
4. Add 50 μL of CellTiter-Glo® Luminescent Cell Viability Assay to each well (ratio 1/1) and mix for 2 min with an orbital plate shaker (*see* **Note 24**).
5. Incubate plate for 10 min at room temperature.
6. Measure luminescence of each well with a microplate reader (0.25–1 s integration time per well). Calculate final luminescence values by subtracting the average medium blank value of each luminescence value. For normalization set untreated controls as 100% and plot relative viability of each control and treated sample.

3.3.3 MTT Assay for Determination of Cellular IC_{50} Values of HDACi

1. Add 10 μL 5 mg/mL MTT stock solution to each well (cells and medium blank) and mix gently.
2. Incubate 96-well plate for 1 h at 37 °C (*see* **Note 25**).
3. Completely discard cell medium and MTT reagent mixture.
4. For denaturation of cells add 50 μL DMSO per well and mix gently to dissolve crystallized structures.
5. Measure absorbance of each well at 570 nm and 620 nm (reference wavelength) with a microplate reader. Subtract values of reference wavelength from 570 nm values and calculate final absorbance values by subtracting the average medium blank value of each absorbance value.
6. Plot inhibitor concentration (x axis) against average absorbance values (y axis). For normalization set DMSO solvent control as 100%.
7. Approximate cellular IC_{50} values by nonlinear regression analyses (*see* **Note 20**).

3.3.4 Colony Forming Assay

1. Prepare 6 cm dishes (UCCs and HEK-293) or 6-well plates (urothelial control cells) with 5 or 2 mL cell culture medium for specific cell type containing 100 μg/mL pen/strep in duplicates per treatment option (*see* Subheading 2.1 and **Notes 1** and **10**).
2. Wash cells with PBS buffer and detach cells with 300 μL specific detachment solution (*see* Subheading 2.1).

3. Resuspend detached cells in 1 mL medium and collect cell suspension in collecting tubes.
4. Transfer 10 μL each of well resuspended cells (500–1500 cells) into 6 cm dishes or 6-well plates and mix thoroughly to spread cells evenly.
5. Culture cells for 7–21 days and observe colony formation. The incubation time depends strongly on the cell line and can be significantly longer especially for urothelial control cells.
6. When clearly visible colonies have formed, stain with Giemsa staining solution: Wash dishes or plates with PBS and subsequently with 50% methanol in PBS, fix colonies with 100% methanol for 10 min at room temperature and stain colonies with Giemsa staining solution for 2–5 min at room temperature.
7. Remove Giemsa staining solution and remove background staining of Giemsa plates by washing the plates for 30 min in tap water.
8. Document colony formation by scanning the plates (*see* **Note 11**).

3.3.5 Flow Cytometry

Cell Cycle Distribution

1. Remove cell culture medium and wash cells with PBS buffer. Collect both in flow cytometer tubes to include death and detached cells from the supernatant.
2. Detach cells with 300 μL specific detachment solution (*see* Subheading 2.1).
3. Resuspend detached cells in 1 mL cell culture medium and add cell suspension to the flow cytometer tubes (*see* **Note 26**).
4. Pellet cells by centrifugation step at 200 × *g* for 5 min at room temperature. Discard supernatant, wash cell pellet with 1 mL PBS buffer, and repeat centrifugation step.
5. Add 300–500 μL Nicoletti buffer to the cells, resuspend cells by vortexing, cover them with aluminum foil and incubate for 30 min at room temperature.
6. Store stained cells on ice and vortex cells again immediately before measuring cell cycle distribution with a flow cytometer.

Annexin V/PI Staining

1. Remove cell culture medium and wash cells with PBS. Collect both medium and wash buffer in flow cytometer tubes to include dead and detached cells from the supernatant.
2. Detach cells with 300 μL specific detachment solution (*see* Subheading 2.1).
3. Resuspend detached cells in 1 mL cell culture medium and add cell suspension to the flow cytometer tubes.

4. Pellet cells by a centrifugation step at 200 × *g* for 5 min at room temperature. Discard supernatant, wash cells with 1 mL Annexin V binding buffer and repeat centrifugation step.
5. Resuspend cells well in 70 μL Annexin V binding buffer by vortexing thoroughly.
6. Add 5 μL Annexin V FITC conjugate and 7.5 μL PI stock to the cells, mix thoroughly, cover them with aluminum foil and incubate for 15 min at room temperature.
7. Add 500 μL Annexin V binding buffer to the cells and vortex cells immediately before determining the amount of apoptotic and necrotic cells with a flow cytometer.

3.3.6 Caspase Activity Assay

1. Wash cells with PBS and detach cells with 300 μL specific detachment solution (*see* Subheading 2.1).
2. Resuspend detached cells in 1 mL cell culture medium and collect cell suspension in collecting tubes.
3. Transfer 50 μL of each cell suspension in quadruplicates into a new 96-well microplate. Additionally, prepare 50 μL of medium in quadruplicates as a blank for background luminescence measurement (*see* **Note 23**).
4. Add 50 μL of Caspase-Glo® 3/7 assay to each well (ratio 1/1) and mix for 30 s with an orbital plate shaker (*see* **Note 24**).
5. Incubate plate for 1 h at room temperature.
6. Measure luminescence of each well with a microplate reader. Calculate final luminescence values by subtracting the average medium blank value of each luminescence value. For normalization, set untreated controls as 100% and plot relative caspase activity of each control and treated sample in a bar graph (*see* **Note 27**).

3.3.7 LDH Assay

The LDH assay is performed as described in the manufacturer's protocol (*see* **Note 15**).

1. Fill 10 μL of 10× lysis buffer into the kit internal maximum LDH activity control wells, mix gently, and incubate the cells for further 45 min at 37 °C in the cell incubator (5% CO_2).
2. Pipette 50 μL medium of each sample into a new 96-well microplate including medium of kit internal controls, medium of untreated and HDACi-treated cells, and medium of cells treated with Bortezomib and Actinomycin D as apoptosis and necrosis control, respectively (*see* **Note 28**).
3. Additionally add 50 μL of LDH positive control in quadruplicates into the new 96-well microplate.

4. Add 50 μL of prepared reaction mix to each sample, mix gently, and incubate the plate in the dark for 30 min on room temperature.
5. Stop the reaction by adding 50 μL of stop solution to each reaction well and mix gently.
6. Measure absorbance of each well at 490 nm and 680 nm (reference wavelength) with a microplate reader. Subtract values of reference wavelength from 490 nm values to calculate corrected absorbance values (cABS).
7. For calculation of the relative LDH release of damaged cells use the formula below (taken from the kit instructions) and plot relative LDH release of each control and treated sample (for reference *see* **Note 15**):

$$\text{Relative LDH release} = \frac{\text{cABS sample LDH activity} - \text{cABS spontaneous LDH activity control}}{\text{cABS maximum LDH activity control} - \text{cABS spontaneous LDH activity control}} \times 100$$

3.3.8 Histone Extraction and Determination of Concentration by BCA Protein Assay

The procedure is adapted from Shechter et al. 2007 [44].

1. Wash cells with PBS buffer, detach cells with specific detachment solution, and resuspend the cells in medium (*see* Subheading 2.1, **Note 29**).
2. Add cells to collection tubes and pellet cells by a centrifugation step at 200 × *g* (rcf) for 5 min at room temperature. Discard supernatant, wash cell pellet with PBS buffer, and repeat centrifugation step.
3. Discard supernatant (*see* **Note 30**) and resuspend cell pellet in 1 mL ice-cold hypotonic lysis buffer. Transfer cell solution into 1.5 mL microliter tubes.
4. Rotate cell solution with a rotating shaker for 1 h at 4 °C.
5. Pellet intact nuclei at 10,000 g (rcf) for 10 min at 4 °C and discard supernatant completely.
6. Resuspend nuclei in 400 μL 0.2 M H_2SO_4 very well and vortex if necessary.
7. Rotate nuclei solution with a rotating shaker overnight at 4 °C.
8. To remove nuclear waste pellet samples at 16,000 g (rcf) for 10 min at 4 °C and transfer the supernatant into new 1.5 mL microliter tubes.
9. Precipitate histones by adding 132 μL of 100% TCA drop by drop and repeatedly inverting the solution. Incubate milky solution for 4 h on ice.

10. Pellet histones at 16,000 g (rcf) for 10 min at 4 °C.
11. Carefully discard supernatant and wash with ice-cold 100% acetone without destroying the histone pellet.
12. Pellet histones at 16,000 g (rcf) for 5 min at 4 °C.
13. Repeat **steps 11** and **12** twice more (*see* **Note 31**).
14. Carefully remove supernatant completely and dry histone pellet for 20 min at room temperature.
15. Dissolve histone pellet in 100 μL ultrapure water and transfer lysates to new 1.5 mL microliter tubes (*see* **Note 32**).
16. Prepare BSA standard dilution set in ultrapure water with 2000, 1000, 500, 250, 125, 62.5, and 31.25 μg/mL final BSA concentrations (*see* **Note 18**), by successive dilution steps.
17. Pipette 10 μL of BSA standard dilution set (2×), extracts (2×), and blank (4×) (*see* **Notes 18** and **33**) into a 96-well microplate.
18. Add 200 μL of staining solution to each well using a stepper pipette, mix 2 min on an orbital plate shaker, and incubate for 30 min at 37 °C.
19. Measure absorbance of each well at 562 nm with a microplate reader, subtract the average blank value of each absorbance value, and calculate histone concentration (*see* **Note 34**).

3.3.9 Immunofluorescence Staining

1. Prepare DNA double-strand break positive control: Incubate 6-well plates without their lid with cells grown on cover slips in a UV crosslinker instrument (100 mJ/cm^2) and then incubate the plates for 1 h in a cell incubator.
2. Preparation of positive controls and HDACi-treated and untreated cells grown on cover slips: Remove media from 6-well plates and wash cells with PBS buffer. Incubate cells with fixation solution for 10 min and wash twice for 5 min with PBST washing buffer (*see* **Note 35**). Afterwards, permeabilize cells with permeabilization solution for 10 min and wash with PBST washing buffer twice for 10 min. Perform all steps at room temperature and during washing steps use an orbital plate shaker.
3. Before antibody staining block cells with blocking solution for 1 h.
4. Double staining with primary antibodies: Prepare 50 μL of primary antibody solution per coverslip by adding 1/100 pH2A.X and 1/250 53-BP1 antibody to antibody dilution buffer (*see* **Note 21**). Fix a plastic paraffin film large enough for all cover slips in a big glass container. Cover the edge of the glass container with wet towels to prevent cover slips from drying out during primary antibody incubation. Pipette

50 μL of primary antibody solution per cover slip onto the film and maintain a certain minimum distance between the drops. Take out the cover slips from blocking solution, carefully remove excess solution and place the cover slips cells downward on the primary antibody solution. Cover the glass container with aluminum foil and incubate cells at 4 °C overnight. After incubation, return the cover slips to the 6-well plates with cells upwards and wash cells four times for 10 min with PBST washing buffer.

5. Double staining with secondary antibodies: Prepare 50 μL of secondary antibody solution per coverslip by adding 1/500 Alexa Fluor 488 Goat Anti-Rabbit IgG and 1/250 TRITC-Goat Anti-Mouse IgG (H + L) Conjugate to antibody dilution buffer. Pipette 50 μL of secondary antibody solution per cover slip onto a plastic paraffin film and place the cover slips with cells down on the secondary antibody solution after carefully removing the excess solution. Cover the paraffin film with a nontransparent box to protect the cover slips from light and incubate at room temperature for 1 h. After incubation return the cover slips into the 6-well plates with cells up and wash three times for 10 min with PBST washing buffer.
6. Counterstain nuclei with 1/4000 DAPI in PBS buffer for 3 min at room temperature and wash two times for 10 min with PBST washing buffer.
7. Add a drop of mounting medium to microscope slides (*see* **Note 36**) and place the cover slips cells downwards onto the drop. Avoid air bubbles and carefully remove the excess solution of cover slips before mounting. Store microscope slides at 4 °C.
8. Document the signals using a fluorescence microscope (*see* **Note 37**).

4 Notes

1. For most listed nonmalignant control cells, coating with collagen IV is required. For this purpose cell culture flasks or plates are coated with 50 μg/mL collagen IV dissolved in 0.1% acetic acid for 30 min at room temperature or overnight at 4 °C and washed twice with PBS buffer before seeding of cells.
2. HBLAK cells and medium required for cultivation can be purchased from CELLnTEC. Other media for cultivation of the epithelial HBLAK cells are not established in our laboratory. We have recently published a comprehensive characterization of HBLAK cells as a urothelial cell culture model [46].

3. We perform isolation of NUCs from ureters after nephrectomy via a protocol based on Southgate et al. 1994 as modified by Swiatkowski et al. 2003 [47, 48].
4. Supplemented KSFM can only be used for 2 weeks. For this reason, medium should be supplemented only in needed amounts and long storage should be avoided.
5. For cell culture we basically use sterile premixed PBS buffer without $CaCl_2$ and $MgCl_2$ and low endotoxin. For all other applications where sterility is optional we use premixed PBS buffer powder dissolved in ultrapure water.
6. Control wells were treated with DMSO only to a maximum of 0.1%. Most HDACis are soluble in DMSO and can be used and stored as a 10 mM DMSO stock. Due to higher cellular IC_{50} values for some inhibitors it is necessary to use a 50 mM DMSO stock in order not to exceed the maximum concentration of DMSO during cell treatment with IC_{50} concentrations.
7. For more detailed information and reference specific for the CellTiter-Glo® Luminescent Cell Viability Assay see the technical bulletin from Promega (www.promega.com/protocols).
8. For luminescence-based applications special 96-well microplates with black well walls and a transparent bottom are optimal to avoid interference by signals of neighboring wells.
9. The sizes of cell culture vessels need to be adjusted for specific cell lines because control cells often have to be used at a higher density for optimal colony growth.
10. For optimal colony formation of nonmalignant control cells collagen IV coating is required (*see* **Note 1**). Especially for colony forming assay with HEK-293 cells a coating is particularly important because the grown colonies detach very easily from cell culture vessels during Giemsa staining. For this reason, we recommend subtle handling during the entire dyeing process.
11. Colony forming assays can be quantitatively and statistically evaluated for number and size of grown colonies manually or automatically using special programs and plugins e.g., ImageJ (https://imagej.nih.gov/ij/).
12. PI is a toxic intercalating molecule that should be handled very carefully.
13. Nicoletti buffer without PI can be stored at 4 °C for a long time. PI should be added always freshly before each experiment.
14. For more detailed information's and reference specific for the Caspase-Glo® 3/7 assay see the technical bulletin (www.promega.com/protocols). The Caspase-Glo® 3/7 reagent is very

sensitive to contaminations with caspases or luciferin. For this reason, any contaminations with other solutions e.g., through reusing pipette tips should be avoided.

15. Substrate mix, assay buffer, and reaction mix should be stored protected from light at −20 °C. 10× lysis buffer, stop solution and LDH positive control should be stored at 4 °C. For more detailed information and reference specific for Pierce™ LDH Cytotoxicity Assay Kit see the user guide (www.thermofisher.com).
16. Serum in cell culture medium can induce strong background signals during measurement of LDH activity. The supplier recommends using a reduced serum amount during the treatment of cells for the LDH assay. It should be tested before, which minimal serum amount can be used without affecting cell viability.
17. The following components should be added just directly before using the hypotonic lysis buffer: DTT, PMSF and protease and phosphatase inhibitor cocktail.
18. For histone extracts ultrapure water should be used for blank (BCA assay) or as diluent for BSA standard set and extracts for BCA assay and SDS-PAGE.
19. For more detailed information and reference specific for Pierce BCA Protein Assay Kit see the supplier's instructions (www.thermofisher.com).
20. For HDACi whose cellular activity is determined for the first time we recommend to refer to IC_{50} values already published for other cell lines to choose an appropriate concentration range. At least eight different inhibitor concentrations within the relevant range and four replicates per concentration with an appropriate standard deviation should be available to perform a reliable regression analyses and IC_{50} determination.
21. In addition to staining of a DNA double-strand break positive control we further use a negative control without primary antibody to check for secondary antibody nonspecific binding and false positive signals.
22. Morphological characteristics frequently observed after pharmacological modulation of HDAC activity in UCCs and control cells are apoptotic features (blebbing, detachment, granularity, and vacuolation), senescence-like features (increase in cell and nuclear size, granulation, and flattening) and cell elongation with fibroblastoid morphology.
23. When using a normal 96-well microplate (*see* **Note 8**) leave at least one well empty between the different sample quadruplicates.

24. Basically, this assay can also be performed in 96-well formats by seeding and treating cells with HDACi directly into 96-well plates. This eliminates steps like detachment and distribution of cells, so that the substrate only has to be added to the cells at a 1:1 ratio.
25. For some cell lines, a shorter or longer incubation period might be necessary. To check, observe the formation of crystals with a microscope.
26. Cells from this experiment can also easily be used for documentation of morphology, combined measurement of cell viability, caspase activity and colony forming capability (*see* Subheading 3.3). If cells are additionally to be used for these experiments the treatment medium and PBS buffer should be collected separately from the cell suspension and later combined for centrifugation in flow cytometer tubes since only the cell suspension is used for these additional assays. For determination of cell cycle distribution at least 20,000 cells are measured in duplicates.
27. For relative determination of caspase activity, we normalize total caspase activity to total viability of cells assessed by ATP assay (*see* Subheading 3.3.2) using aliquots of the same cell suspension.
28. As an additional control, viability of cells should be measured simultaneously by ATP assay (*see* Subheading 3.3.2) or MTT assay (*see* Subheading 3.3.3) using the same 96 cell culture plate after transfer of 50 μL sample medium to the 96-well microplate.
29. 5×10^6 cells should be used per treatment condition and preparation.
30. Cell pellets can be stored until further processing at −80 °C.
31. These three washing steps are very important because acetone removes TCA from the protein pellet.
32. To resolve the extracted histones that are normally precipitated at the tube wall, pipette ultrapure water up and down along the tube wall and remove insoluble components by centrifugation. The volume of ultrapure water should be adapted to the number of used cells, e.g., 100 μL for 5×10^6 cells. Histone extracts in ultrapure water should be stored at −80 °C.
33. Use 10 μL of a 1/5 or 1/10 extract dilution to ensure that absorbance values of the samples are in the range of the BSA standard dilution set. For values that are not within the standard range measurement should be adjusted and repeated.
34. In order to calculate the histone concentrations first prepare a calibration curve from the BSA standard values. Multiply the calculated concentrations by the dilution factor 5× or 10× if

diluted extracts were used for the assay. Additionally to BCA assay efficacy of histone extraction can be easily checked by SDS-PAGE and Coomassie gel staining. In our hands, PVDF membranes appear to be more convenient for transfer of histones following SDS-PAGE than nitrocellulose membranes. For optimal transfer of histones the methanol concentration of the transfer buffer should be 20%.

35. After cell fixation, cover slips can be stored for several weeks in PBS buffer at 4 °C.
36. Before mounting, slides should be thoroughly cleaned with ethanol and labeled.
37. Number of signals of pH2A.X and 53-BP1 foci can be evaluated for statistical analysis with special programs e.g., ImageJ (https://imagej.nih.gov/ij/).

Acknowledgements and Conflicts of Interest

The HDAC project including the PhD position for M.P. was supported by grants from the Deutsche Forschungsgemeinschaft (NI 1398/1-1), the Forschungskommission of the Medical Faculty of the Heinrich-Heine-University (42/2015) and the Brigitte-und-Dr.-Konstanze-Wegener-Stiftung (project number 11) to G. N.. Further, G. N. reports receiving a commercial research grant (provision of experimental compound 4SC-202, publication costs) from 4SC.

References

1. TCGA (2014) Comprehensive molecular characterization of urothelial bladder carcinoma. Nature 507:315–322. doi:10.1038/nature12965
2. Niegisch G, Retz M, Thalgott M, Balabanov S, Honecker F, Ohlmann CH, Stockle M, Bogemann M, Vom Dorp F, Gschwend J, Hartmann A, Ohmann C, Albers P (2015) Second-line treatment of advanced urothelial cancer with paclitaxel and everolimus in a German phase II trial (AUO trial AB 35/09). Oncology 89:70–78. doi:10.1159/000376551
3. Krege S, Rexer H, vom Dorp F, de Geeter P, Klotz T, Retz M, Heidenreich A, Kuhn M, Kamradt J, Feyerabend S, Wulfing C, Zastrow S, Albers P, Hakenberg O, Roigas J, Fenner M, Heinzer H, Schrader M (2014) Prospective randomized double-blind multicentre phase II study comparing gemcitabine and cisplatin plus sorafenib chemotherapy with gemcitabine and cisplatin plus placebo in locally advanced and/or metastasized urothelial cancer: SUSE (AUO-AB 31/05). BJU Int 113(3):429–436. doi:10.1111/bju.12437
4. Gallagher DJ, Milowsky MI, Gerst SR, Ishill N, Riches J, Regazzi A, Boyle MG, Trout A, Flaherty AM, Bajorin DF (2010) Phase II study of sunitinib in patients with metastatic urothelial cancer. J Clin Oncol 28(8):1373–1379. doi:10.1200/JCO.2009.25.3922
5. Oudard S, Culine S, Vano Y, Goldwasser F, Theodore C, Nguyen T, Voog E, Banu E, Vieillefond A, Priou F, Deplanque G, Gravis G, Ravaud A, Vannetzel JM, Machiels JP, Muracciole X, Pichon MF, Bay JO, Elaidi R, Teghom C, Radvanyi F, Beuzeboc P (2015) Multicentre randomised phase II trial of gemcitabine+platinum, with or without trastuzumab, in advanced or metastatic urothelial carcinoma overexpressing Her2. Eur J Cancer 51(1):45–54. doi:10.1016/j.ejca.2014.10.009

6. Miller K, Morant R, Stenzl A, Zuna I, Wirth M (2016) A phase II study of the central European society of anticancer-drug research (CESAR) group: results of an open-label study of gemcitabine plus cisplatin with or without concomitant or sequential gefitinib in patients with advanced or metastatic transitional cell carcinoma of the urothelium. Urol Int 96(1):5–13. doi:10.1159/000381589
7. Knievel J, Schulz WA, Greife A, Hader C, Lubke T, Schmitz I, Albers P, Niegisch G (2014) Multiple mechanisms mediate resistance to sorafenib in urothelial cancer. Int J Mol Sci 15(11):20500–20517. doi:10.3390/ijms151120500
8. Nawroth R, Stellwagen F, Schulz WA, Stoehr R, Hartmann A, Krause BJ, Gschwend JE, Retz M (2011) S6K1 and 4E-BP1 are independent regulated and control cellular growth in bladder cancer. PLoS One 6(11):e27509. doi:10.1371/journal.pone.0027509
9. Guo G, Sun X, Chen C, Wu S, Huang P, Li Z, Dean M, Huang Y, Jia W, Zhou Q, Tang A, Yang Z, Li X, Song P, Zhao X, Ye R, Zhang S, Lin Z, Qi M, Wan S, Xie L, Fan F, Nickerson ML, Zou X, Hu X, Xing L, Lv Z, Mei H, Gao S, Liang C, Gao Z, Lu J, Yu Y, Liu C, Li L, Fang X, Jiang Z, Yang J, Li C, Chen J, Zhang F, Lai Y, Zhou F, Chen H, Chan HC, Tsang S, Theodorescu D, Li Y, Zhang X, Wang J, Yang H, Gui Y, Cai Z (2013) Whole-genome and whole-exome sequencing of bladder cancer identifies frequent alterations in genes involved in sister chromatid cohesion and segregation. Nat Genet 45(12):1459–1463. doi:10.1038/ng.2798
10. Schulz WA, Koutsogiannouli EA, Niegisch G, Hoffmann MJ (2015) Epigenetics of urothelial carcinoma. Methods Mol Biol 1238:183–215. doi:10.1007/978-1-4939-1804-1_10
11. Pinkerneil M, Hoffmann MJ, Kohlhof H, Schulz WA, Niegisch G (2016) Evaluation of the therapeutic potential of the novel isotype specific HDAC inhibitor 4SC-202 in urothelial carcinoma cell lines. Target Oncol 11 (6):783–798. doi:10.1007/s11523-016-0444-7
12. Pinkerneil M, Hoffmann MJ, Deenen R, Kohrer K, Arent T, Schulz WA, Niegisch G (2016) Inhibition of class I histone deacetylases 1 and 2 promotes urothelial carcinoma cell death by various mechanisms. Mol Cancer Ther 15(2):299–312. doi:10.1158/1535-7163.MCT-15-0618
13. Niegisch G, Knievel J, Koch A, Hader C, Fischer U, Albers P, Schulz WA (2013) Changes in histone deacetylase (HDAC) expression patterns and activity of HDAC inhibitors in urothelial cancers. Urol Oncol 31(8):1770–1779. doi:10.1016/j.urolonc.2012.06.015
14. Lehmann M, Hoffmann MJ, Koch A, Ulrich SM, Schulz WA, Niegisch G (2014) Histone deacetylase 8 is deregulated in urothelial cancer but not a target for efficient treatment. J Exp Clin Cancer Res 33:59. doi:10.1186/s13046-014-0059-8
15. Rosik L, Niegisch G, Fischer U, Jung M, Schulz WA, Hoffmann MJ (2014) Limited efficacy of specific HDAC6 inhibition in urothelial cancer cells. Cancer Biol Ther 15(6):742–757. doi:10.4161/cbt.28469
16. Pinkerneil M, Hoffmann MJ, Schulz WA, Niegisch G (2017) HDACs and HDAC inhibitors in urothelial carcinoma - perspectives for an antineoplastic treatment. Curr Med Chem:2017. Epub ahead of print
17. Fischle W, Dequiedt F, Hendzel MJ, Guenther MG, Lazar MA, Voelter W, Verdin E (2002) Enzymatic activity associated with class II HDACs is dependent on a multiprotein complex containing HDAC3 and SMRT/N-CoR. Mol Cell 9(1):45–57. doi:10.1016/S1097-2765(01)00429-4
18. Lahm A, Paolini C, Pallaoro M, Nardi MC, Jones P, Neddermann P, Sambucini S, Bottomley MJ, Lo Surdo P, Carfi A, Koch U, De Francesco R, Steinkuhler C, Gallinari P (2007) Unraveling the hidden catalytic activity of vertebrate class IIa histone deacetylases. Proc Natl Acad Sci U S A 104 (44):17335–17340. doi:10.1073/pnas.0706487104
19. Martin M, Kettmann R, Dequiedt F (2007) Class IIa histone deacetylases: regulating the regulators. Oncogene 26(37):5450–5467. doi:10.1038/sj.onc.1210613
20. Valenzuela-Fernandez A, Cabrero JR, Serrador JM, Sanchez-Madrid F (2008) HDAC6: a key regulator of cytoskeleton, cell migration and cell-cell interactions. Trends Cell Biol 18 (6):291–297. doi:10.1016/j.tcb.2008.04.003
21. Wang Z, Zang C, Cui K, Schones DE, Barski A, Peng W, Zhao K (2009) Genome-wide mapping of HATs and HDACs reveals distinct functions in active and inactive genes. Cell 138 (5):1019–1031. doi:10.1016/j.cell.2009.06.049
22. Yang PH, Zhang L, Zhang YJ, Zhang J, Xu WF (2013) HDAC6: physiological function and its selective inhibitors for cancer treatment. Drug Discov Ther 7(6):233–242. doi:10.5582/ddt.2013.v7.6.233
23. Oehme I, Linke JP, Bock BC, Milde T, Lodrini M, Hartenstein B, Wiegand I, Eckert C, Roth

W, Kool M, Kaden S, Grone HJ, Schulte JH, Lindner S, Hamacher-Brady A, Brady NR, Deubzer HE, Witt O (2013) Histone deacetylase 10 promotes autophagy-mediated cell survival. Proc Natl Acad Sci U S A 110(28): E2592–E2601. doi:10.1073/pnas.1300113110

24. Chen J, Sahakian E, Powers J, Lienlaf M, Perez-Villarroel P, Knox T, Villagra A (2016) Functional analysis of histone deacetylase 11 (HDAC11). Methods Mol Biol 1436:147–165. doi:10.1007/978-1-4939-3667-0_11
25. Deubzer HE, Schier MC, Oehme I, Lodrini M, Haendler B, Sommer A, Witt O (2013) HDAC11 is a novel drug target in carcinomas. Int J Cancer 132(9):2200–2208. doi:10.1002/ijc.27876
26. Li Y, Seto E (2016) HDACs and HDAC inhibitors in cancer development and therapy. Cold Spring Harb Perspect Med 6(10). doi:10.1101/cshperspect.a026831
27. Ozawa A, Tanji N, Kikugawa T, Sasaki T, Yanagihara Y, Miura N, Yokoyama M (2010) Inhibition of bladder tumour growth by histone deacetylase inhibitor. BJU Int 105(8):1181–1186. doi:10.1111/j.1464-410X.2009.08795.x
28. Ozdag H, Teschendorff AE, Ahmed AA, Hyland SJ, Blenkiron C, Bobrow L, Veerakumarasivam A, Burtt G, Subkhankulova T, Arends MJ, Collins VP, Bowtell D, Kouzarides T, Brenton JD, Caldas C (2006) Differential expression of selected histone modifier genes in human solid cancers. BMC Genomics 7:90. doi:10.1186/1471-2164-7-90
29. Poyet C, Jentsch B, Hermanns T, Schweckendiek D, Seifert HH, Schmidtpeter M, Sulser T, Moch H, Wild PJ, Kristiansen G (2014) Expression of histone deacetylases 1, 2 and 3 in urothelial bladder cancer. BMC Clin Pathol 14(1):10. doi:10.1186/1472-6890-14-10
30. Junqueira-Neto S, Vieira FQ, Montezuma D, Costa NR, Antunes L, Baptista T, Oliveira AI, Graca I, Rodrigues A, Magalhaes JS, Oliveira J, Henrique R, Jeronimo C (2015) Phenotypic impact of deregulated expression of class I histone deacetylases in urothelial cell carcinoma of the bladder. Mol Carcinog 54(7):523–531. doi:10.1002/mc.22117
31. Xu XS, Wang L, Abrams J, Wang G (2011) Histone deacetylases (HDACs) in XPC gene silencing and bladder cancer. J Hematol Oncol 4:17. doi:10.1186/1756-8722-4-17
32. Moser MA, Hagelkruys A, Seiser C (2014) Transcription and beyond: the role of mammalian class I lysine deacetylases. Chromosoma 123(1–2):67–78. doi:10.1007/s00412-013-0441-x
33. Reichert N, Choukrallah MA, Matthias P (2012) Multiple roles of class I HDACs in proliferation, differentiation, and development. Cell Mol Life Sci 69(13):2173–2187. doi:10.1007/s00018-012-0921-9
34. Stengel KR, Hiebert SW (2015) Class I HDACs affect DNA replication, repair, and chromatin structure: implications for cancer therapy. Antioxid Redox Signal 23(1):51–65. doi:10.1089/ars.2014.5915
35. Kelly RD, Cowley SM (2013) The physiological roles of histone deacetylase (HDAC) 1 and 2: complex co-stars with multiple leading parts. Biochem Soc Trans 41(3):741–749. doi:10.1042/BST20130010
36. Hubbert C, Guardiola A, Shao R, Kawaguchi Y, Ito A, Nixon A, Yoshida M, Wang XF, Yao TP (2002) HDAC6 is a microtubule-associated deacetylase. Nature 417(6887):455–458. doi:10.1038/417455a
37. Matsuyama A, Shimazu T, Sumida Y, Saito A, Yoshimatsu Y, Seigneurin-Berny D, Osada H, Komatsu Y, Nishino N, Khochbin S, Horinouchi S, Yoshida M (2002) In vivo destabilization of dynamic microtubules by HDAC6-mediated deacetylation. EMBO J 21(24):6820–6831. doi:10.1093/emboj/cdf682
38. Boyault C, Sadoul K, Pabion M, Khochbin S (2007) HDAC6, at the crossroads between cytoskeleton and cell signaling by acetylation and ubiquitination. Oncogene 26(37):5468–5476. doi:10.1038/sj.onc.1210614
39. Micelli C, Rastelli G (2015) Histone deacetylases: structural determinants of inhibitor selectivity. Drug Discov Today 20(6):718–735. doi:10.1016/j.drudis.2015.01.007
40. Seto E, Yoshida M (2014) Erasers of histone acetylation: the histone deacetylase enzymes. Cold Spring Harb Perspect Biol 6(4):a018713. doi:10.1101/cshperspect.a018713
41. Falkenberg KJ, Johnstone RW (2014) Histone deacetylases and their inhibitors in cancer, neurological diseases and immune disorders. Nat Rev Drug Discov 13(9):673–691. doi:10.1038/nrd4360
42. Gryder BE, Sodji QH, Oyelere AK (2012) Targeted cancer therapy: giving histone deacetylase inhibitors all they need to succeed. Future Med Chem 4(4):505–524. doi:10.4155/fmc.12.3
43. Roche J, Bertrand P (2016) Inside HDACs with more selective HDAC inhibitors. Eur J

Med Chem 121:451–483. doi:10.1016/j.ejmech.2016.05.047

44. Shechter D, Dormann HL, Allis CD, Hake SB (2007) Extraction, purification and analysis of histones. Nat Protoc 2(6):1445–1457. doi:10.1038/nprot.2007.202
45. Oehme I, Deubzer HE, Wegener D, Pickert D, Linke JP, Hero B, Kopp-Schneider A, Westermann F, Ulrich SM, von Deimling A, Fischer M, Witt O (2009) Histone deacetylase 8 in neuroblastoma tumorigenesis. Clin Cancer Res 15(1):91–99. doi:10.1158/1078-0432.CCR-08-0684
46. Hoffmann MJ, Koutsogiannouli E, Skowron MA, Pinkerneil M, Niegisch G, Brandt A, Stepanow S, Rieder H, Schulz WA (2016) The new immortalized uroepithelial cell line HBLAK contains defined genetic aberrations typical of early stage urothelial tumors. Bladder Cancer 2(4):449–463. doi:10.3233/blc-160065
47. Swiatkowski S, Seifert HH, Steinhoff C, Prior A, Thievessen I, Schliess F, Schulz WA (2003) Activities of MAP-kinase pathways in normal uroepithelial cells and urothelial carcinoma cell lines. Exp Cell Res 282(1):48–57. doi:10.1006/excr.2002.5647
48. Southgate J, Hutton KA, Thomas DF, Trejdosiewicz LK (1994) Normal human urothelial cells in vitro: proliferation and induction of stratification. Lab Invest 71(4):583–594
49. Nicoletti I, Migliorati G, Pagliacci MC, Grignani F, Riccardi C (1991) A rapid and simple method for measuring thymocyte apoptosis by propidium iodide staining and flow cytometry. J Immunol Methods 139(2):271–279

Chapter 22

Evaluation of Protein Levels of the Receptor Tyrosine Kinase ErbB3 in Serum

Leandro S. D'Abronzo, Chong-Xian Pan, and Paramita M. Ghosh

Abstract

The epidermal growth factor receptor (EGFR) family of receptor tyrosine kinases (RTK) consists of four members: EGFR1/ErbB1/HER1, ErbB2/HER2, ErbB3/HER3, and HER4/ErbB4. Signaling through these receptors regulates many key cellular activities, such as cell division, migration, adhesion, differentiation, and apoptosis. The ErbB family has been shown to be overexpressed in different types of cancers and is a target of several inhibitors already in clinical trials. ErbB3 lacks a functional tyrosine kinase domain and therefore has not been as extensively studied as the other members of this family, but its importance in activating downstream pathways, such as the PI3K/Akt pathway, makes this RTK a worthy investigation target, especially in urothelial carcinoma where the PI3K/Akt pathway is vital for progression. In recent times, ErbB3 overexpression has been linked to drug resistance and progression of various diseases, especially cancer. ErbB3 levels in the serum were shown in many cases to be reflective of its role in disease progression, and therefore detection of serum ErbB3 levels during treatment may be of importance.

Here we describe two methods for detecting ErbB3 protein in serum from patients who have undergone a clinical trial, utilizing two well-established methods in molecular biology—western blotting and ELISA, focusing on sample preparation and troubleshooting.

Key words EGFR, ERBB3, Serum, Urothelial carcinoma, Western blot, Elisa

1 Introduction

V-Erb-B2 Avian Erythroblastic Leukemia Viral Oncogene Homolog 3 (ErbB3), also known as Human Epidermal Growth Factor Receptor 3 (HER3), is a member of the epidermal growth factor receptor (EGFR) family of receptor tyrosine kinases (RTK) [1]. While both EGFR and HER2/ErbB2, the first two members of this family that were discovered, have been well investigated in various diseases including cancer [2], in cardiac [3] or neural function [4, 5], as well as in other instances; ErbB3 and the fourth member, ErbB4/HER4, were not given due diligence, at least until recently. ErbB3, especially, has been under-investigated in cancer and other diseases because, unlike other members of this family, its tyrosine kinase domain is functionally defective [6]. Both ErbB3

Wolfgang A. Schulz et al. (eds.), *Urothelial Carcinoma: Methods and Protocols*, Methods in Molecular Biology, vol. 1655, DOI 10.1007/978-1-4939-7234-0_22, © Springer Science+Business Media LLC 2018

and ErbB4 are activated by ligand binding with the neuregulin family of growth factors [7], and heterodimerize with other members of the family, especially ErbB2, for complete activation. However, despite the lack of kinase activity, it was discovered that ErbB3 signals effectively to downstream targets, especially the phosphoinositide-3-kinase (PI3K) pathway [8] through binding sites in the intracellular domain. Interest in this RTK really peaked when it was shown that overexpression of ErbB3 caused resistance of various cancers to inhibitors of EGFR and ErbB2 [9]. Since then, monoclonal antibodies to ErbB3 have been developed in an effort to target this RTK [10], and the role of this protein in cancer development and progression was granted a much closer look.

Muscle invasive bladder cancer (MIBC) constitute 33% of initial cases of urothelial carcinoma (UC) while the remainder are classified as non-muscle invasive bladder cancer (NMIBC) [11]. NMIBC is usually treated with transurethral resection of bladder tumor (TURBT) followed by either a single dose of intravesical chemotherapy or intravesical Bacillus Calmette-Guérin (BCG) [12]. In contrast, the majority of patients presenting with MIBC undergo radical cystectomy (RC), alone or following platinum-based neoadjuvant chemotherapy [13, 14]. Upon development of metastases, cytotoxic chemotherapy with the combination of cisplatin and gemcitabine (GC) as a first-line treatment is usually accepted [15].

The urothelium consists of three prominent layers—the superficial urothelium (umbrella cell layer), intermediate urothelial cells and basal urothelial cells. In the normal urothelium, ErbB3 is expressed primarily on the superficial cells but lower expression of ErbB3 may be seen in the other layers as well [16]. Multiple studies demonstrated a positive association between ErbB3 and tumor size, number, and histological grade [17–22]. Furthermore, ErbB3 was found to be a good predictor of first tumor recurrence [17]. ErbB3 expression may moreover be a good biomarker to detect the efficacy of ErbB inhibitors [23]. A phase II study of 59 patients with MIBC to determine the efficacy of the dual EGFR/ErbB2 inhibitor lapatinib as a second-line therapy following disease progression on prior platinum-based chemotherapy found that overall survival (OS) was significantly prolonged in patients with ErbB3 overexpressing tumors ($p = 0.001$) [24].

There are several ErbB3 transcripts that are transcribed in various tissues to form protein isoforms of different sizes. Full-length human ErbB3 is a 180 kDa glycoprotein [25]. As described in more detail in a previous publication [26], this RTK consists of an extracellular ligand-binding domain consisting of four subdomains (I, II, III, IV), a transmembrane domain (TM) and a cytoplasmic region consisting of a tyrosine kinase domain (TKD) and a C-terminal domain (CTD) [25, 26] (Fig. 1). *ErbB3* has been shown to encode two other alternate forms resulting from

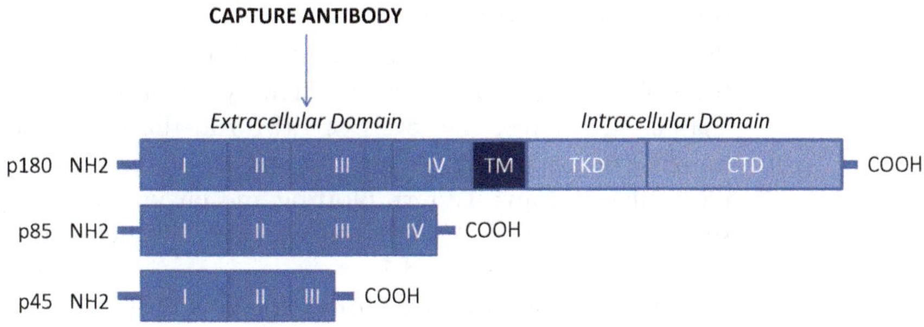

Fig. 1 Schematic representation of different splice variants of ErbB3 (p180, p85 and p45). Full-length ErbB3 consists of an extracellular ligand-binding domain consisting of four subdomains (I, II, III, IV), a transmembrane domain (TM) and a cytoplasmic region consisting of a tyrosine kinase domain (TKD) and a C-terminal domain (CTD). The p85 isoform of ErbB3 is formed by subdomains I, II and III and part of IV, with addition of 24 unique C-terminal amino acids, whereas the p45 isoform consists of extracellular subdomains I and II and part of domain III, plus 2 unique C-terminal amino acids. Note that all three forms are capable of binding the common ligands of ErbB3—neuregulins 1 and 2, but only the full-length one is capable of transmitting intracellular signals. The capture antibody coated in the 96-well plate recognizes the extracellular domain common to all three isoforms

alternately spliced variants—a p85 protein formed by extracellular subdomains I, II, and III and part of IV, with addition of 24 unique C-terminal amino acids [27], and a p45 form that consists of extracellular subdomains I and II and part of subdomain III, plus 2 unique C-terminal amino acids [28, 29] (Fig. 1). Because these forms lack the transmembrane and cytoplasmic domains, they are easily secreted outside the cell and are labeled soluble ErbB3 (sErbB3). The p85 and p45 forms, similar to full-length ErbB3, bind neuregulins, but are unable to transduce signals to downstream targets inside the cell. Many investigators have therefore thought of these truncated forms of ErbB3 as negative regulators of neuregulin signaling; however, studies show that p45ErbB3 is a bone metastasis factor [30].

Significantly, it was found that many of these isoforms of ErbB3 could be detected in the serum or plasma [27, 30, 31]. Since ErbB3 overexpression has been associated with resistance to a large number of therapies in some cancers [32–34], whereas other cancers are thought to be sensitized to certain therapies by ErbB3 expression [35, 36], a blood marker of ErbB3 expression would be useful, as it is noninvasive and can be detected relatively easily. Therefore, we determined to identify methods for detecting ErbB3 levels in the serum, especially in patients undergoing therapy for cancer.

Here we describe techniques to detect ErbB3 levels in samples obtained from patients on a clinical trial at the UC Davis Comprehensive Cancer Center. The blood from these patients was collected at the time of treatment and separated into two parts—one was fractionated to serum and the other to plasma and peripheral blood mononuclear cells (PBMC). Our laboratory received samples of separated serum for analysis. The serum samples were frozen immediately following collection and stored at −80 °C in aliquots of 0.5 mL or less, to avoid freeze–thaw cycles, until the time of the analysis. To detect the levels of ErbB3 in the serum samples we utilized two methods of protein detection commonly used in molecular biology: western blotting and enzyme-linked immunosorbent assays (ELISA). These are described in detail in the protocols in Subheadings 2 and 3.

ELISAs were developed for the detection of a target substance within a liquid sample, in this specific case ErbB3 protein in the serum following outlines described by others [37]. ELISAs rely upon relatively specific antibody–antigen interactions, and reporter-linked antibodies for detection and quantification of the analyte. It is therefore a rapid test to quantify or detect a specific antibody (Ab) or antigen (Ag).

There are four types of ELISAs: direct, indirect, competitive, and sandwich:

1. In a direct ELISA, the antigen-coated plate is detected by an antibody that is already conjugated with an enzyme ready for detection.
2. In an indirect ELISA, an unlabeled antibody is used first to bind to the antigen-coated plate, and then a secondary antibody, now conjugated with an enzyme, binds to the first antibody.
3. In competitive ELISA, the solution is pre-mixed with a known amount of enzyme-conjugated antigen that will then compete in the plate for the coated capture antibody.
4. In a sandwich ELISA, the plate is coated with the Ab against the desired Ag, the sample is added and then the detection Ab is allowed to bind to any captured Ag; next, a secondary enzyme-linked Ab is added to the mix and allows the substrate to be chromatographically detected.

Of the four, the sandwich ELISA was deemed by us to be the most sensitive for our current needs (Fig. 2). It utilizes two primary antibodies—the detection antibody and the antibody against the desired antigen, the "capture" antibody. Because one capture antibody can bind to multiple detection antibodies, this assay amplifies the signal, making it extremely sensitive. Such a sensitive assay would be needed for the detection of small amounts of protein in serum samples.

While ELISA is easy to use, it has certain disadvantages. The single biggest problem is that if the antibody recognizes more than one isoform of the protein, as is the case for a multi-isoform protein such as ErbB3, it is impossible to determine which isoform is being expressed. The capture antibody in the ELISA used above is directed against the N-terminal region of ErbB3, so theoretically

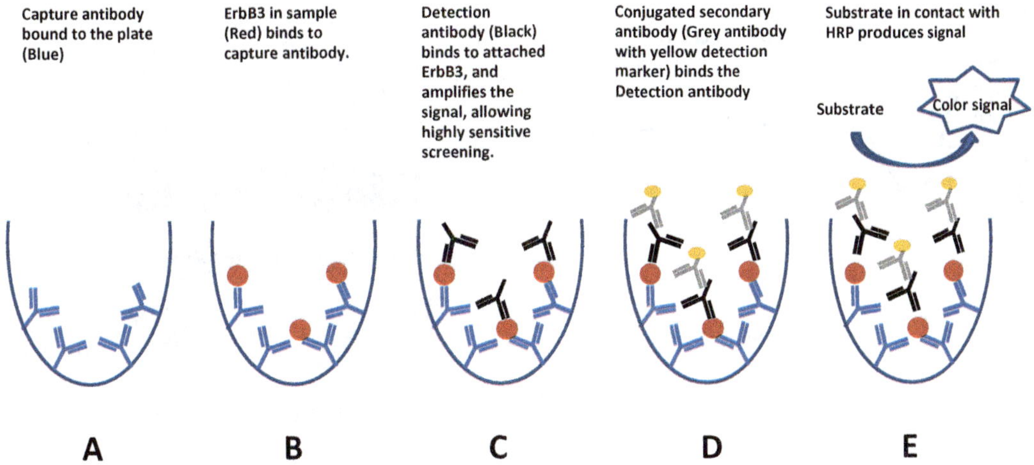

Fig. 2 Schematic representation of a sandwich ELISA using a pre-coated plate with the capture antibody. (**a**) The walls of the well are pre-coated with the antibody. (**b**) Sample is added to the wells and the antigen binds to capture antibodies. (**c**) After washing nonattached antigens, a primary detection antibody (biotinylated anti-human ErbB3) is added to amplify the signal (**d**) followed by the conjugated secondary antibody (HRP-conjugated streptavidin). (**e**) The TMB substrate solution is added to each well developing a color signal with intensity proportional to the amount of bound ErbB3 from the sample

it would recognize all three isoforms identified in Fig. 1. To distinguish between the three isoforms of ErbB3 in the serum, we used Western blotting. Western blotting or simply immunoblotting is an easy method to analyze the presence of specific proteins in a tissue lysate or sample extract. This method utilizes electrophoresis to separate proteins in a polyacrylamide gel based on their isoelectric point, molecular weight or electric charge in a one-dimension gel or combination of these properties in a two-dimension gel. These proteins are then transferred onto a nitrocellulose or polyvinylidene difluoride (PVDF) membrane for detection. In our laboratory, we utilize molecular weight to identify specific proteins in a membrane and the steps for this protocol will be discussed below.

Comparison of the results for ErbB3 levels over time from a single patient shown in Fig. 3 illustrates that ELISA and Western blotting yield similar results. The ELISA capture and detection antibodies were against the N-terminal ErbB3 where all three isoforms had identical sequences. Therefore, the ELISA would not distinguish between the three isoforms. In contrast, the Western blot analysis revealed the three isoforms, however, the similarity between the 180 kDa band of ErbB3 in the Western blot with the ELISA, but not the other two isoforms, indicates that the ELISA is detecting p180 ErbB3 and not the other isoforms.

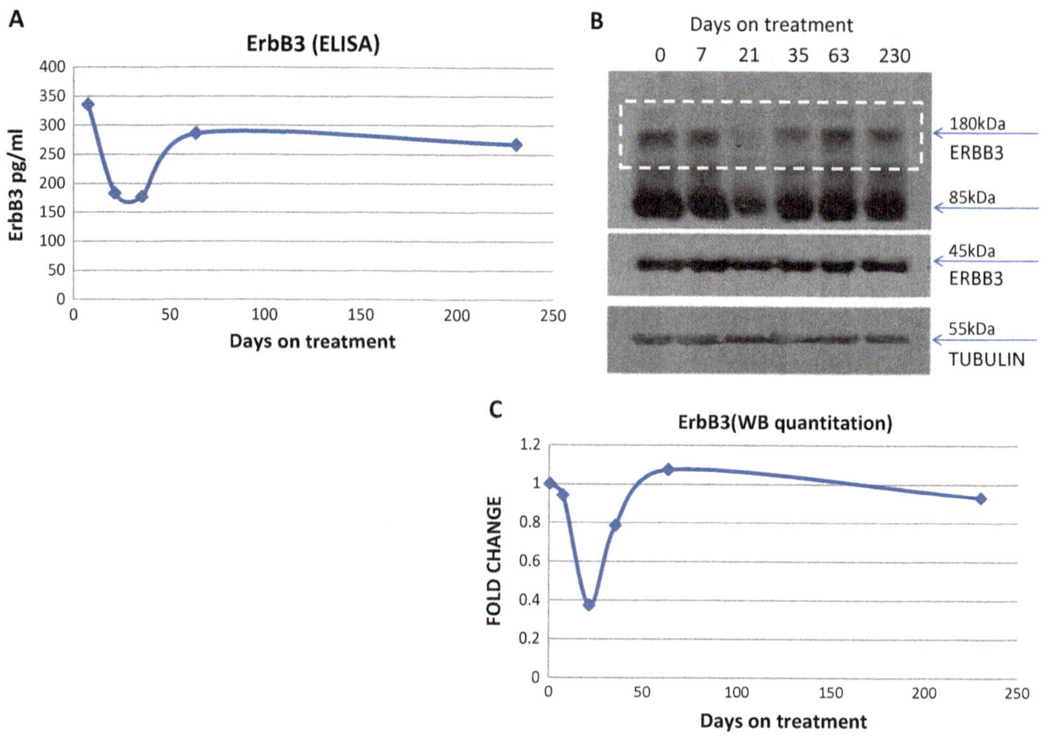

Fig. 3 Graphic representation of two different results to detect (**a**) ErbB3 levels in one patient collected on different days of treatment. (**b**) Western blots of serum from the same patient immunoblotted for ErbB3. (**c**) Graphic representation of fold change from western blot results using tubulin as a control and imageJ for quantification

2 Materials

2.1 Determination of Protein Concentrations

1. Pierce bicinchoninic acid assay (BCA assay).
2. Spectrophotometer with capacity to read 450 nm.
3. 96-well plate.
4. 4× Laemmli Sample Buffer Stock; 10 mL separating buffer, 40 mL glycerol, 10 g sodium dodecyl sulfate (SDS), water to complete 100 mL. Aliquoted in 1.5 mL tubes and kept at −20 °C.

2.2 Enzyme-Linked Immunosorbent Assay (ELISA) for ErbB3

We identified a sandwich ELISA kit from Abcam (ErbB3 Human ELISA kit ab100511) that had specifically been optimized for serum samples. In this kit is included:

1. ErbB3-coated plate: A 96-well plate coated with an anti-ErbB3 antibody that recognizes extracellular portion of the ErbB3 protein (the capture antibody).
2. 20× wash buffer (*see* TBST).

3. Assay diluents A and B (for serum/plasma (diluent A) or cells in suspension/urine (diluent B), respectively. Since we did not use diluent B for our serum experiments, all reference to diluents are for diluent A).
4. Biotinylated anti-human ErbB3: This is the detection antibody.
5. Recombinant ErbB3 standards,
6. 200× horseradish peroxidase (HRP)-Streptavidin concentrate,
7. Tetramethylbenzidine (TMB) one-step stop solution.

2.3 Western Blotting

All reagents are kept in room temperature unless stated otherwise. Water used must be deionized water.

1. 30% Acrylamide.
2. Sodium dodecyl sulfate (SDS) (10% solution in water).
3. Ammonium persulfate (APS) (40% solution in water).
4. Glycerol (50% solution in water).
5. Tetramethylethylenediamine (TEMED).
6. Mini PROTEAN spacer plates and casting frame stand.
7. Isobutanol.
8. Bromophenol blue.
9. 2-Mercaptoethanol.
10. Stacking Buffer; 60.6 g Tris (0.5 M), 4 g SDS (0.4%), water to 1 L, pH 6.8.
11. Separating Buffer; 181.8 g Tris (1.5 M), 4 g SDS (0.4%), water to 1 L, pH 8.8.
12. 10× stock Running Buffer, 30.3 g Tris, 144 g glycine, 10 g SDS in 1 L water, pH 8.3 (if adjustment is needed). Dilute to 1× in water before use.
13. 10× stock Transfer Buffer; 24.2 g Tris, 45 g glycine in 1 L of water. Dilute to 1× and add 20% methanol before use. Store in 4 °C.
14. 4× Laemmli Sample Buffer Stock; 10 mL separating buffer, 40 mL glycerol, 10 g SDS; water to 100 mL. Aliquoted in 1.5 mL tubes and kept at −20 °C.
15. 20× Tris-buffered saline stock with Tween (TBST); 242.2 g Tris, 210.4 g NaCl in 2 L of water, pH 7.4. Dilute to 1× in water before use. Add 10% Tween.
16. Skim milk powder.
17. Polyvinylidene difluoride (PVDF) membrane.
18. Chromatography paper.
19. Mini-PROTEAN 3 Electrophoresis Cell and Mini Trans-Blot Electrophoretic Transfer Cell ® with all accessories.

20. Pre-stained protein standards.
21. X-Ray film.
22. Supersignal West Femto maximum sensitivity Substrate (ThermoFisher scientific).

3 Methods

3.1 Determination of Protein Concentrations

The bicinchoninic acid assay (BCA assay) kit is used to estimate protein content in the serum samples. This assay determines protein concentrations from a standard curve with known protein contents.

1. Prepare the BCA standards by diluting the known protein sample (provided in the kit, typically bovine serum albumin). The solvent in which the standards are diluted is also provided as part of the kit and is used as the blank controls in the assay. The standards (0–2 μg/mL) are loaded in triplicate in a 96-well plate alongside the blanks which receive the solvent alone. It is advisable to have at least 5–6 standards with known protein concentrations in order to be able to accurately estimate the unknowns.
2. Serum samples are serially diluted in 1× Laemmli sample buffer to match the protein range compatible with the standards (*see* **Note 1** below). Run triplicates of the undetermined samples on the same 96-well plate as the standards. As a general rule of thumb, samples in different plates cannot usually be correlated. A different set of standards should therefore be used for each plate. Read the 96-well plate using a spectrophotometer (Powerwave X plate reader, BioTek, Winooski, VT, USA) at 450 nm.
3. Determine the samples' protein concentration by calculating the mean of the triplicates of each standard and subtracting the average value of the blanks from this mean. Plot the results against the corresponding known concentration. The slope of the plot and the y-intercept can be calculated from the data (demonstrated in Fig. 4a). These parameters can then be used to determine the total protein concentrations of the unknown samples (Fig. 4b). Based on this concentration, the volume of sample required for each assay can be calculated and the samples can be used for ELISA or for Western blotting.

3.2 Enzyme-Linked Immunosorbent Assay (ELISA) for ErbB3

1. Dilute all reagents from concentrate to 1× before starting. The 50 ng/mL stock solution is prepared by adding 400 μL of 1× Diluent A into the **recombinant human ErbB3 standard**. Standards are prepared by serial dilution in diluent A as described in Fig. 5. Diluent A alone is used as control.

A

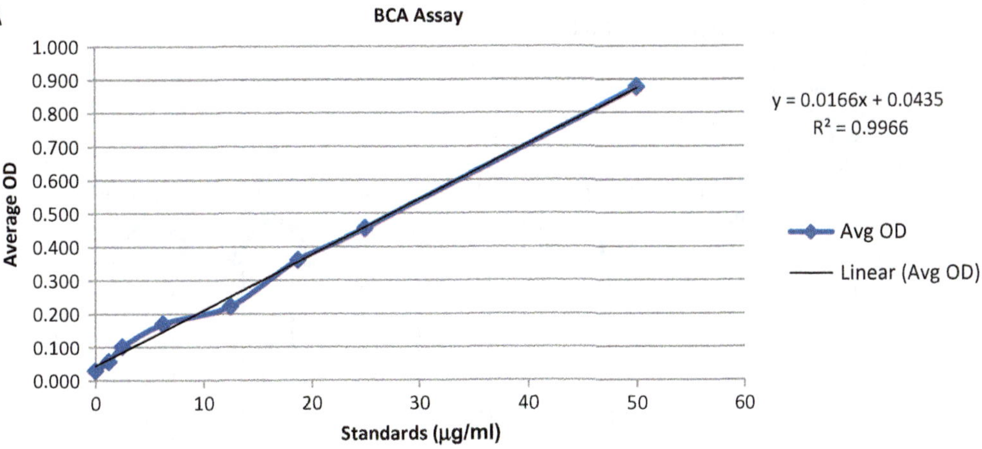

B

Background = 0.030

Sample	OD-1	OD-2	OD-3	Avg OD	Avg-bkgd	Conc (µg/µl)
S - 0001	1.202	1.234	1.225	1.220	1.190	69.066
S – 0002	0.997	1.029	1.014	1.013	0.983	56.596
S – 0003	1.115	1.140	1.143	1.133	1.102	63.785
S – 0004	0.743	0.756	0.748	0.749	0.719	40.673
S – 0005	0.934	0.944	0.932	0.937	0.906	51.978
S – 0006	0.514	0.512	0.513	0.513	0.483	26.456
S – 0007	0.812	0.835	0.828	0.825	0.795	45.251
S – 0008	1.104	1.095	1.120	1.106	1.076	62.199
S – 0009	0.429	0.433	0.436	0.433	0.402	21.616
S - 0010	1.654	1.667	1.636	1.652	1.622	95.090

Fig. 4 Methodology to calculate protein concentrations. (**a**) Graphic demonstration of BCA assay data plotted in a scatter graph with average optic density (OD) in *y* and Standards concentration (µg/mL) in *x* axis. A trend line can be drawn from the points yielding an equation (**b**) Table showing individual readings from samples, average OD, average OD with background substracted and the concentration obtained from the trend line equation

2. Serum samples should be diluted in diluent A to ensure the sample protein contents are in the range of the standards used. 100 µL of each standard and diluted samples should be added into appropriate wells (*see* **Note 2** below), considering that at least three (or four) replicates/duplicates should be used for each standard and samples. Incubate the plate at 4 °C on a rocker overnight (*see* **Note 3** below).
3. The next morning, discard the solution and wash each well by adding 200–300 µL of 1× wash buffer (diluted from 20× supplied), discarding the buffer and inverting the plate onto absorbent paper to remove the remaining buffer (*see* **Note 4** below). The washing process should be repeated three times.
4. Add 100 µL of 1× **Biotinylated ErbB3 detection antibody** to each well and incubate for 1 h at room temperature on a shaker (*see* **Note 5** below).

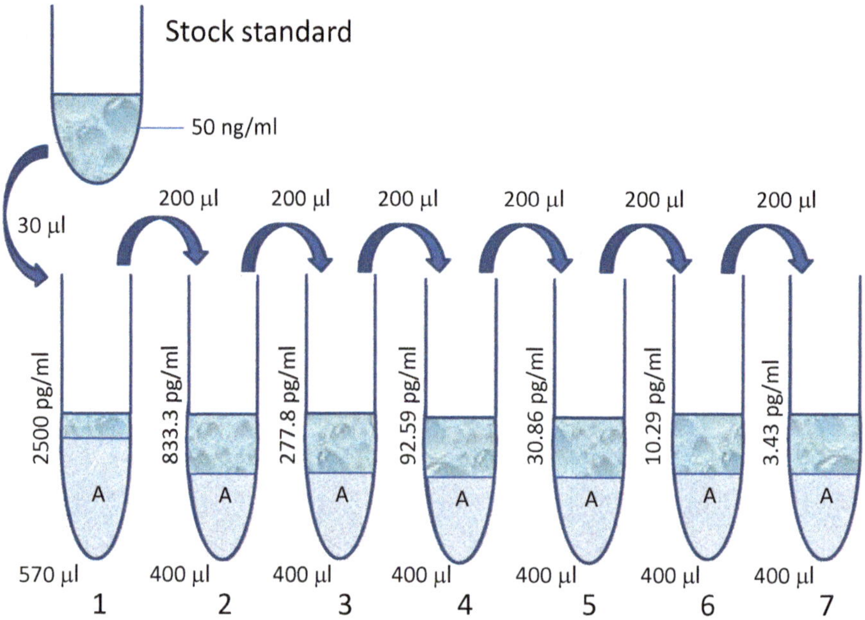

Fig. 5 Dilution of recombinant human ErbB3 standard stocks for ELISA. The 50 ng/mL stock solution is prepared through serial dilution of the **recombinant human ErbB3 standard** with 1× diluent A. Label seven [7] tubes from 1 to 7, adding 570 μL of assay diluent A into tube #1 and 400 μL of diluent A into tubes #2–7. Prepare standard #1 by adding 30 μL of stock standard (to 600 μL) and mixing thoroughly (2500 pg/mL). Prepare standard #2 by adding 200 μL of standard #1 into tube #2 (which already has 400 μL, bringing the volume to 600 μL) and mixing it (833.3 pg/mL). Prepare tubes #3 to #7 by repeating the process of adding 200 μL from the previous one until tube #7

5. Discard the solution and repeat the washing steps.
6. Add 100 μL of **HRP-Streptavidin solution** to each well and incubate for 45 min at room temperature on a shaker, followed by three washing steps.
7. Add 100 μL of the One-step substrate reagent to each well and incubate for 30 min in the dark with light shaking. Do not discard this mixture.
8. Follow by adding 50 μL of TMB **stop solution** onto each well and immediately reading the preparation at 450 nm.
9. To analyze the data, the readings from the spectrophotometer are plotted against the corresponding concentrations for the standards (0–2500 pg/mL). Protein concentrations are calculated from the standard curve as explained above for BCA.

3.3 Western Blotting

Polyacrylamide gels have two phases, a stacking phase where the proteins are packed in one band and a separating phase where the proteins are separated by molecular weight. These gels can have different polyacrylamide concentrations associated with large or small pores to separate proteins of different sizes. Full-length ErbB3 runs at 180 kDa. Therefore we recommend 6–8% SDS gels.

1. To cast a 6% resolution gel (*see* **Note 6** below), add 2 mL of 30% acrylamide, 2.45 mL of Separating buffer, 5.4 mL of water, 0.1 mL of 10% SDS solution in water, 0.04 mL of 50% glycerol solution in water, 0.0135 mL of 40% APS solution in water, and 0.01 mL of TEMED to a 50 mL tube (*see* **Note 7** below). Mix by inverting the tube and dispense the solution with a pipette between the plates in the casting stand leaving enough space for the casting gels and well combs. For more than one gel, adjust quantities accordingly.
2. To assure even polymerization, add 200–300 μL of water or isobutanol to the top of the gel and wait until gel sets.
3. In a separate tube, prepare the stacking gel by mixing 0.95 mL of 30% acrylamide, 1.25 mL of stacking buffer, 3 mL of water, 0.1 mL of 10% SDS solution, 0.005 mL of 50% glycerol solution, 0.01 mL 40% APS solution and 0.01 mL of TEMED and mix it by inversion. After dispensing the water or isobutanol from the top of the resolution gel, dispense the stacking gel on top of the separating gel and place the desired well comb to form the loading wells, allowing it to set.
4. Once gel has set, remove the plates from the casting stand and slowly remove the well combs, place the plates with the gel in the Mini-PROTEAN 3 Electrophoresis Cell and fill the chamber to indicated amount with 1× running buffer (*see* **Note 8** below).
5. Prepare each sample by mixing the predetermined amount of serum sample to load 30–50 μg of protein (*see* **Note 9** below) from the BCA assay with 1× sample buffer to bring volume to 19 μL and then adding 1 μL of bromophenol blue mixed in 2-mercaptoethanol (dip a clean pipette tip in bromophenol blue and mix in 400 μL of 2-mercaptoethanol.
6. Vortex the samples and heat at 95 °C for 5 min (*see* **Note 10** below). Load the samples into the wells with appropriate protein standards and run electrophoresis at 150 V for 2 h or until desired protein standard separation.
7. Following electrophoresis, separate the plates and remove the stacking gel portion with the preformed combs and move the gel into a container with 1× transfer buffer (*see* **Note 11** below). Label a 2.5″ × 3.5″ PVDF membrane and soak it in 100% pure methanol for 1 min, discard the methanol and keep it in transfer buffer.
8. Set up the transfer by placing the gel and PVDF membrane in between two 3” × 4” filter paper and sponges inside a cassette accordingly to manufactures directions, and slide inside transfer cell stand. Fill the chamber with 1× transfer buffer, adding the cooling unit and running the electrophoretic transfer at stable 200 mA in 4 °C room for 2 h.

9. Next remove the membrane from the apparatus and place it in a container for 5 min washes with TBST. Repeat the washes five times.
10. Block the membrane by submerging it in 10 mL of 5% skim milk dissolved in TBST for 1 h on a rocker followed by five TBST washes. The membrane is now ready to receive desired primary antibody (Santa Cruz (SC-285)) diluted as indicated by the manufacturer overnight on a rocker at 4 °C (*see* **Note 12–14** below).
11. Next day take the primary antibody off the membrane and wash it with TBST five more times.
12. Prepare the secondary antibody (Jackson Immunoresearch goat anti-rabbit IgG (111–035-045)) at 1:10,000 dilution in 2.5% skim milk solution in TBST and incubate on rocker for 1–2 h at room temperature. Wash blots once again with TBST five times.
13. To visualize the transferred proteins, mix in a 10 mL tube 1:1 parts of the two substrates found in the Supersignal West Femto kit and dilute it with water to 1:10 dilution to complete to 5 mL total volume (*see* **Note 15, 16** for adjusting concentration). Allow the substrate to bind for 2 min on a rocker and place the membrane in between plastic sheets inside the cassette. In a dark room, place the x-ray film on top of the membrane for 1 min and pass it through the developer. Adjust time of exposure accordingly. (*see* **Note 17** for quantitative analysis of western blots).

4 Notes

1. For ELISA. Serum samples should be diluted in 1× sample buffer prior to use. We find that a 1:20–1:40 dilution provides best readings from the plate and it is within the protein range of the standards provided with the Abcam kit.
2. Using a reagent vessel helps facilitate the washes and reagent distribution if using a multichannel pipette.
3. Seal the plate with sealing film to avoid evaporation of reagents when incubating overnight.
4. In each wash, keep a stack of paper towels to blot the plate upside down after dispensing the wash buffer, making sure to remove all washing buffer from the wells before going into the next steps.
5. Try to avoid forming bubbles when adding the reagents by touching the side of the well when dispensing reagents into each well.

6. When putting the plates together for casting the gel, it is a good way to seal the bottom and sides of the plates using laboratory film before installing it into the clips and onto the stand. Simply cut a strip of the film and stretch it on the bottom of the plates making a seal, and then sliding it into the clips.
7. Polymerization of the gels is more even and faster if the 40% APS solution in water is freshly made. Prepare aliquots in small 0.5 mL tubes and replace them often.
8. For all buffers prepared, add half the amount of water to the graduated cylinder before starting to add any powder reagent. Allow the magnetic stir bar to stably stir and add reagents in small portions. Wear a mask when weighting powdered reagents.
9. Different well combs will produce different well sizes, and we found that a final sample amount of 20 μL fit most wells
10. Heat the samples at 95 °C for about 5 min before you load them into the gel, spinning them briefly afterwards to collect the entire sample in the bottom of the tube. Plan to load 2–3 μL less than final volume to account for pipetting errors.
11. Transfer buffer takes 20% pure methanol, which should be added right before preparing the transfer. Dilute the 20× transfer buffer in water to 1× leaving space enough for 20% methanol and allow it to cool down before using.
12. For primary antibodies dilution, start at 1:1000 in TBST and test the strength of the signal shown in the x-ray film. Adjust the concentration accordingly to save antibody. Secondary antibody dilution should be adjusted as well if too much background is found on the film.
13. Serum samples will show a lot of background on western blots. There are kits to clean up IgG and albumin background that will appear around 50 and 65 kDa, respectively. Since we were looking for ErbB3, which is 180 kDa, we had no background influence in the desired bands. Also we suggest using a loading control that is away from the range of IgG and albumin sizes.
14. When dealing with small sample quantity, a membrane which was already blotted for a specific primary can be blotted for another primary even if the size bands are similar. For that purpose, we recommend using a stripping solution such as Restore from ThermoFisher and incubating at 37 °C for 15 min completely submerged and then washing with TBST five times before incubating with new antibody.
15. The 1:1 developing solution diluted to 1:10 in water should be adjusted depending on the signal strength of the primary antibody. If not sure of how strong the signal is, start the final dilution at 1:40 and increase as necessary.

16. When preparing the 1:1 developing solution, it is best to mix them inside the dark room since it is light sensitive. Keeping the solution in a dark place while working allows reuse of the solution for several membranes.
17. For Western blot quantitative analysis, we suggest the use of image quantification software such as ImageJ that can relatively quantify individual bands in a single gel to show fold increase/decrease in band intensity. To quantify the bands, open the image in ImageJ then with the rectangular tool make a selection including all bands you wish to quantify. Go to *Analyze > gels > Select first lane* to highlight the selection. Then go to *Analyze > gels > Plot lanes*. A Plot with all the selected lanes will appear in a separate box. If the bands are well separated, there will be a clear depression in between the bands indicating the limits of each band. With the straight line tool, draw a line from the lower part of the peaks and the bottom of the graph. Then using the wand tool, click in each individual peak representing each band. A new window will open with the quantification values, which can be used for times fold calculations.

Acknowledgement

This work was supported by Biomedical Laboratory Research & Development (BLRD) Merit Awards (I01BX000400, PMG; I01BX001784, CXP) from the Department of Veterans Affairs, and by the National Institutes of Health (Awards R01CA133209 and R01CA185509, PMG).

References

1. Jones RB, Gordus A, Krall JA, MacBeath G (2006) A quantitative protein interaction network for the ErbB receptors using protein microarrays. Nature 439(7073):168–174
2. Gschwind A, Fischer OM, Ullrich A (2004) The discovery of receptor tyrosine kinases: targets for cancer therapy. Nat Rev Cancer 4 (5):361–370
3. Negro A, Brar BK, Lee KF (2004) Essential roles of Her2/erbB2 in cardiac development and function. Recent Prog Horm Res 59:1–12
4. Corfas G, Roy K, Buxbaum JD (2004) Neuregulin 1-erbB signaling and the molecular/cellular basis of schizophrenia. Nat Neurosci 7 (6):575–580
5. Garratt AN, Ozcelik C, Birchmeier C (2003) ErbB2 pathways in heart and neural diseases. Trends Cardiovasc Med 13(2):80–86
6. Guy PM, Platko JV, Cantley LC, Cerione RA, Carraway KL III (1994) Insect cell-expressed p180erbB3 possesses an impaired tyrosine kinase activity. Proc Natl Acad Sci U S A 91 (17):8132–8136
7. Carraway KL 3rd, Cantley LC (1994) A neu acquaintance for erbB3 and erbB4: a role for receptor heterodimerization in growth signaling. Cell 78(1):5–8
8. Hynes NE, MacDonald G (2009) ErbB receptors and signaling pathways in cancer. Curr Opin Cell Biol 21(2):177–184

9. Arteaga CL, Engelman JA (2014) ERBB receptors: from oncogene discovery to basic science to mechanism-based cancer therapeutics. Cancer Cell 25(3):282–303
10. Baselga J, Swain SM (2009) Novel anticancer targets: revisiting ERBB2 and discovering ERBB3. Nat Rev Cancer 9(7):463–475
11. Amsellem-Ouazana D, Bièche I, Tozlu S, Botto H, Debré B, Lidereau R (2006) Gene expression profiling of ERBB receptors and ligands in human transitional cell carcinoma of the bladder. J Urol 175(3):1127–1132
12. Brincks EL, Risk MC, Griffith TS (2013) PMN and anti-tumor immunity–the case of bladder cancer immunotherapy. Semin Cancer Biol 23 (3):183–189
13. Vishnu P, Mathew J, Tan WW (2011) Current therapeutic strategies for invasive and metastatic bladder cancer. Onco Targets Ther 4:97–113
14. Winquist E, Kirchner TS, Segal R, Chin J, Lukka H (2004) Genitourinary cancer disease site group CCOPiE-bCPGI. Neoadjuvant chemotherapy for transitional cell carcinoma of the bladder: a systematic review and meta-analysis. J Urol 171(2 Pt 1):561–569
15. Zachos I, Konstantinopoulos PA, Tzortzis V et al (2010) Systemic therapy of metastatic bladder cancer in the molecular era: current status and future promise. Expert Opin Investig Drugs 19(7):875–887
16. Chow NH, Liu HS, Yang HB, Chan SH, Su IJ (1997) Expression patterns of erbB receptor family in normal urothelium and transitional cell carcinoma. An immunohistochemical study. Virchows Arch 430(6):461–466
17. Chow NH, Chan SH, Tzai TS, Ho CL, Liu HS (2001) Expression profiles of ErbB family receptors and prognosis in primary transitional cell carcinoma of the urinary bladder. Clin Cancer Res 7(7):1957–1962
18. Dyrskjot L, Kruhoffer M, Thykjaer T et al (2004) Gene expression in the urinary bladder: a common carcinoma in situ gene expression signature exists disregarding histopathological classification. Cancer Res 64(11):4040–4048
19. Lee JS, Leem SH, Lee SY et al (2010) Expression signature of E2F1 and its associated genes predict superficial to invasive progression of bladder tumors. J Clin Oncol 28 (16):2660–2667
20. Modlich O, Prisack HB, Pitschke G et al (2004) Identifying superficial, muscle-invasive, and metastasizing transitional cell carcinoma of the bladder: use of cDNA array analysis of gene expression profiles. Clin Cancer Res 10 (10):3410–3421
21. Sanchez-Carbayo M, Socci ND, Lozano J, Saint F, Cordon-Cardo C (2006) Defining molecular profiles of poor outcome in patients with invasive bladder cancer using oligonucleotide microarrays. J Clin Oncol 24 (5):778–789
22. NCI (2013) The Cancer Genome Atlas - Bladder Urothelial Carcinoma DNA Copy Number Data In: Insititue TNc, ed. http://tcga-data.nci.nih.gov/tcga/: Oncomine
23. Mooso BA, Vinall RL, Mudryj M, Yap SA (2015) deVere white RW, Ghosh PM. The role of EGFR family inhibitors in muscle invasive bladder cancer: a review of clinical data and molecular evidence. J Urol 193(1):19–29
24. Wulfing C, Machiels JP, Richel DJ et al (2009) A single-arm, multicenter, open-label phase 2 study of lapatinib as the second-line treatment of patients with locally advanced or metastatic transitional cell carcinoma. Cancer 115 (13):2881–2890
25. Sithanandam G, Anderson LM (2008) The ERBB3 receptor in cancer and cancer gene therapy. Cancer Gene Ther 15(7):413–448
26. Jathal MK, Chen L, Mudryj M, Ghosh PM (2011) Targeting ErbB3: the new RTK(id) on the prostate cancer block. Immunol Endocr Metab Agents Med Chem 11(2):131–149
27. Lee H, Akita RW, Sliwkowski MX, Maihle NJ (2001) A naturally occurring secreted human ErbB3 receptor isoform inhibits heregulin-stimulated activation of ErbB2, ErbB3, and ErbB4. Cancer Res 61(11):4467–4473
28. Lin SH, Lee YC, Choueiri MB et al (2008) Soluble ErbB3 levels in bone marrow and plasma of men with prostate cancer. Clin Cancer Res 14(12):3729–3736
29. Chen N, Ye XC, Chu K et al (2007) A secreted isoform of ErbB3 promotes osteonectin expression in bone and enhances the invasiveness of prostate cancer cells. Cancer Res 67 (14):6544–6548
30. Lin SH, Cheng CJ, Lee YC et al (2008) A 45-kDa ErbB3 secreted by prostate cancer cells promotes bone formation. Oncogene 27 (39):5195–5203
31. Bei R, Masuelli L, Moriconi E et al (1999) Immune responses to all ErbB family receptors detectable in serum of cancer patients. Oncogene 18(6):1267–1275
32. Morrison MM, Williams MM, Vaught DB et al (2016) Decreased LRIG1 in fulvestrant-treated luminal breast cancer cells permits ErbB3 upregulation and increased growth. Oncogene 35(9):1143–1152
33. Ghasemi R, Rapposelli IG, Capone E et al (2014) Dual targeting of ErbB-2/ErbB-3

results in enhanced antitumor activity in preclinical models of pancreatic cancer. Oncogene 3:e117

34. Zhu S, Belkhiri A, El-Rifai W (2011) DARPP-32 increases interactions between epidermal growth factor receptor and ERBB3 to promote tumor resistance to gefitinib. Gastroenterology 141(5):1738–48 e1–2
35. Liu W, Barnette AR, Andreansky S, Landgraf R (2016) ERBB2 overexpression establishes ERBB3-dependent hypersensitivity of breast cancer cells to Withaferin A. Mol Cancer Ther 15(11):2750–2757
36. Chen JY, Chen YJ, Yen CJ, Chen WS, Huang WC (2016) HBx sensitizes hepatocellular carcinoma cells to lapatinib by up-regulating ErbB3. Oncotarget 7(1):473–489
37. Butler JE (2000) Enzyme-linked immunosorbent assay. J Immunoass 21(2–3):165–209

Chapter 23

Targeting the PI3K/AKT/mTOR Pathway in Bladder Cancer

Anuja Sathe and Roman Nawroth

Abstract

The PI3K/AKT/mTOR signaling pathway shows frequent molecular alterations and increased activity in cancer. Given its role in the regulation of cell growth, survival and metastasis, molecules within this pathway are promising targets for pharmacologic intervention. Metastatic bladder cancer (BLCA) continues to have few treatment options. Although various molecular alterations in PI3K/AKT/mTOR signaling have been described in BLCA, clinical trials with small molecule inhibitors have not met their endpoints. In this article, we summarize results from preclinical studies and clinical trials that examined PI3K pathway inhibitors in BLCA focusing on technical challenges that might result in contradictory findings in preclinical studies. Based on published data from our group, we also address challenges that need to be overcome to optimize PI3K inhibition in BLCA and enable its successful translation into the clinic.

Key words Bladder cancer, PI3K/AKT/mTOR

1 Introduction

The phosphoinositide 3-kinase (PI3K)/AKT/ mammalian target of rapamycin (mTOR) pathway is one of the most investigated therapeutic targets in cancer. Class IA PI3Ks possess a p85 regulatory subunit and a p110 catalytic subunit, with various isoforms p110α, p110β, p110γ, and p110δ. These PI3Ks can phosphorylate phosphatidylinositol-4,5 bisphosphate (PI-4,5-P2) to produce phosphatidylinositol-3,4,5-trisphosphate (PIP3), while the phosphatase and tensin homolog (PTEN) can reverse this reaction [1, 2] (Fig. 1). PIP3 acts as a second messenger by recruiting molecules such as AKT and phosphoinositide-dependent kinase 1 (PDK1) via their pleckstrin homology domains resulting in their translocation to the cell membrane and subsequent activation [3]. Functional activation of AKT requires phosphorylation at two distinct sites, namely threonine 308 by PDK1 and serine 473 by mTORC2. mTORC2 is a protein complex consisting of the kinase mTOR and various scaffolding proteins including rictor. AKT is an oncogenic serine/threonine kinase and has the potential to regulate

Wolfgang A. Schulz et al. (eds.), *Urothelial Carcinoma: Methods and Protocols*, Methods in Molecular Biology, vol. 1655, DOI 10.1007/978-1-4939-7234-0_23, © Springer Science+Business Media LLC 2018

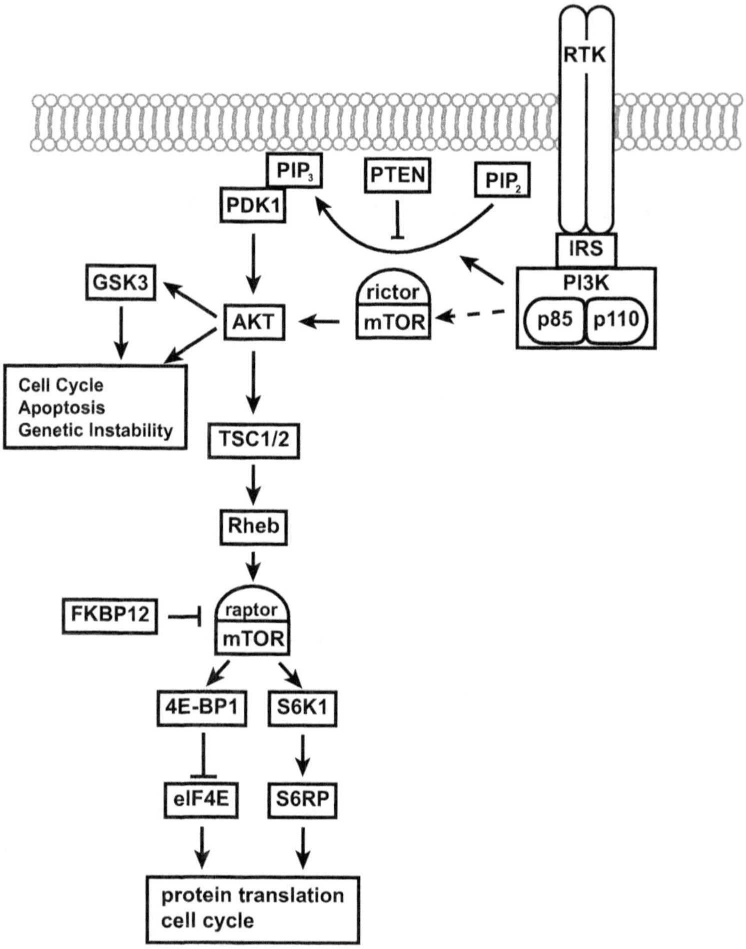

Fig. 1 PI3K/AKT/mTOR signaling. Schematic representation of the PI3K/AKT/mTOR pathway

multiple downstream effectors and signaling pathways. One major effector is the mTORC1 complex which is activated by AKT via TSC1 and TSC2 [3]. mTORC1 also contains the mTOR kinase together with associated proteins such as raptor. Two important mTORC1 substrates are ribosomal protein S6 kinase β1 (S6 K1) and eukaryotic translation initiation factor 4E–binding protein 1 (4EBP1), which regulate mRNA translation and protein synthesis [4].

Frequent overactivation of the PI3K signaling pathway in muscle-invasive or metastatic bladder cancer (BLCA) has been demonstrated in multiple independent studies. Mutations in *PIK3CA* (encoding for the p110α subunit of PI3K) are present in 21–25% of muscle-invasive BLCA [5–7]. Although PTEN mutations are found in only 3–4% [5, 6], loss of PTEN expression is commonly observed in 39–94% patients [7–11]. Loss of heterozygosity (LOH) leading to decreased expression of TSC1 or TSC2 is also present in 40–50% and 15% of BLCA respectively [7, 12]. Activating mutations in *AKT1* are rare and observed in only 2–3% of the cases [6, 13]. Deregulation of PI3K signaling can also result from molecular alterations in upstream components including receptor tyrosine kinases (RTKs) such as the ERRB family of proteins (2–11%), FGFR3 (3–11%), or RAS proteins (1–5%). According to recent data from the Cancer Genome Atlas, the RTK/RAS/PI3K/AKT/mTOR pathway is altered in 72% of BLCA (Network, 2014). This high frequency of deregulation of PI3K pathway signaling, as well as the possibility to inhibit it by several available small molecule inhibitors, makes it an attractive therapeutic target in BLCA.

Progress in the treatment of metastatic BLCA has been limited and the average survival of patients is only 12–14 months with standard chemotherapy regimens. Despite over 30 years of research, the first FDA approval for second line therapy following platinum-based chemotherapy in these patients occurred only in 2016, for anti-PD-L1 immunotherapy [14, 15]. Therapeutic targeting of the PI3K/AKT/mTOR pathway thus represents a novel and much-needed approach for improving the outcome of patients with metastatic BLCA.

Here, we review the various preclinical and clinical studies examining the effect of PI3K pathway inhibition in BLCA and discuss the challenges in the successful translation of this treatment into the clinic. We also highlight the experimental methodology to conduct preclinical studies examining PI3K pathway inhibition in BLCA.

2 Preclinical and Clinical Studies Examining PI3K Pathway Inhibition in BLCA

The PI3K signaling pathway can be targeted by different classes of compounds that inhibit PI3K, AKT, mTORC1, mTORC1 and mTORC2, PI3K ,and mTOR [16]. These agents have the potential to induce distinct therapeutic effects and need to be examined individually in preclinical models.

2.1 mTORC1 Inhibitors

Rapamycin analogs or rapalogs function as allosteric inhibitors of the mTORC1 complex by binding to the FKBP-12 protein domain [17]. They were historically the first inhibitors of the PI3K pathway and have been tested in both preclinical and clinical settings in BLCA. Rapalogs have a proven safety record and have been approved for the treatment of renal cell carcinoma, mantle cell lymphoma and neuroendocrine tumors [18]. In BLCA, at biochemically relevant concentrations these compounds exhibit a limited effect on cell viability in the large majority of tested cell lines [19–24]. One explanation for this weak activity is that rapalogs, unlike ATP competitive mTOR inhibitors such as Torin or PP242, can induce dephosphorylation only of S6K1 but importantly not of 4E-BP1 and thus no inactivation of its downstream targets [19, 25, 26]. For an effective reduction in cell growth and viability the inactivation of both factors is required [19, 22]. Additionally, rapalogs also result in an S6K1-IRS1-PI3K-mediated feedback phosphorylation of AKT, which can hamper their anti-tumor efficacy [19, 27]. In this context, it is interesting to note that using an shRNA targeting mTOR also affects only S6K1 but not 4E-BP1 phosphorylation (Fig. 2).

In clinical trials for BLCA as second line therapy for metastatic disease the majority of patients had either progressive disease (PD) or stable disease (SD), suggesting that rapalogs have limited utility in BLCA (Table 1). However, a subset of patients exhibited partial (PR) or complete responses (CR). These responses were retrospectively correlated to genomic alterations in tumors in some of these trials. By targeted deep sequencing, a patient with CR to everolimus was found to have a TSC1 mutation, together with an NF2 mutation. However, three other patients with TSC1 mutations had only minor responses to everolimus with 7–24% tumor regression [28]. This was also reflected in a preclinical study, where only 1 out of 3 TSC1 mutant cell lines responded to rapamycin [23]. Meanwhile, in another cohort, PTEN deficiency was associated with PD, suggesting that this alteration might correlate with resistance to treatment [29]. In a clinical trial that examined the effect of everolimus in different solid tumor entities, a BLCA patient with CR was determined to have an activating mTOR mutation by whole-exome sequencing [30]. While the characterization of exceptional response to rapalogs provides valuable insights, there is a need for in-depth evaluation of the determinants of sensitivity, which remain incompletely defined. These data are important because they demonstrate that besides the use of novel technologies such as next generation sequencing (NGS), an understanding of the molecular mechanism underlying drug activity is crucial in order to identify a panel of effective predictive stratifying biomarkers.

2.2 AKT Inhibitors

The effects of AKT inhibition in BLCA have been examined in two independent studies using an ATP-competitive inhibitor, MK-2206, and an allosteric inhibitor, AZ7328, respectively. Results from our group with MK-2206 demonstrate that AKT inhibition induces apoptosis and reduces cell viability only in cells that possess helical domain-activating *PIK3CA* mutations [31]. This relationship was confirmed not only by correlation in a panel of different cell lines, but also by genetic manipulation of the *PIK3CA* mutation status. Cells with alterations in PTEN, TSC1 or RAS remained resistant. Interestingly, AKT inhibition also failed to reduce 4E-BP1 phosphorylation and regulated only S6K1, similar to the results obtained with rapalogs in our group (Fig. 2a). Sensitivity to

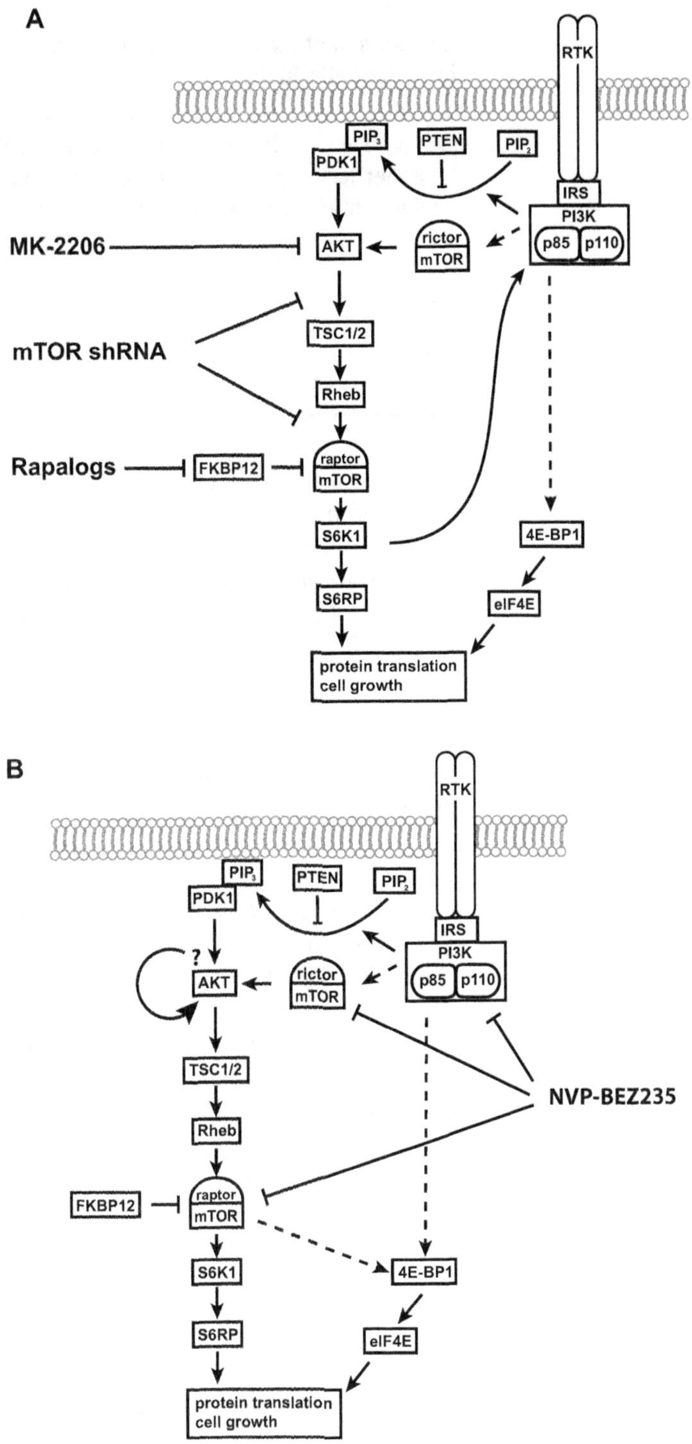

Fig. 2 Effect of PI3K pathway inhibitors on downstream signaling in BLCA. (**a**) AKT or mTORC1 inhibitors as well as mTOR shRNA reduce only S6K1 but not 4E–BP1 phosphorylation. (**b**) Dual PI3K/mTOR inhibitors result in dephosphorylation of both S6K1 and 4E–BP1 but also lead to AKT rephosphorylation

Table 1
Comparison of various clinical trials using rapalogs as second line therapy for metastatic BLCA

Reference number for clinical trial	No. of patients assessed	Complete response (CR)	Partial response (PR)	Stable disease (SD)	Progressive disease (PD)
[50]	24	0	5	9	10
[51]	37	1	1	23	20
[52]	14	0	0	4	10
[29]	37	0	2	8	27

AZ7328 also correlated with *PIK3CA* mutations, but a direct role of those mutations on the activity of this compound was not addressed [32]. Additionally, this study also demonstrated that AKT inhibition induces autophagy, which prevents cell death and limits its efficacy. Activating mutations in the *PIK3CA* gene occur in 20–25% of bladder cancer patients [5]. These data strongly support the implementation of a clinical trial that would stratify patients for *PIK3CA* mutations as an inclusion criterion.

2.3 PI3K Inhibitors

A recent study evaluated the effects of the PI3K inhibitor, GDC-0941, in a panel of BLCA cell lines [33]. Similar to findings with AKT inhibitors, this study demonstrated that cells with activating *PIK3CA* mutations were sensitive to PI3K inhibition. Cells with rare *PIK3CA* mutations or coexistent *TSC1* or *PTEN* mutations were less sensitive, while single *TSC1* or *PTEN* alterations or co-occurring *AKT1* or *RAS* alterations were associated with resistance. Moreover, shRNA-mediated silencing of *PIK3CA* in *PIK3CA* mutant cells was accompanied by reduced anchorage-independent growth and motility. Preliminary data from a phase II trial that examined the PI3K inhibitor BKM-120 as second line therapy for metastatic BLCA in 13 patients demonstrated SD and PR in 6 and 1 patients, respectively [34]. One patient with SD and PR harbored a *TSC1* mutation, while patients with *PIK3CA* mutations showed PD. Despite the limited single agent activity of BKM-120 and its poor functional characterization, this trial is currently in an expansion phase with inclusion based on genetic alterations in the PI3K pathway (NCT01551030, https://clinicaltrials.gov/). There are no publications that thoroughly characterize the biochemical downstream effects upon PI3K inhibition in BLCA and further studies are needed to enable a reasonable stratification of patients.

2.4 Dual PI3K/mTOR Inhibitors

mTOR is a member of the PI3K-related kinase family and shares structural similarity with the various PI3K isoforms. This has led to the development of dual PI3K/mTOR inhibitors that act as

ATP-competitive inhibitors of both PI3K and mTOR kinases. They also have the theoretical advantage of suppressing the S6K1-IRS1-PI3K-mediated feedback rephosphorylation of AKT that is seen with rapalogs, due to the direct additional inhibition of PI3K [18]. Unlike rapalogs or AKT inhibitors, dual PI3K/mTOR inhibitors such as NVP-BEZ235 suppress the phosphorylation of not only S6K1 but also of 4E–BP1 [19] (Fig. 2b). They also reduce cell growth to a much greater extent than rapalogs [19, 35]. NVP-BEZ235 leads to a G1 arrest, reduction in S phase fraction of BLCA cell lines and promotes autophagy. However, no significant effect on apoptosis can be induced by dual PI3K/mTOR inhibition [19, 36]. We have previously demonstrated that despite an initial dephosphorylation after 1 h of treatment, NVP-BEZ235 results in AKT hyperphosphorylation when administered for 24 h in vitro [19]. This rephosphorylation of AKT might provide a mechanism that prevents induction of cell death by dual PI3K/mTOR inhibition and its functional consequences should be examined in additional detail.

A recent clinical trial examined the effects of NVP-BEZ235 as second line therapy in 20 BLCA patients with locally advanced or metastatic disease after progression with platinum-based therapy [37]. These tumors were also examined for *PTEN* loss or *PI3KCA* mutations. SD and PR were observed in only two and one patient respectively, in tumors without alterations in either *PTEN* or *PI3KCA*. 90% of patients experienced adverse effects, with grade 3–4 adverse effects reported in 50%. In a phase I trial with GSK2126458, another dual PI3K/mTOR inhibitor, SD and PR was observed in one and two patients, respectively, out of a cohort of 14 evaluable patients, neither correlating with *PI3KCA* status [38]. These results demonstrate that dual PI3K/mTOR inhibitors show limited clinical efficacy in BLCA and are accompanied by toxicity. It is thus of utmost importance that additional preclinical studies are conducted to explain these limitations, possibly by using rationally designed combination therapy.

2.5 Long-Term Effects of PI3K Pathway Inhibitors and Crosstalk with the MAPK Signaling Pathway

PI3K pathway inhibition is also influenced by its complicated crosstalk with the mitogen activated protein kinase (MAPK) signaling pathway [18]. Very few preclinical studies are available that have examined PI3K inhibitors in BLCA with a focus on long-term biochemical effects and crosstalk with the MAPK pathway. Observations from our group revealed that the use of the rapalog RAD001 results not only in the described feedback loop involving IRS1 and AKT, but also in the activation of the MAPK signaling pathway [19]. Increased MAPK signaling was also detected with the dual PI3K/mTOR inhibitor NVP-BEZ235. Interestingly, when using the MEK1/2 inhibitor U0126, activation of AKT but not S6K1 could be observed. U0126 increased the fraction of cells arrested in G1 phase with a reduction in S phase, similar to the effects of NVP-BEZ235. Despite the importance of both MAPK and PI3K signaling in regulating the induction of apoptosis, no increase in caspase 3/7 activity could be observed with the use of U0126, NVP-BEZ235 or their combination.

3 Challenges to PI3K Pathway Inhibition in BLCA

Despite the frequent deregulation of PI3K signaling in BLCA, clinical trials using either rapalogs or dual PI3K/mTOR inhibitors have had limited success. There is thus a need to critically reevaluate the potential of therapeutic targeting of this pathway.

Preclinical studies in both BLCA and other tumor entities have revealed the presence of several feedback loops as well as crosstalk with other signaling pathways such as the MAPK or the JAK-STAT pathway [18, 39]. These effects on cell signaling are also specific to the inhibitor used and have the potential to impair the efficacy of PI3K pathway inhibition. A thorough preclinical characterization of the biochemical effects of various PI3K pathway inhibitors has the potential to reveal such effects on cell signaling. It can also aid in devising rationally designed combination target therapies to counter these effects. Two important questions that remain to be answered are the effects of various inhibitors on 4E-BP1 and AKT phosphorylation, given the impact of these activated proteins on tumor growth.

Initial reports have demonstrated synergism of PI3K pathway inhibitors with cisplatin-based chemotherapy or radiotherapy [35, 40]. These effects should be examined in greater detail to enable the translation of these findings into the clinic in the form of combination therapies. The approval of immune checkpoint-based immunotherapy for metastatic BLCA also opens new avenues for examining the effects of combination treatment with PI3K pathway inhibition.

Several examples of the preclinical studies that we have reviewed as well as the genetic profiling of exceptional responders in clinical trials demonstrate that the utility of PI3K pathway inhibition might be limited to tumors with specific genetic alterations. Also, the correlation with only single genetic alterations seems insufficient to identify suitable predictive markers, as has been demonstrated for TSC1 mutations and rapalogs. This is important to note as BLCA possesses tremendous molecular heterogeneity [41]. It is thus necessary that future preclinical and clinical studies are designed rationally to provide realistic estimates on the value of personalized medicine and biomarker-based pre-stratification for BLCA patients receiving PI3K-based therapy. It is also important that studies examining exceptional responses are validated both preclinically and in larger prospective clinical trials undertaking a robust molecular characterization of drug response. The response to target therapy might be influenced by multiple rather than single genetic alterations. The focus should thus also be on the development of biomarker panels and their validation.

4 Methods to Analyze PI3K Pathway Inhibition in BLCA

Examining the effects of PI3K pathway inhibition in a preclinical setting necessitates an extensive use of BLCA cell line models, small molecule inhibitors and molecular biology methods. Functional effects on tumor inhibition can be assessed using a variety of assays that examine cell viability, cell cycle progression, clonogenic growth, apoptosis or senescence. Analyzing the effects on various phosphoproteins in signaling cascades remains a critical method and can be accomplished by immunoblotting, immunofluorescence or high-throughput techniques like mass spectrometry or mass cytometry. Various methods of genetic manipulation of protein expression, including genetic silencing by small interfering RNAs (siRNAs), short hairpin RNAs (shRNAs) or clustered regularly interspaced palindromic repeats (CRISPR) guide RNAs (gRNAs), as well as overexpression by recombinant proteins using plasmid transfection or transduction are also important in assessing the PI3K signaling pathway. Use of each of these methods requires several important considerations that should be studied in detail before starting experiments. Here we would like to highlight some specific experimental aspects that we have experienced during our work with PI3K signaling in BLCA, each of which can impact the final experimental outcome.

4.1 Cell Culture

When characterizing signaling events in cells, the cell culture conditions play a major role in the outcome and reproducibility. One critical aspect is the authentication of cell lines, which is necessary to ensure the correct genetic background of the cells of interest. Several open access databases are available with data on the genetic alterations including mutations and copy number variations of commonly used cell lines (http://cancer.sanger.ac.uk/cell_lines#, https://portals.broadinstitute.org/ccle/home) [42–44]. These databases can provide useful information in order to select cell lines bearing relevant genetic alterations in order to answer a particular research question.

Several practical aspects of cell culture influence the ability of cells to change their properties during serial passages. One of these is the influence of temperature during passaging of cells. It should be ensured that cell culture reagents such as media, PBS and trypsin are adequately warmed to 37 °C before use. Cells should also be handled at room temperature for a minimum amount of time and returned to their 37 °C incubator environment at the earliest. Trypsinization is also a stressful process for cells and the time of

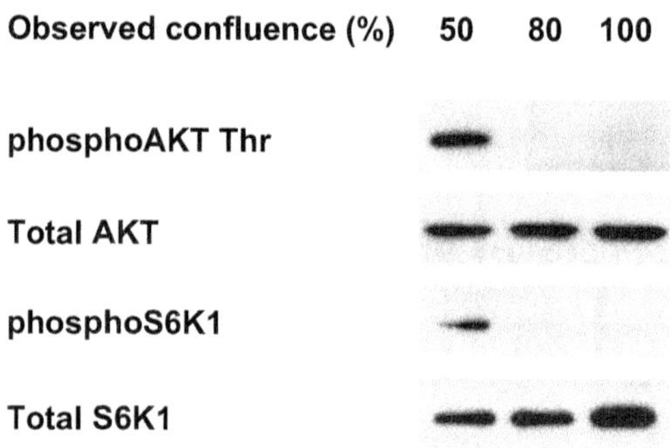

Fig. 3 Influence of cell confluence on protein phosphorylation. RT112 cells were seeded at 0.2×10^6, 0.3×10^6 or 0.4×10^6 cells per well in a 6-well plate and lysates were prepared the following day and subjected to immunoblotting. All methods were performed as described previously [19]. Briefly, cells were lysed for 15 min on ice in lysis buffer (150 mM NaCl, 50 mM Tris–HCl, pH 7.2, 1% Triton X-100, 0.05% SDS, 5 mM EDTA) containing freshly added protease and phosphatase inhibitors. Protein lysates were quantified and subjected to SDS-PAGE, followed by transfer onto a PVDF membrane. Membranes were blocked in 5% nonfat milk in washing buffer (0.05 M Tris–HCl, pH 7.6 with 0.1% Tween-20) for 1 h at room temperature, followed by washing and overnight incubation with respective primary antibodies. Membranes were then incubated with peroxidase conjugated IgG for 30 min at room temperature, which was detected by recording the chemiluminescent signal on autoradiography films

exposure to trypsin or similar agents should be minimized and has to be optimized not only for a given cell line but also be controlled in each experiment.

Another important variable is the degree of confluence of cells. We have observed that the protein phosphorylation level of several molecules within the PI3K pathway is influenced by the degree of confluence of cells. For example, phosphorylated AKT and S6K1 levels decrease in cells with increasing confluence (Fig. 3). Due to these observations, our group controls the confluence status of cells during routine cell culture as well as during individual experiments stringently. The condition of cells during culture influences signaling events to a large extent. It is imperative that cell culture conditions are properly controlled to ensure reproducibility.

4.2 Cell Viability Assays

The ideal measure of the effect of a small molecule inhibitor on tumor growth is the number of viable cells relative to a solvent control. However, cell counting is a cumbersome process and cell viability assays are commonly used as a surrogate measure to enable comparatively high-throughput experiments. However, it is important to consider the underlying principle of these assays. For instance, several of these assays detect the reduction of tetrazolium or resazurin salts or the production of ATP [45]. Hence, it is necessary to conduct preliminary experiments which can verify the

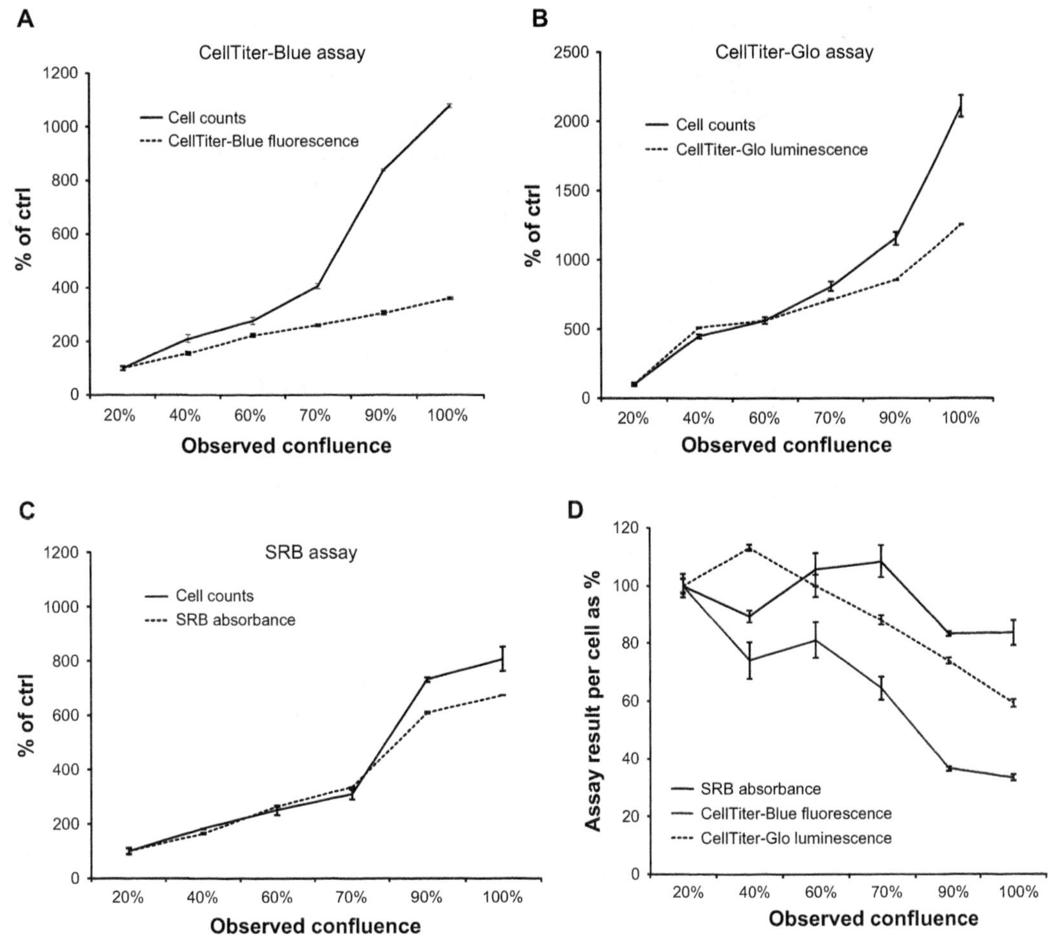

Fig. 4 Influence of cell confluence on cell viability assays. RT112 cells were seeded at 3000, 5000, 8000, 10,000, 20,000 or 30,000 cells per well in a 96-well plate. Cell confluence was estimated the next day. Cells were counted using trypan blue exclusion or the CellTiter-Blue (**a**), CellTiter-Glo (**b**) or SRB (**c**) assay, respectively. All assays were performed according to the manufacturer's protocol or as described previously [49]. Results were expressed as percentage of the lowest cell number (ctrl). The respective readout for each assay was divided by the corresponding cell number to yield the assay value per cell (**d**), which was expressed as percentage. *Error bars* indicate standard error. Results are representative of two independent experiments

correlation of these assay readouts with cell number. It is also possible that specific conditions such as cell confluence can influence the results of such assays.

We examined the influence of cell confluence on results of the CellTiter-Blue, CellTiter-Glo and sulforhodamine B (SRB) assays, in comparison to cell counts detected by trypan blue exclusion. The CellTiter-Blue assay correlated with the cell counts only when cells were between 20 and 60% confluent (Fig. 4a). At higher confluence, the assay underestimated the cell counts by 35–65%. This reduction was also seen when calculating the fluorescent signal per cell (Fig. 4d). The CellTiter-Glo assay correlated well with the number of viable cells at a confluence between 20 and 70% (Fig. 4b). However, once cells reached 90–100% confluence, this assay also showed a 25–40% reduction in the luminescence detected per cell and underestimated the number of viable cells (Fig. 4d). Among the three assays examined, the SRB assay correlated best with cell numbers (Fig. 4c). At 90–100% confluence, the absorbance per cell was reduced by around 16% and this assay also underestimated the number of viable cells (Fig. 4d). However, this assay is more time consuming and not often used for high-throughput screening. Hence, cell confluence has the potential to act as a confounding factor when using these assays. For instance, such assays would underestimate the effect of a small molecule inhibitor if the control cells were allowed to reach confluence.

Recent studies have compared the effects of two large-scale pharmacogenomics studies, both of which analyzed the effect of small molecule inhibitors on various cell lines in relation to their genetic alterations, but yielded differing results. According to these studies, this variability arose not from differences in genomic data but from variations in cell culture conditions, seeding density and the viability assays that were used [46, 47]. These examples once again stress the importance of controlling cell culture conditions and viability assays in order to ensure reproducible results.

4.3 Chemical Inhibition via Small Molecule Inhibitors

Small molecule inhibitors are an important resource for translational projects involving cell signaling. The choice of inhibitors should be guided by a thorough study of their properties and described effects. An important consideration is the range of specificity of such inhibitors relative to the concentration used in an assay. It should thus always be confirmed that the inhibitor engages with its proposed target and does not exhibit off-target effects. This can be ensured by examining the dose-dependency of the effect of these inhibitors on the biochemical activity of their target, for example, by analyzing its downstream effectors. Owing to the propensity for off-target effects, it is important to stay within this biochemically relevant concentration range when analyzing the functional effects of inhibitors on cell growth and proliferation. Specific phenotypes that are observed should also be confirmed by using multiple small molecule inhibitors against the same target to increase confidence in the specificity of the effect. In addition, this approach can also be combined with data from genetic manipulation of the target.

4.4 Genetic Inhibition or Activation of Target Molecules

Various methods of either genetic silencing via siRNAs, shRNAs or gRNAs, or protein overexpression via cDNA or gRNAs can be used to confirm findings from an experiment using a small molecule inhibitor. However, such oligonucleotide-based strategies are also prone to off-target effects [48]. It is thus important to use multiple oligonucleotide constructs against a single gene of interest to generate reliable data. Following genetic knockdown by siRNAs or shRNAs, the specificity of the induced phenotype can be confirmed by reversing it by reintroducing the protein of interest via cDNA transfection. In order to ensure that the siRNA or shRNA does not silence the expression of the reconstituted protein, it can be designed to target untranslated (UTR) regions of the gene of interest, which are usually not included in cDNA expression constructs. We have recently used this strategy to examine the effect of *PI3KCA* mutations on AKT inhibition in BLCA [31]. Lastly, while a comparison of chemical and genetic inhibition can provide useful insights, it should also be remembered that these two methods have the potential to lead to distinct effects on cell signaling and these results should be critically analyzed.

References

1. Engelman JA, Luo J, Cantley LC (2006) The evolution of phosphatidylinositol 3-kinases as regulators of growth and metabolism. Nat Rev Genet 7(8):606–619. doi:10.1038/nrg1879
2. Franke TF (2008) PI3K/Akt: getting it right matters. Oncogene 27(50):6473–6488. doi:10.1038/onc.2008.313
3. Laplante M, Sabatini DM (2009) mTOR signaling at a glance. J Cell Sci 122(Pt 20):3589–3594. doi:10.1242/jcs.051011
4. Mamane Y, Petroulakis E, LeBacquer O, Sonenberg N (2006) mTOR, translation initiation and cancer. Oncogene 25 (48):6416–6422. doi:10.1038/sj.onc.1209888
5. Cancer Genome Atlas Research N (2014) Comprehensive molecular characterization of urothelial bladder carcinoma. Nature 507 (7492):315–322. doi:10.1038/nature12965
6. Iyer G, Al-Ahmadie H, Schultz N, Hanrahan AJ, Ostrovnaya I, Balar AV, Kim PH, Lin O, Weinhold N, Sander C, Zabor EC, Janakiraman M, Garcia-Grossman IR, Heguy A, Viale A, Bochner BH, Reuter VE, Bajorin DF, Milowsky MI, Taylor BS, Solit DB (2013) Prevalence and co-occurrence of actionable genomic alterations in high-grade bladder cancer. J Clin Oncol 31(25):3133–3140. doi:10.1200/JCO.2012.46.5740
7. Platt FM, Hurst CD, Taylor CF, Gregory WM, Harnden P, Knowles MA (2009) Spectrum of phosphatidylinositol 3-kinase pathway gene alterations in bladder cancer. Clin Cancer Res 15(19):6008–6017. doi:10.1158/1078-0432.CCR-09-0898. [pii]
8. Calderaro J, Rebouissou S, de Koning L, Masmoudi A, Herault A, Dubois T, Maille P, Soyeux P, Sibony M, de la Taille A, Vordos D, Lebret T, Radvanyi F, Allory Y (2014) PI3K/AKT pathway activation in bladder carcinogenesis. Int J Cancer 134(8):1776–1784. doi:10.1002/ijc.28518
9. Cappellen D, Gil Diez de Medina S, Chopin D, Thiery JP, Radvanyi F (1997) Frequent loss of heterozygosity on chromosome 10q in muscle-invasive transitional cell carcinomas of the bladder. Oncogene 14(25):3059–3066. doi:10.1038/sj.onc.1201154
10. Aveyard JS, Skilleter A, Habuchi T, Knowles MA (1999) Somatic mutation of PTEN in bladder carcinoma. Br J Cancer 80 (5–6):904–908. doi:10.1038/sj.bjc.6690439
11. Tsuruta H, Kishimoto H, Sasaki T, Horie Y, Natsui M, Shibata Y, Hamada K, Yajima N, Kawahara K, Sasaki M, Tsuchiya N, Enomoto K, Mak TW, Nakano T, Habuchi T, Suzuki A (2006) Hyperplasia and carcinomas in Pten-deficient mice and reduced PTEN protein in human bladder cancer patients. Cancer Res 66 (17):8389–8396. doi:10.1158/0008-5472.CAN-05-4627
12. Knowles MA, Habuchi T, Kennedy W, Cuthbert-Heavens D (2003) Mutation spectrum of the 9q34 tuberous sclerosis gene TSC1 in transitional cell carcinoma of the bladder. Cancer Res 63(22):7652–7656
13. Askham JM, Platt F, Chambers PA, Snowden H, Taylor CF, Knowles MA (2010) AKT1 mutations in bladder cancer: identification of a novel oncogenic mutation that can co-operate with E17K. Oncogene 29 (1):150–155. doi:10.1038/onc.2009.315
14. Alfred Witjes J, Lebret T, Comperat EM, Cowan NC, De Santis M, Bruins HM, Hernandez V, Espinos EL, Dunn J, Rouanne M, Neuzillet Y, Veskimae E, van der Heijden AG, Gakis G, Ribal MJ (2017) Updated 2016 EAU

guidelines on muscle-invasive and metastatic bladder cancer. Eur Urol 71:462–475. doi:10.1016/j.eururo.2016.06.020
15. Ratner M (2016) Genentech's PD-L1 agent approved for bladder cancer. Nat Biotechnol 34(8):789–790. doi:10.1038/nbt0816-789
16. Dienstmann R, Rodon J, Serra V, Tabernero J (2014) Picking the point of inhibition: a comparative review of PI3K/AKT/mTOR pathway inhibitors. Mol Cancer Ther 13 (5):1021–1031. doi:10.1158/1535-7163.MCT-13-0639
17. Shimobayashi M, Hall MN (2014) Making new contacts: the mTOR network in metabolism and signalling crosstalk. Nat Rev Mol Cell Biol 15(3):155–162. doi:10.1038/nrm3757
18. Fruman DA, Rommel C (2014) PI3K and cancer: lessons, challenges and opportunities. Nat Rev Drug Discov 13(2):140–156. doi:10.1038/nrd4204
19. Nawroth R, Stellwagen F, Schulz WA, Stoehr R, Hartmann A, Krause BJ, Gschwend JE, Retz M (2011) S6K1 and 4E-BP1 are independent regulated and control cellular growth in bladder cancer. PLoS One 6(11):e27509. doi:10.1371/journal.pone.0027509
20. Chiong E, Lee IL, Dadbin A, Sabichi AL, Harris L, Urbauer D, McConkey DJ, Dickstein RJ, Cheng T, Grossman HB (2011) Effects of mTOR inhibitor everolimus (RAD001) on bladder cancer cells. Clin Cancer Res 17 (9):2863–2873. doi:10.1158/1078-0432.CCR-09-3202
21. Lin JF, Lin YC, Yang SC, Tsai TF, Chen HE, Chou KY, Hwang TI (2016) Autophagy inhibition enhances RAD001-induced cytotoxicity in human bladder cancer cells. Drug Des Devel Ther 10:1501–1513. doi:10.2147/DDDT.S95900
22. Kyou Kwon J, Kim SJ, Hoon Kim J, Mee Lee K, Ho Chang I (2014) Dual inhibition by S6K1 and Elf4E is essential for controlling cellular growth and invasion in bladder cancer. Urol Oncol 32(1):51 e27-35. doi:10.1016/j.urolonc.2013.08.005
23. Guo Y, Chekaluk Y, Zhang J, Du J, Gray NS, Wu CL, Kwiatkowski DJ (2013) TSC1 involvement in bladder cancer: diverse effects and therapeutic implications. J Pathol 230 (1):17–27. doi:10.1002/path.4176
24. Seront E, Pinto A, Bouzin C, Bertrand L, Machiels JP, Feron O (2013) PTEN deficiency is associated with reduced sensitivity to mTOR inhibitor in human bladder cancer through the unhampered feedback loop driving PI3K/Akt activation. Br J Cancer 109(6):1586–1592. doi:10.1038/bjc.2013.505
25. Thoreen CC, Kang SA, Chang JW, Liu Q, Zhang J, Gao Y, Reichling LJ, Sim T, Sabatini DM, Gray NS (2009) An ATP-competitive mammalian target of rapamycin inhibitor reveals rapamycin-resistant functions of mTORC1. J Biol Chem 284(12):8023–8032. doi:10.1074/jbc.M900301200
26. Feldman ME, Apsel B, Uotila A, Loewith R, Knight ZA, Ruggero D, Shokat KM (2009) Active-site inhibitors of mTOR target rapamycin-resistant outputs of mTORC1 and mTORC2. PLoS Biol 7(2):e38. doi:10.1371/journal.pbio.1000038
27. Efeyan A, Sabatini DM (2010) mTOR and cancer: many loops in one pathway. Curr Opin Cell Biol 22(2):169–176. doi:10.1016/j.ceb.2009.10.007
28. Iyer G, Hanrahan AJ, Milowsky MI, Al-Ahmadie H, Scott SN, Janakiraman M, Pirun M, Sander C, Socci ND, Ostrovnaya I, Viale A, Heguy A, Peng L, Chan TA, Bochner B, Bajorin DF, Berger MF, Taylor BS, Solit DB (2012) Genome sequencing identifies a basis for everolimus sensitivity. Science 338 (6104):221. doi:10.1126/science.1226344
29. Seront E, Rottey S, Sautois B, Kerger J, D'Hondt LA, Verschaeve V, Canon JL, Dopchie C, Vandenbulcke JM, Whenham N, Goeminne JC, Clausse M, Verhoeven D, Glorieux P, Branders S, Dupont P, Schoonjans J, Feron O, Machiels JP (2012) Phase II study of everolimus in patients with locally advanced or metastatic transitional cell carcinoma of the urothelial tract: clinical activity, molecular response, and biomarkers. Ann Oncol 23 (10):2663–2670. doi:10.1093/annonc/mds057
30. Wagle N, Grabiner BC, Van Allen EM, Hodis E, Jacobus S, Supko JG, Stewart M, Choueiri TK, Gandhi L, Cleary JM, Elfiky AA, Taplin ME, Stack EC, Signoretti S, Loda M, Shapiro GI, Sabatini DM, Lander ES, Gabriel SB, Kantoff PW, Garraway LA, Rosenberg JE (2014) Activating mTOR mutations in a patient with an extraordinary response on a phase I trial of everolimus and pazopanib. Cancer Discov 4 (5):546–553. doi:10.1158/2159-8290.CD-13-0353
31. Sathe A, Guerth F, Cronauer MV, Heck MM, Thalgott M, Gschwend JE, Retz M, Nawroth R (2014) Mutant PIK3CA controls DUSP1-dependent ERK 1/2 activity to confer response to AKT target therapy. Br J Cancer 111 (11):2103–2113. doi:10.1038/bjc.2014.534
32. Dickstein RJ, Nitti G, Dinney CP, Davies BR, Kamat AM, McConkey DJ (2012) Autophagy limits the cytotoxic effects of the AKT inhibitor AZ7328 in human bladder cancer cells. Cancer

Biol Ther 13(13):1325–1338. doi:10.4161/cbt.21793

33. Ross RL, McPherson HR, Kettlewell L, Shnyder SD, Hurst CD, Alder O, Knowles MA (2016) PIK3CA dependence and sensitivity to therapeutic targeting in urothelial carcinoma. BMC Cancer 16:553. doi:10.1186/s12885-016-2570-0
34. Gopa Iyer CMT, Garcia-Grossman IR, Scott SN, Boyd ME, McCoy AS, Berger MF, Al-Ahmadie H, Solit DB, Rosenberg JE, Bajorin DF (2015) Phase 2 study of the pan-isoform PI3 kinase inhibitor BKM120 in metastatic urothelial carcinoma patients. J Clin Oncol 33 (suppl 7):abstr 324
35. Moon du G, Lee SE, Oh MM, Lee SC, Jeong SJ, Hong SK, Yoon CY, Byun SS, Park HS, Cheon J (2014) NVP-BEZ235, a dual PI3K/mTOR inhibitor synergistically potentiates the antitumor effects of cisplatin in bladder cancer cells. Int J Oncol 45(3):1027–1035. doi:10.3892/ijo.2014.2505
36. Li JR, Cheng CL, Yang CR, Ou YC, Wu MJ, Ko JL (2013) Dual inhibitor of phosphoinositide 3-kinase/mammalian target of rapamycin NVP-BEZ235 effectively inhibits cisplatin-resistant urothelial cancer cell growth through autophagic flux. Toxicol Lett 220(3):267–276. doi:10.1016/j.toxlet.2013.04.021
37. Seront E, Rottey S, Filleul B, Glorieux P, Goeminne JC, Verschaeve V, Vandenbulcke JM, Sautois B, Boegner P, Gillain A, van Maanen A, Machiels JP (2016) Phase II study of dual phosphoinositol-3-kinase (PI3K) and mammalian target of rapamycin (mTOR) inhibitor BEZ235 in patients with locally advanced or metastatic transitional cell carcinoma. BJU Int 118(3):408–415. doi:10.1111/bju.13415
38. Munster P, Aggarwal R, Hong D, Schellens JH, van der Noll R, Specht J, Witteveen PO, Werner TL, Dees EC, Bergsland E, Agarwal N, Kleha JF, Durante M, Adams L, Smith DA, Lampkin TA, Morris SR, Kurzrock R (2016) First-in-human phase I study of GSK2126458, an oral pan-class I phosphatidylinositol-3-kinase inhibitor, in patients with advanced solid tumor malignancies. Clin Cancer Res 22 (8):1932–1939. doi:10.1158/1078-0432.CCR-15-1665
39. Rodon J, Dienstmann R, Serra V, Tabernero J (2013) Development of PI3K inhibitors: lessons learned from early clinical trials. Nat Rev Clin Oncol 10(3):143–153. doi:10.1038/nrclinonc.2013.10
40. Nassim R, Mansure JJ, Chevalier S, Cury F, Kassouf W (2013) Combining mTOR inhibition with radiation improves antitumor activity in bladder cancer cells in vitro and in vivo: a novel strategy for treatment. PLoS One 8(6): e65257. doi:10.1371/journal.pone.0065257
41. Knowles MA, Hurst CD (2015) Molecular biology of bladder cancer: new insights into pathogenesis and clinical diversity. Nat Rev Cancer 15(1):25–41. doi:10.1038/nrc3817
42. Nickerson ML, Witte N, Im KM, Turan S, Owens C, Misner K, Tsang SX, Cai Z, Wu S, Dean M, Costello JC, Theodorescu D (2017) Molecular analysis of urothelial cancer cell lines for modeling tumor biology and drug response. Oncogene 36:35–46. doi:10.1038/onc.2016.172
43. Barretina J, Caponigro G, Stransky N, Venkatesan K, Margolin AA, Kim S, Wilson CJ, Lehar J, Kryukov GV, Sonkin D, Reddy A, Liu M, Murray L, Berger MF, Monahan JE, Morais P, Meltzer J, Korejwa A, Jane-Valbuena J, Mapa FA, Thibault J, Bric-Furlong E, Raman P, Shipway A, Engels IH, Cheng J, Yu GK, Yu J, Aspesi P Jr, de Silva M, Jagtap K, Jones MD, Wang L, Hatton C, Palescandolo E, Gupta S, Mahan S, Sougnez C, Onofrio RC, Liefeld T, MacConaill L, Winckler W, Reich M, Li N, Mesirov JP, Gabriel SB, Getz G, Ardlie K, Chan V, Myer VE, Weber BL, Porter J, Warmuth M, Finan P, Harris JL, Meyerson M, Golub TR, Morrissey MP, Sellers WR, Schlegel R, Garraway LA (2012) The cancer cell line encyclopedia enables predictive modelling of anticancer drug sensitivity. Nature 483 (7391):603–607. doi:10.1038/nature11003
44. Forbes SA, Beare D, Gunasekaran P, Leung K, Bindal N, Boutselakis H, Ding M, Bamford S, Cole C, Ward S, Kok CY, Jia M, De T, Teague JW, Stratton MR, McDermott U, Campbell PJ (2015) COSMIC: exploring the world's knowledge of somatic mutations in human cancer. Nucleic Acids Res 43(Database issue): D805–D811. doi:10.1093/nar/gku1075
45. Riss TL, Moravec RA, Niles AL, Duellman S, Benink HA, Worzella TJ, Minor L (2004) Cell viability assays. In: Sittampalam GS, Coussens NP, Nelson H et al (eds) Assay guidance manual. Eli Lilly & Company and the National Center for Advancing Translational Sciences, Bethesda (MD)
46. Haverty PM, Lin E, Tan J, Yu Y, Lam B, Lianoglou S, Neve RM, Martin S, Settleman J, Yauch RL, Bourgon R (2016) Reproducible pharmacogenomic profiling of cancer cell line panels. Nature 533(7603):333–337. doi:10.1038/nature17987
47. Haibe-Kains B, El-Hachem N, Birkbak NJ, Jin AC, Beck AH, Aerts HJ, Quackenbush J (2013) Inconsistency in large pharmacogenomic studies. Nature 504(7480):389–393. doi:10.1038/nature12831

48. Boettcher M, McManus MT (2015) Choosing the right tool for the job: RNAi, TALEN, or CRISPR. Mol Cell 58(4):575–585. doi:10.1016/j.molcel.2015.04.028
49. Vichai V, Kirtikara K (2006) Sulforhodamine B colorimetric assay for cytotoxicity screening. Nat Protoc 1(3):1112–1116. doi:10.1038/nprot.2006.179
50. Niegisch G, Retz M, Thalgott M, Balabanov S, Honecker F, Ohlmann CH, Stockle M, Bogemann M, Vom Dorp F, Gschwend J, Hartmann A, Ohmann C, Albers P (2015) Second-line treatment of advanced Urothelial cancer with paclitaxel and Everolimus in a German phase II trial (AUO trial AB 35/09). Oncology 89 (2):70–78. doi:10.1159/000376551
51. Milowsky MI, Iyer G, Regazzi AM, Al-Ahmadie H, Gerst SR, Ostrovnaya I, Gellert LL, Kaplan R, Garcia-Grossman IR, Pendse D, Balar AV, Flaherty AM, Trout A, Solit DB, Bajorin DF (2013) Phase II study of everolimus in metastatic urothelial cancer. BJU Int 112(4):462–470. doi:10.1111/j.1464-410X.2012.11720.x
52. Gerullis H, Eimer C, Ecke TH, Georgas E, Freitas C, Kastenholz S, Arndt C, Heusch C, Otto T (2012) A phase II trial of temsirolimus in second-line metastatic urothelial cancer. Med Oncol 29(4):2870–2876. doi:10.1007/s12032-012-0216-x

Chapter 24

Visualization and Quantitative Measurement of Drug-Induced Platinum Adducts in the Nuclear DNA of Individual Cells by an Immuno-Cytological Assay

Margarita Melnikova and Jürgen Thomale

Abstract

Immunocytological staining with adduct-specific antibodies allows the visualization and measurement of structurally defined types of DNA damage in the nuclei of individual cells. Here we describe an immunocytological assay (ICA) procedure for the localization and quantification of such damage, in particular induced by platinum-based anticancer drugs, in cell lines, in primary cell suspensions and in frozen tissue sections.

Key words DNA adducts, Cisplatin, Monoclonal antibody, Immunofluorescence, Single cell analysis, Quantitative image analysis

1 Introduction

Platinum-based anticancer drugs like cis-, carbo-, or oxaliplatin play a major role in chemotherapeutic regimen for a broad spectrum of solid tumors including urothelial carcinoma [1]. These drugs mediate their antineoplastic activity by forming platination products, so called adducts, in the nuclear DNA of tumor cells [2, 3]. The relative chemosensitivity/-resistance of cells is closely correlated to the amount of adducts induced and to their persistence in the nucleus [4]. To determine these critical parameters in experimental cell systems as well as in clinical specimen we have developed a sensitive immunoanalytical procedure based on an adduct-specific monoclonal antibody [5]. The ICA method described here allows the quantitative analysis of Pt-adduct levels in the nuclear DNA of individual cells and has successfully been applied in various cell lines [6, 7], in mouse models [8–10], and in clinical cell samples like primary tumor tissue [11], ascites fluids, or circulating tumor cells from peripheral blood [12]. Other types of structural DNA damage such as specific alkylation products [13], oxidative damage [14], or

Wolfgang A. Schulz et al. (eds.), *Urothelial Carcinoma: Methods and Protocols*, Methods in Molecular Biology, vol. 1655, DOI 10.1007/978-1-4939-7234-0_24,

UV-induced lesions [15] can similarly be detected where suitable antibodies are available.

2 Materials

2.1 Sample Preparation

1. Microscopic slides for sample preparation: strictly use "Superfrost Plus Gold" slides (*see* **Note 1**).

2.2 Immunostaining

Prepare all solutions using ultrapure water (at least double distilled water, ddH_2O) and analytical-grade reagents. Prepare and store all reagents at room temperature (unless indicated otherwise).

1. Alkali solution: Prepare 70 mM NaOH (2.8 g/L) + 140 mM NaCl (8.2 g/L), store solution at 4 °C, before use mix 60: 40 (v/v) with methanol, cool to 0 °C in ice bath.
2. PBS: Na_2HPO_4 $2H_2O$ (1.44 g/L), KH_2PO4 (0.2 g/L), NaCl (8 g/L), KCl (0.2 g/L). Dissolve in ddH_2O, adjust to pH 7.2 with HCl, autoclave for storage.
3. PBST: mix 0.25% Tween 20 (2.5 mL/L) in PBS.
4. PBS-Glycine: dissolve 0.2% glycine (2 mg/L) in PBS.
5. Blocking solution: dissolve 5% (w/v) skim milk powder (50 mg/mL) in PBS.
6. Pepsin solution: Use pepsin from Thermo Scientific (10 FIP-U/mg), prepare stock solution of 1 mg/mL in ddH_2O and store aliquots at −20 °C. Working concentration: 100–800 μg/mL ddH_2O (*see* **Note 2**).
7. Proteinase K buffer: 20 mM Tris base, 2 mM $CaCl_2$, dissolve in ddH_2O, adjust to pH 7.5 with HCl, store at 4 °C.

   Proteinase K solution: Use proteinase K from Thermo Scientific (30 U/mg), prepare stock solution of 1 mg/mL in proteinase K buffer, store aliquots at −20 °C. Working concentration: 100–800 μg/mL in proteinase K buffer (*see* **Note 2**).
8. Primary antibody: Monoclonal antibody R-C18 (rat, specific for the major DNA platination product Pt-[GpG]) [5], prepare stock solution of 50 μg/mL in PBS/BSA (5% w/v) and store at −20 °C.
9. Secondary antibody: Use, e.g., Cy3-labeled goat anti-(rat Ig) from Dianova (dilution 1: 200).
10. DAPI solution: Dissolve 4′,6-diamidino-2-phenylindole dihydrochloride (DAPI) in ddH_2O for stock solution of 100 μg/mL store at −20 °C in dark.
11. Mounting solution with low auto-fluorescence.

2.3 Instruments

1. Fluorescence microscope or laser-scanning confocal microscope.
2. Image analysis system.

3 Methods

3.1 Preparation of Samples

3.1.1 Carry Out All Steps at Room Temperature Unless Specified Otherwise

1. Seed cells (e.g., in 6-well plates), grow over night, and treat with cisplatin, e.g., for 4 h (include an untreated control), continue with **step 3**.
2. For repair kinetics: remove cisplatin from cells after 2 or 4 h of exposure and replace by fresh, pre-warmed medium, further incubate cells for different periods.
3. Trypsinize cells in one or two well(s) per time point or treatment condition.
4. Count cells to allow corrections for adduct dilution by de novo DNA synthesis during replication if necessary (*see* **Note 3**).
5. Spin cells down and wash 2× with PBS (to get rid of protein before placing cells onto slides).
6. Resuspend cells at a density of 1×10^6/mL in PBS.
7. Place a drop of 10 μL (about 10^4 cells) for each concentration/ time point onto "Superfrost Plus Gold" slides, Apply up to right spots per slide, include an untreated control (*see* Fig. 1). Label slides with pencil (don't use ink marker).
8. Let cells adhere and completely air-dry at room temperature (RT).
9. Keep slides frozen at −20 °C in box (no wrapping with foil, *see* **Note 4**) until analysis or shipment.

3.1.2 Cells in Suspension

Same procedure as for adherent cells but spin down cells in **step 2** and omit **step 3**.

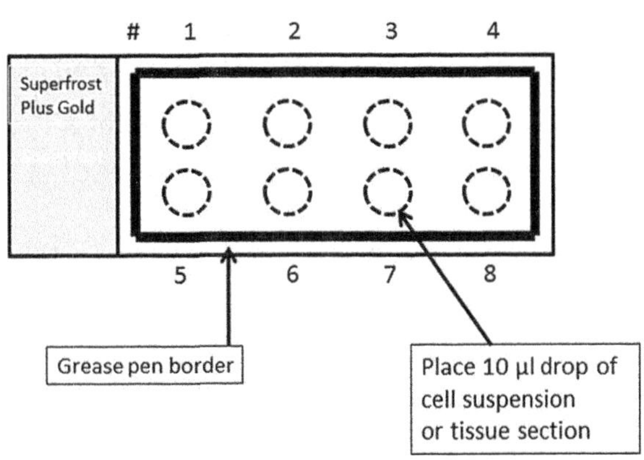

Fig. 1 Application of cell samples/tissue sections onto microscopic slides

3.1.3 Tissue Sections

1. Embed small samples of fresh tissue in freezing solution (e.g., OTC, Leica), shock-freeze in liquid N_2 and store at −80 °C (*see* **Note 5**).
2. Prepare frozen sections (7–9 μm) at suitable freezing temperature (−18 to −25 °C, depending on tissue type) and place onto "Superfrost Plus Gold" slides.

3.2 Staining Procedure

1. Let slides warm up to room temperature (*see* **Note 4**).
2. Fix samples in cooled methanol (−20 °C) in a container for at least 30 min.
3. Wash slides in PBS for 5 min at RT in container.
4. Alkali denaturation step: Mix 60% 70 mM NaOH/140 mM NaCl and 40% methanol (v/v) in container and cool in ice bath, immerse slides for exactly 5 min at 0 °C.
5. Wash in PBS (2 × 5 min with buffer change, RT, container), wipe edges dry, and encircle samples with grease pen.
6. Digest with warmed pepsin (100–800 μg/mL in ddH_2O, for activation add 10 μL 2 M HCl/mL) by carefully overlying slides with 1 mL solution and incubate 10 min at 37 °C. Perform this and all following incubations in a moist chamber.
7. Wash in PBS for 5 min at RT.
8. Digest with warmed proteinase K (100–800 μg/mL proteinase K buffer; 1 mL solution per slide) for 10 min at 37 °C (as in **step 6**).
9. Wash slides in PBS-glycine (10 min, RT).
10. Blocking step: Incubate in PBS + 5% skim milk powder (w/v) for 30 min at RT in container.
11. Incubate with anti-(Pt-[GpG]) antibody (RC-18, concentration 0.01 to 0.1 μg/mL), carefully place 1 mL solution onto each slide, incubate at 4 °C overnight.
12. Wash in PBS-Tween (5 min) and in PBS (5 min, RT).
13. Incubate with secondary antibody (e.g., goat anti-[rat Ig]-Cy3, diluted 1:200), 500 μL per slide) for 1 h at 37 °C in dark.
14. Wash in PBST (5 min, RT) and in PBS (5 min, RT) in dark.
15. Counterstain with DAPI (1 μg/mL PBS in container, 30 min, RT) in dark.
16. Wash with PBS (5 min, RT) in dark.
17. Carefully and slowly cover with antifade mounting solution and with coverslips, seal coverslips with nail polish (*see* **Note 6**).
18. Keep at 4 °C in dark until measurement.

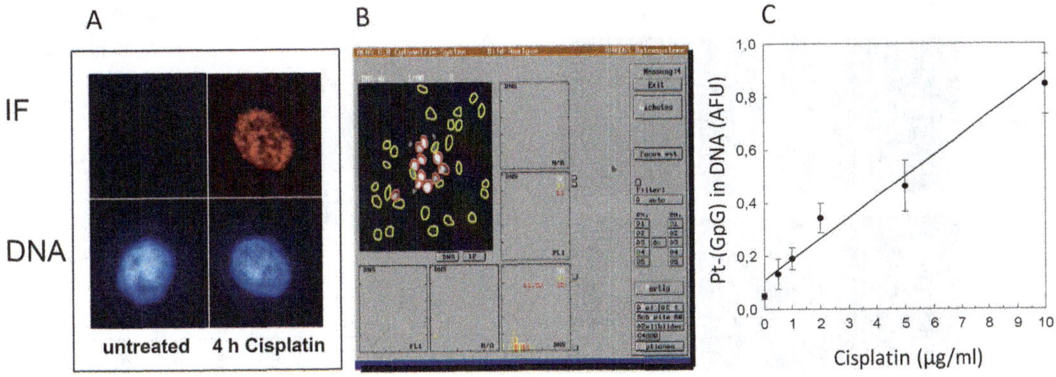

Fig. 2 Visualization and measurement of platinum adducts in the nuclear DNA of single cells. **(a)** Fluorescence micrographs of ICA-stained cells untreated or exposed to cisplatin (5 µg/mL, 4 h). Upper part: Cy3-channel (Pt-[GpG]), lower part: DAPI-channel (DNA). **(b)** Snap shot of the ACAS II image analysis system showing cell images (*upper left*) and integrated signal values from individual cells for DAPI and Cy3. The area of interest (AOI) for each nucleus is defined by the DAPI-derived pixels. Subpopulations of cells can be marked by different colors (*yellow, red*). **(c)** Quantitative evaluation of Pt-(GpG) adduct levels from a cisplatin dose response experiment with human A549 lung cancer cells. Plotted are calculated mean AFU (Arbitrary Fluorescence Units) values +/− SD from 100 nuclei analyzed per dose

3.3 Quantification of Adduct Levels as Arbitrary Fluorescence Units, (AFU)

For evaluation use a fluorescence microscope or a laser scanning microscope with appropriate filter sets coupled to an image analyzer (e.g., ACAS 2 Image Analysis System, Ahrens Electronics, Bargteheide) to determine integrated fluorescence signals from DAPI and from antibody separately for individual nuclei. Pixels from areas of interest (AOI) are defined by the DAPI stain (*see* Fig. 2). Then calculate relative adduct concentration per cell by dividing antibody-derived values by DAPI values of each nucleus resulting in Arbitrary Fluorescence Units (AFUs). From these, calculate mean values (with standard deviations or 95% confidence intervals) which represent relative adduct levels. In dose-response experiments this should result in an approximately linear correlation between adduct values and cisplatin exposure (*see* Fig. 2). Subtract AFU values of untreated controls (if any detectable) and finally correct for DNA de novo synthesis rates if necessary (*see* **Note 3**). Figure 3 illustrates typical results obtained by this technique in our own experiments.

4 Notes

1. For sample preparation use "Superfrost Plus Gold" adhesion slides (Thermo Scientific or Menzel) to prevent loss of cells during the rather harsh alkali step and protease digestions during the staining procedure.

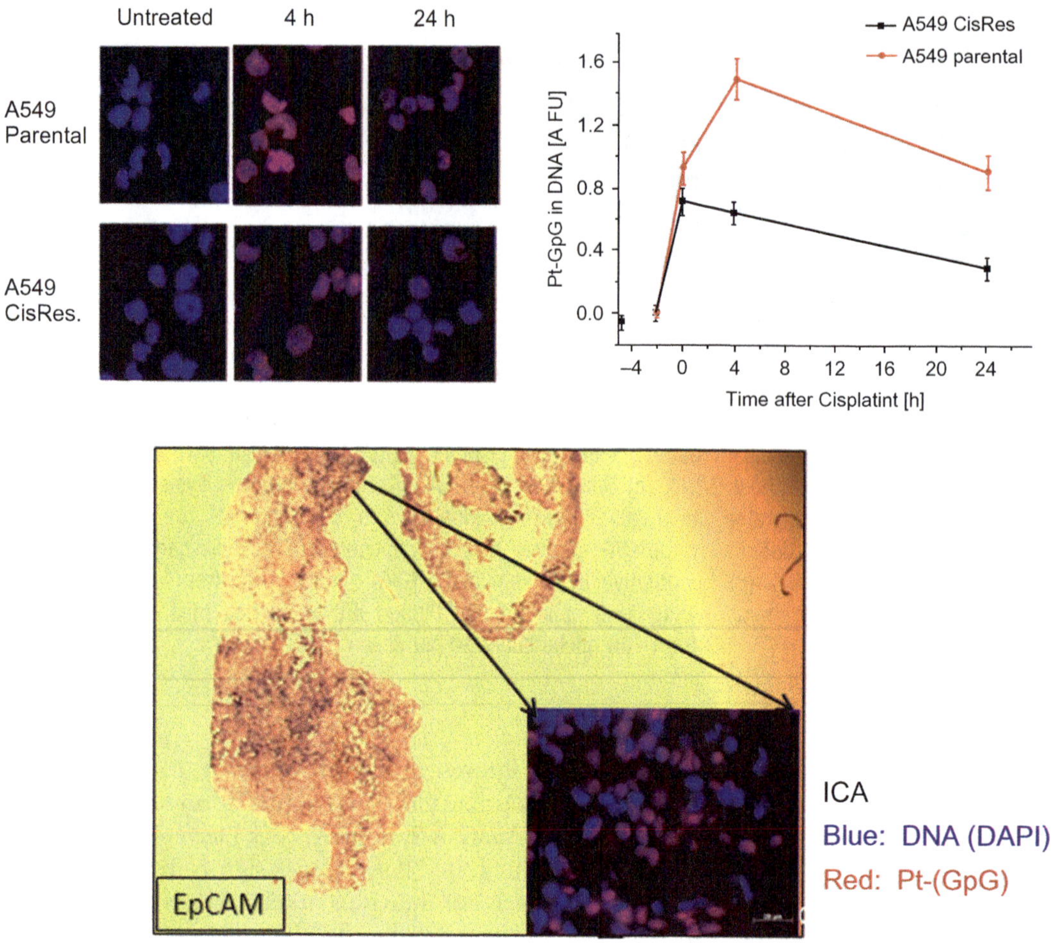

Fig. 3 Application of ICA analysis for the measurement of DNA repair kinetics and of adduct levels in primary tumor tissue. *Upper left*: Fluorescence images (matched Cy3- and DAPI-derived signals) from parental A549 cells and from a cisplatin-resistant variant (CisRes) at different time points after exposure to cisplatin (10 μg/mL 2 h). *Upper right*: Pt-adduct kinetics of both cell lines during 24 h after exposure. Note the different peak adduct formations but similar repair rates in both cell lines. *Bottom*: Visualization of Pt adducts in a sample of ovarian cancer tissue taken from a patient immediately after high dose, high temperature intraperitoneal perfusion with cisplatin (HIPEC, Lit). Shown are the EpCAM-staining of tumor cells (*yellow/brown*) and the ICA-staining (*insert*: matched Cy3 and DAPI signals) from a tumor cell-rich area. Note the distinct intercellular heterogeneity of DNA platination (*see* **Note 7**)

2. Concentrations of proteases (proteinase K and pepsin) as given above are good starting points but have to be optimized for each type of cells or tissue to get rid of unspecific staining in untreated controls on one hand and to minimize structural damage of nuclei and cell loss on the other. Be aware that specific activities of the enzymes often vary grossly between different batches and providers.

3. Calculated mean AFU values can be corrected for adduct dilution due to de novo DNA synthesis during replication (e.g., in

the run of repair kinetics) by multiplying the respective values, e.g., by a factor of two in case the cell number has doubled since t0 (end of drug exposure). By this, proper repair rates can be calculated for a given cell type.

4. Do not wrap slides in aluminum or plastic foil during freezing but store in slide boxes to strictly avoid moistening of samples by condensed/frozen water. Slides must be completely dry before fixation in methanol.
5. The usage of sections from formalin-fixed tissue in paraffin blocks is not recommended as the unmasking of the antigens in DNA for antibody staining is complicated and doesn't give reproducible results.
6. Be very careful with the overlay of the mounting solution and the placement of the coverslips as the nuclei are rather fragile after digestion.
7. Specific types of cells (e.g., tumor or stem cells) in heterogeneous populations can be addressed in this assay by immunostaining relevant (surface) marker prior to the ICA procedure. Fluorescence images and x-y-positions for cells of interest on the slide can be stored electronically by using, e.g., the Tango scanning table system (Märzhäuser, Wetzlar) or any other suitable device. Do not cover slides after cell type staining with mounting medium but place a drop of glycerine/PBS (1:1) onto the slides before putting on a cover slip very carefully. After image storage remove the slip by immersing the slide slowly and in horizontal position in PBS to avoid disturbance of cell positions. During the subsequent ICA staining procedure it is recommended to perform all washing steps and incubations following **step 4** (alkali denaturation) with slides in horizontal position, e.g., in a Petri dish within a moist chamber.

Acknowledgement

We thank Maria Eynck (IFZ) for excellent technical assistance.

References

1. Wheate NJ, Walker S, Craig GE et al (2010) The status of platinum anticancer drugs in the clinic and in clinical trials. Dalton Trans 39:8113–8127
2. Wang D, Lippard SJ (2005) Cellular processing of platinum anticancer drugs. Nat Rev Drug Discov 4:307–320
3. Ziehe M, Esteban-Fernández D, Hochkirch U et al (2012) On the complexity and dynamics of in vivo Cisplatin-DNA adduct formation using HPLC/ICP-MS. Metallomics 4:1098–1104
4. Galluzzi L, Vitale I, Michels J et al (2014) Systems biology of cisplatin resistance: past, present and future. Cell Death Dis 5:e1257
5. Liedert B, Pluim D, Schellens J et al (2006) Adduct-specific monoclonal antibodies for the measurement of cisplatin-induced DNA lesions

in individual cell nuclei. Nucleic Acids Res 34: e47

6. Liedert B, Materna V, Schadendorf D et al (2003) Overexpression of cMOAT (MRP2/ ABCC2) is associated with decreased formation of platinum-DNA adducts and decreased G2-arrest in melanoma cells resistant to cisplatin. J Invest Dermatol 121:172–176
7. Barr M, Gray SG, Hoffmann AC et al (2013) Generation and characterization of cisplatin-resistant non-small cell lung cancer cell lines displaying a stem-like signature. PLoS One 8: e54193
8. Dzagnidze A, Katsarava Z, Makhalova J et al (2007) Repair capacity for platinum-DNA adducts determines the severity of cisplatin-induced peripheral neuropathy. J Neurosci 27:9451–9457
9. Oliver TG, Mercer KL, Sayles LC et al (2010) Chronic cisplatin treatment promotes enhanced damage repair and tumor progression in a mouse model of lung cancer. Genes Dev 24:837–852
10. Jokić M, Vlašić I, Rinneburger M et al (2016) Ercc1 deficiency promotes tumorigenesis and increases Cisplatin sensitivity in a Tp53 context-specific manner. Mol Cancer Res 14:1110–1123
11. Zivanovic O, Abramian A, Kullmann M et al (2015) HIPEC ROC I: a phase i study of cisplatin administered as hyperthermic intraoperative intraperitoneal chemoperfusion followed by postoperative intravenous platinum-based chemotherapy in patients with platinum-sensitive recurrent epithelial ovarian cancer. Int J Cancer 136:699–708
12. Nel I, Gauler TC, Eberhardt WE et al (2013) Formation and repair kinetics of Pt-(GpG) DNA adducts in extracted circulating tumor cells and response to platinum treatment. Br J Cancer 109:1223–1329
13. Sorg UR, Kleff V, Fanaei S et al (2007) O6-methylguanine-DNA-methyltransferase (MGMT) gene therapy targeting haematopoietic stem cells: studies addressing safety issues. DNA Repair (Amst) 6:1197–1209
14. Thomas JP, Lautermann J, Liedert B et al (2006) High accumulation of platinum–DNA adducts in strial marginal cells of the cochlea is an early event in cisplatin but not carboplatin ototoxicity. Mol Pharmacol 70:23–29
15. Kobayashi N, Katsumi S, Imoto K et al (2001) Quantitation and visualization of ultraviolet-induced DNA damage using specific antibodies: application to pigment cell biology. Pigment Cell Res 14:94–102

Check for updates

Erratum to: Urinary Protein Markers for the Detection and Prognostication of Urothelial Carcinoma

Tibor Szarvas, Péter Nyirády, Osamu Ogawa, Hideki Furuya, Charles J. Rosser, and Takashi Kobayashi

Erratum to:
Chapter 19 in: Wolfgang A. Schulz et al. (eds.), *Urothelial Carcinoma: Methods and Protocols*, Methods in Molecular Biology, vol. 1655, https://doi.org/10.1007/978-1-4939-7234-0_19

The original version of this chapter was inadvertently published with incorrect order of authors. The correct order is updated in the current version as Tibor Szarvas, Péter Nyirády, Osamu Ogawa, Hideki Furuya, Charles J. Rosser, and Takashi Kobayashi.

The updated original online version of this chapter can be found at https://doi.org/10.1007/978-1-4939-7234-0_19

Wolfgang A. Schulz et al. (eds.), *Urothelial Carcinoma: Methods and Protocols*, Methods in Molecular Biology, vol. 1655, https://doi.org/10.1007/978-1-4939-7234-0_25, © Springer Science+Business Media LLC 2018

INDEX

Wolfgang A. Schulz et al. (eds.), *Urothelial Carcinoma: Methods and Protocols*, Methods in Molecular Biology, vol. 1655, DOI 10.1007/978-1-4939-7234-0, © Springer Science+Business Media LLC 2018

L

M

N

O

P

Q

R

MIX
Papier aus verantwortungsvollen Quellen
Paper from responsible sources
FSC® C105338

Printed by Books on Demand, Germany